PATIENT-CENTERED DIAGNOSIS

Methodologies to Predict Individually Tailored Outcomes
of Current Diagnostic Tests and to Create New Tests

James R. Miller III, PhD
Mohammed Kashani-Sabet, MD
and Richard W. Sagebiel MD

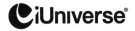

PATIENT-CENTERED DIAGNOSIS
METHODOLOGIES TO PREDICT INDIVIDUALLY TAILORED OUTCOMES OF
CURRENT DIAGNOSTIC TESTS AND TO CREATE NEW TESTS

iUniverse books may be ordered through booksellers or by contacting:

iUniverse
1663 Liberty Drive
Bloomington, IN 47403
www.iuniverse.com
1-800-Authors (1-800-288-4677)

ISBN: 978-1-4917-7949-1 (sc)
ISBN: 978-1-4917-7950-7 (e)

Library of Congress Control Number: 2015917893

Print information available on the last page.

iUniverse rev. date: 12/14/2015

CONTENTS

PREFACE

The practice of medicine is both an art and a science.

Underlying the practice of medicine as an art is the clear recognition that no two human beings are exactly alike. Preventative procedures, diagnoses, prognoses, and treatment selection decisions cannot be carried out as if individual differences did not exist. They abound! Even identical twins gradually develop small differences in their DNA due to mutations relating to their separate life paths.

It therefore makes sense to practice medicine in an experience-based manner. A physician's personal experience frequently provides a sensitive and effective guide to tailoring medical care to individual patient needs. The many and varied dissimilarities among individual patient personalities, their cultural and religious backgrounds, and their unique life situations render sole reliance on scientific generalizations inadequate.

Underlying the practice of medicine as a science is the equally clear recognition that human beings constitute a particular biological species. Most of us possess a single head, two arms, and two legs; a single heart and two separate kidneys; a brain with two separate but highly interconnected hemispheres; and so forth. These anatomical regularities and their many biological implications amply justify treating medicine as a science.

It therefore makes equal sense to practice medicine in an evidence-based manner. The collective experience of many physicians is typically superior to that of any single physician. We can exploit what we come to know as common among many or most human beings if we collect patient data and organize our medical practice in a systematic, scientific manner.

The prediction of interesting end points in medicine requires identifying useful indicators of a patient's future state of health. Prognostic research is carefully designed to discover such indicators.

An indicator is called a prognostic factor when it can be shown to influence, systematically, salient patient outcomes, such as the future course of cancer and other progressive diseases. Explaining the exact manner in which and the exact pathways through which an underlying factor exerts its influence is an equally important goal of prognostic research.

On the other hand, an indicator can be prognostically useful even if it merely predicts salient patient outcomes. This may happen without understanding fully the exact nature of its biological linking mechanisms and pathways. For example, just the size of a primary tumor in the initial diagnosis of colorectal cancer, breast cancer, and melanoma matters. Smaller tumors generally portend more favorable patient outcomes. Only the existence and the direction of this simple predictive relationship are fully understood.

A similar distinction can be drawn between understanding in detail the mechanisms and pathways linking newly discovered biomarkers to disease outcomes and using what knowledge we have already accumulated about these biomarkers to make simple directional predictions. To understand and explain in full detail the complex and frequently interactive biological roles played by particular genes in the same and in different disease contexts will require substantial additional research.

We shall characterize prognostic research that focuses primarily on the underlying factors, mechanisms, and pathways influencing salient patient outcomes as factor-centered. Patients are viewed as carriers of these factors and the salient outcomes to which they are linked. Detailed, sometimes quantitative models are constructed to connect factors with outcomes via mechanisms and pathways. However, in the factor-centered approach research conclusions are about the factors themselves. They describe common linkage pathways and associated biological mechanisms that exist in selected patient populations. They do not constitute separate conclusions about each individual patient.

We shall characterize prognostic research that focuses primarily on making separate, individually tailored predictions of salient patient outcomes as patient-centered. Prognostic factors serve as the basis for making individually tailored predictions. Research conclusions are therefore based on at least a partial understanding of underlying mechanisms and pathways; but they are never about the factors, mechanisms, or pathways themselves. In the patient-centered approach research conclusions are always about individual patients. They apply separately to each patient. They are designed to facilitate tailored patient management decisions and individual lifestyle choices.

The flavor of factor-centered prognostic research is perhaps more comfortably allied with viewing medicine as a science. The flavor of patient-centered prognostic research is perhaps more comfortably allied with viewing medicine as an art.

Our view is that these two flavors are not properly considered as competing with one another. They are inescapably complementary. Conventional methodology developed in the service of factor-centered research (e.g., analysis of clinical trials) does not, itself, make individual patient predictions. It does, however, serve to identify prognostic factors, linkage mechanisms, and pathways that are essential to predicting individual patient outcomes. The accuracy of such predictions can be improved by modifying conventional methodology in certain selective ways. Selective modification for this purpose is exactly what our Patient-Centered Methodology (PCM) seeks to accomplish. Simultaneously, some but not all of the selective modifications can be useful in drawing traditional, factor-centered conclusions.

This is the second in a series of books about making predictions of individual patient outcomes more accurate. Our first book introduced PCM. It described the selective modifications (analytical devices) that facilitate greater predictive accuracy. It showed how these modifications (devices) separately and in combination improve predictive accuracy at the individual patient level.

PCM was applied first to a sample of 1,222 melanoma patients from the United States and then to a sample of 1,225 patients from Finland diagnosed with invasive breast cancer. Disease-specific death within five years of initial diagnosis served as the common end point to be predicted. Substantial improvements in accuracy compared to conventional prognostic methodology were achieved in both samples.

More details about our first book and the previously published medical journal article introducing the same material and presenting the same results appear as entries 1 and 2 in "ANNOTATED REFERENCES" at the end of this second book.

The results reported in our first book were promising but not definitive. The book ended with the suggestion that some centralized organization with significant resources attempt to replicate the apparently superior predictive accuracy offered by PCM. This would mean selecting a particular progressive disease, such as a specific cancer, and launching a large-scale replication project. The situation seemed similar to where promising results had been achieved in phase I and phase II clinical trials and where the next step was to achieve definitive results in phase III.

So far, no organization has taken our suggestion. That is too bad. Successful replication would justify putting up on the Internet a service useful both to patients and to their physicians. PCM could provide individually tailored probabilistic predictions of many salient patient outcomes relating to many progressive diseases derived from the centrally collected, centrally maintained, and regularly updated medical records of many patients.

Successful replication would require validating that PCM's individually tailored probabilistic predictions really were more accurate than whatever predictions could be obtained from conventional prognostic methodology. That would justify replacing conventional methodology with PCM for this purpose.

This second book has been designed to support two assertions.

1. PCM's superior predictive accuracy at the individual patient level can be exploited both to reduce the cost and to increase the triage efficiency of certain existing diagnostic procedures. A sentinel lymph node biopsy (SLNB), administered to melanoma and to breast cancer patients, serves as a first illustrative example. An FDG-PET/CT scan, administered to patients with many forms of cancer, serves as a second illustrative example. Cost savings of at least 40 percent and triage efficiency improvements of at least 66 percent appear attainable.
2. PCM's accuracy-improving analytical devices can be incorporated within a novel diagnostic procedure developed some years ago. The procedure was first utilized to discriminate between malignant melanomas and benign nevi (moles). It is called the Discriminator Selection and Sequencing Algorithm (DSSA). Without PCM, DSSA achieved a differential diagnosis with a sensitivity of 91 percent and with a specificity of 95 percent. It made 92 percent correct discriminations. Modified by PCM, DSSA reanalyzed exactly the same data. This improved DSSA's diagnostic performance to a sensitivity of 97 percent and to a specificity of 98 percent, allowing it to make 97 percent correct discriminations.

A detailed description of DSSA and its application to the differential diagnosis of primary lesions obtained from 699 melanoma patients is presented in sections 4 and 5 of this book. Section 5 describes the complete reanalysis. The original analysis (see entry 13 in "ANNOTATED REFERENCES") was noteworthy:

1. because it pioneered the use of five gene-based molecular markers to facilitate the diagnosis of melanoma;
2. because it showed that differences in the intensity of expression of all five genes between the top and bottom regions of a primary lesion were especially useful in making accurate differential diagnoses; and
3. because it introduced DSSA and showed that its discriminating efficacy compared quite favorably with alternative diagnostic procedures.

Convincing physicians that PCM's predictive accuracy can actually improve the practice of medicine will likely continue to be a hard sell.

For one thing, the fundamental concept lacks the proper medical aroma. It is nothing like a breakthrough surgical procedure or a modern wonder drug. It is based on statistical ideas and computer-driven data analysis techniques. Neither is a familiar concept in the experience of very many physicians. Neither topic is accorded more than cursory treatment in a typical medical education. So how could a statistician or a computer person make a significant contribution to medicine?

There is historical precedent for such skepticism. Few physicians in the middle of the nineteenth century could accept that living microorganisms existed with the capacity to infect and sometimes to kill human beings. Louis Pasteur's germ theory was widely rejected for several decades. After all, Pasteur was not a physician. He was a chemist. The potentially fatal microbes whose existence he proposed were not based on familiar concepts. Neither did allegations of their existence emanate from a seemingly credible source.

Contrast that with today where thoroughly disinfecting one's hands and sterilizing one's medical instruments between successive patients and between successive procedures have become incorporated in the standard of care. Biology and immunology have come a long way since Pasteur's time. More importantly, the behavior of practicing physicians has changed.

For another thing, a sustained behavioral change may require more than mere evidence of improvement. A case in point occurred during the 1840s. This was a decade before Louis Pasteur proposed the existence of microbes. Dr. Ignaz Semmelweis then practiced medicine in Vienna. Two maternity wards at the hospital where he worked displayed startlingly different rates of death among mothers due to what was then called childbed fever.

Dr. Semmelweis pursued several false leads in trying to explain the difference. He eventually came to suspect that the problem might lie in the failure of physicians in the higher-mortality ward to wash their hands and clean their instruments between successive procedures. It was not uncommon for them to deliver a baby right after performing an autopsy. Babies in the lower-mortality ward were delivered by midwives and nurses, none of whom performed autopsies. Dr. Semmelweis therefore guessed that physicians in the higher-mortality ward might be transferring some kind of unknown "death substance" from cadavers to delivering mothers.

To verify his guess physicians in the higher-mortality ward were persuaded to soak their hands and their instruments in a chlorine solution between procedures. A chlorine solution was known to eliminate the stench of death. It was hoped that it might likewise eliminate the imagined "death substance."

Death due to childbed fever in the higher-mortality ward soon dropped to about the same rate as death in the lower-mortality ward (temporarily to a slightly lower rate). Regrettably, however, the change in physician behavior was not permanent. Nobody understood exactly how or why the chlorine solution worked. It was later realized that chlorine kills sepsis-inducing bacteria (Dr. Semmelweis' hypothesized "death substance"), but not until much later.

Physicians in the higher-mortality ward returned to their previous practices. The rate of death due to childbed fever returned to its previous higher level.

Adopting PCM to make individually tailored patient predictions could suffer a similar fate. PCM is most useful in situations where the existence and direction of predictive relationships are well known, but where the detailed linking mechanisms and pathways are not. This can breed understandable skepticism. For example, one of PCM's accuracy-improving devices is the unusual way it searches for and sometimes identifies an apparent signal in missing observations. Inferring any meaningful connection from missing data strikes some as an inappropriate "stretch." Consequently, even after a convincing demonstration of its superior accuracy, endorsement by a credible source and inducement by a governmental or paying agency might still be required to bring about any permanent change in physician behavior.

ACKNOWLEDGEMENTS

The melanoma data set collected from 1,340 University of California at San Francisco (UCSF) patients between 1987 and 2007 was produced, verified, and corrected many times largely by the three authors; by Stanley P. L. Leong, MD; and by Mehdi Nosrati, BS. Of these patients, 1,039 underwent sentinel lymph node biopsies (SLNBs), while 301 did not. Dr. Leong was the surgeon performing the lion's share of the biopsies. Many additional UCSF personnel contributed substantially. Noteworthy among them were Robert E. Allen, MD, and Mark Singer, MD, who also performed many SLNBs; and Serena Mraz-Gernhard, MD, who collected much of the early SLNB patient data.

The melanoma data set collected from 699 University of California at San Francisco (UCSF) patients prior to and during 2006 was produced, verified, and corrected largely by the three authors; by Javier Rangel, MD; by Sima Torabian, MD; and by Mehdi Nosrati, BS. Special thanks are due to Javier Rangel for his diligent efforts in obtaining and verifying these 699 medical records. Other UCSF personnel also contributed substantially to creating the multi-marker assay to distinguish malignant melanomas from benign nevi. Christopher Haqq, MD, PhD, and Mohammed Kashani-Sabet, MD, were principally responsible for the pioneering research effort identifying various genes implicated in the development and differential diagnosis of melanoma. David M. Jablons, MD, steered our research efforts toward the single most discriminating gene (WNT2). Jeffry P. Simco, MD, PhD, provided a useful concordance check on our pathologist's diagnoses, although it was our pathologist (Dr. Sagebiel) who discovered the importance of top-to-bottom differences in expression of all five of the genes in making differential diagnoses. Finally, Dan H. Moore, PhD, performed an alternative statistical analysis (RPART) related to DSSA'S original diagnostic conclusions.

The melanoma data set collected from 269 California Pacific Medical Center (CPMC) patients between 2007 and 2014 was also verified and corrected by the three authors and by Maria Danielsen, a medical student at the University of Copenhagen. Special recognition is due to Maria Danielsen for her diligent efforts in obtaining and verifying medical records both from the 173 CPMC patients who underwent FDG-PET/CT scans and from the ninety-six plausible candidates for that procedure who did not. Other CPMC personnel also contributed substantially to the production and verification of the data. Noteworthy among them were Stanley P. L. Leong, MD; Mark Wu, MD; Karin L. Petersen, MD; and Lea Martineau, RN, BSN.

Special thanks are due to Mehdi Nosrati, BS, currently at the California Pacific Medical Center Research Institute, for producing the ten figures presented in this book.

1.0   INTRODUCTION

A Patient-Centered Methodology (PCM) has been designed to improve the accuracy of individually tailored prognoses in dealing with progressive diseases such as cancer and heart disease. Alternative ways to use PCM are also possible.

A particularly beneficial alternative use is to predict the individually tailored outcome of undergoing a given diagnostic test procedure. There are always attendant costs. There may also be potential complications. If the test result can be predicted with sufficient accuracy, the likelihood of making two kinds of mistakes can be reduced. Both the attendant costs and the potential complications can be avoided by some patients who did not really need to take the test, while test benefits can actually be realized by other patients who did not initially appear to be reasonable candidates to undergo that procedure.

The early portion of this book demonstrates how substituting reliance on PCM-generated, individually tailored probabilities that a test result will be positive for contemporary, guideline-based triage criteria can reduce the prevalence of both kinds of mistakes.

Selecting patients to undergo a sentinel lymph node biopsy (SLNB) will provide a first illustrative context. An SLNB is a surgical procedure given to some cancer patients to diagnose the current extent of their disease progression. It indicates whether or not the cancer has already penetrated their lymphatic system. SLNB surgery is an appropriate illustrative context both because it has substantial attendant costs and because it may produce unwanted side effects.

Selecting patients to undergo an FDG-PET/CT scan will provide a second context to illustrate PCM's ability to avoid both kinds of mistakes. PET/CT scans are also undertaken to ascertain disease progression in several types of cancer.

A brief summary of PCM as originally developed for prognostic purposes follows.

What does it mean for a prognostic methodology to be "patient-centered"? The answer, of course, lies in "patient-centered compared to what?" Let us begin by distinguishing between becoming patient-centered in making focused predictions of patient outcomes and remaining factor-centered. The factor-centered approach is the established paradigm in traditional prognostic research. Based both on its historical success and on its role as a necessary precursor to becoming patient-centered this is a fortunate state of affairs.

Becoming patient-centered is an extension of already being factor-centered. It enhances an existing methodological orientation. It is not a competing alternative orientation. One cannot become effectively patient-centered without having first achieved substantial factor-centered success.

Both the factor-centered and the patient-centered methodological orientations are being viewed here strictly from an evidence-based perspective.

1.1   A Ten-Step Individually Tailored Prognostic Methodology

If individually tailored patient prognoses are to be evidence-based, one may:

1. begin with a targeted individual patient, and then choose some salient state, event, situation or outcome as the focal end point of interest;
2. identify a group of patients similar to the targeted patient in certain

respects relevant to predicting that patient's focal end point;
3. identify a set of prognostic factors that are known to be useful in predicting the focal end point within the specific group identified as similar patients;
4. gather observations on these prognostic factors from a sample of these similar patients;
5. pick a prognostic model (e.g., a regression model) that predicts the focal end point based on each patient's prognostic factor observations;
6. use the sample data to train the model—to estimate via an appropriate statistical technique (e.g., likelihood maximization) the specific numeric model parameters that best fit the observations gathered in the sample of similar patients;
7. assess how well the model fits the data, each prognostic factor's statistical significance, in which direction each factor points, the "shape" of each predictive relationship, and each factor's relative predictive potency, typically involving successive model refinements;
8. if the refined prognostic model statistically fitted to the sample data achieves at least minimal adequacy, derive from it an explicit prognostic algorithm whose inputs (independent variables) relate to observations on the set of prognostic factors and whose output (dependent variable) is a prediction of the focal end point;
9. apply the prognostic algorithm to each patient in the sample to obtain individually tailored predictions of the focal end point; and
10. assess the accuracy of the resulting individual patient predictions.

Traditional prognostic research tends to focus on step seven as just outlined. Executing steps eight, nine, and ten is only carried out to generate some measure of the factors' collective explanatory efficacy (e.g., R-squared, their coefficient of determination). The point of the research is not to make any statements about any particular patient. It is to generate conclusions about the role and the usefulness of various prognostic factors that may be generalized to some prespecified population of interesting patients.

Research conclusions are statistical inferences concerning the prespecified population. Inferences are drawn from careful analysis of sample observations. However, from a deductive perspective, the population must be specified first. Then both the sample of patients on which statistical inferences are based and the targeted individual patient must belong to that prespecified population.

More widely generalizable research conclusions (e.g., more widely encompassing definitions of the prespecified population) are typically judged as an indicator of higher-quality research.

Designing, executing, and evaluating prognostic research in this traditional manner has several important implications.

First, research conclusions based on isolated or otherwise limited samples (e.g., on patients drawn from a single institution) are frequently criticized as "biased,""unrepresentative," or "not population-based." They are suspected not to be representative of some more comprehensive and, therefore, more interesting overall patient population.

Second, research conclusions are presented as attributes of the prognostic factors rather than as attributes of individual patients. They are displayed in tables organized factor-by-factor, not patient-by-patient. They characterize the prognostic factors. They say nothing, directly, about individual patients.

Thus, conclusions from a Cox (proportional hazards) regression analysis are typically tabled values of the estimated regression coefficients, their corresponding relative risks (hazard ratios), and their corresponding p values and calculated confidence intervals. The table contains a separate row for each prognostic factor. Individually tailored survival curves, although easily producible from these tabled values, are rarely graphed or even mentioned.

Conclusions from a logistic regression analysis are also presented as tabled values of the estimated regression coefficients, their corresponding odds ratios, and their corresponding p values and calculated confidence intervals. Individually tailored focal end point probabilities, although easily computable from these tabled values, are rarely produced, displayed, or even mentioned.

Third, the subsequent operations required to move from step seven to step ten, as just outlined, are either omitted or not emphasized. This is because the reason to execute them and their interpretation are not considered "general."

Empirical science is sometimes characterized as the search for relationships among critical variables within some general context. Except for starting with a targeted patient, steps one through seven are consistent with this traditional scientific view of prognostic modeling. Steps eight, nine, and ten then translate an evidence-based prognostic model into something useful to the artful practice of medicine.

Notice, however, that medicine is actually practiced as a skillful art. Doctors do their thing patient-by-patient, not factor-by-factor. Most importantly, translating a prognostic model into useful medical practice interchanges the means-ends relationship between prognostic factors and individual patients.

While trying to establish predictive relationships between prognostic factors and focal states, events, and situations during steps one through seven, data obtained from individual patients are used to draw conclusions about prognostic factors. This is a factor-centered reasoning process. Conclusions are about the factors. Individual patient data serve as a means of (a basis for) drawing such conclusions. Individual patients are freely added to or removed from the similar-patient sample as a matter of analytical convenience, according to their role in contributing to appropriate conclusions about the factors. A patient who is not from the prespecified population or who possesses missing values of any prognostic factor is frequently deleted from the analysis.

While trying to draw a specific conclusion about an individual patient during steps eight, nine, and ten, prognostic factors provide the data source. This is a patient-centered reasoning process. Conclusions are about each separate patient. Conclusions are generated by executing an explicit prognostic algorithm applied, separately, to each patient. This time it is the particular prognostic factors that are added to or removed from the algorithm as a matter of analytical convenience, according to their role in contributing to accurate predictions about individual patients. The very idea of completely ignoring (i.e., drawing no conclusion about) any patient because of missing data on one or more (but not all) prognostic factors is fundamentally antithetical to the goal of becoming patient-centered.

It seems fruitless to debate whether the prognostic factors or the individual patients constitute the "proper" or "more important" focus of medical research. It has just been demonstrated that a detailed consideration of each is necessary to draw evidence-based conclusions about the other.

Notice that the ten-step PCM does not begin by specifying any particular population. It begins instead by targeting an individual patient. We can think of it as the next patient freshly diagnosed with a particular cancer. For purposes of statistical inference, then, the relevant population is specified in steps one and two according to certain attributes of this next patient. The population includes all patients similar to this next patient—similar in terms of our practical ability to make an accurate prediction of the targeted patient's focal end point. It is just by tailoring the subsequent analysis to each patient, separately, that the methodology becomes patient-centered.

The transition from a factor-centered to a patient-centered approach should be regarded as an important shift in methodology. The shift is to a different, though intimately related research paradigm. Yet nothing is being discarded or replaced. Hence, the transition might best be characterized as a significantly reoriented paradigm enhancement rather than as an abrupt paradigm shift.

1.2 How PCM Differs from Traditional Prognostic Methodology

Although securely rooted in traditional prognostic methodology, PCM possesses six differentiating characteristics.

1. Altered Focus

PCM focuses on individual patients rather than on selected prognostic factors. The analysis begins with a targeted individual patient rather than with an interesting patient population. A sample of similar patients is selected on the basis of that targeted patient's particular characteristics. The analysis then proceeds, separately, for separate samples of similar patients. The analysis ends with specific predictions about targeted patients rather than with general conclusions about the role and relative potency of prognostic factors in some interesting population.

Since PCM's focus is on patients, not on prognostic factors, the ultimate purpose of any PCM analysis is neither to estimate nor to test statistical hypotheses concerning distributional parameters that characterize the impact of various prognostic factors in any population. Producing such estimates and performing such formal hypothesis tests do occur along the way. Nevertheless, these are only penultimate activities. They are the means to deriving separate conclusions about individual patients. The ultimate objective of PCM is to estimate, probabilistically, whether or not and when individual patients will experience specific outcomes. Formal hypothesis tests relate to which of two or more separate analytical procedures produce more accurate estimates and whether or not one such procedure is significantly superior to another in this respect.

PCM's altered focus requires different measures of prognostic success. Novel success measures must be devised. After considering the traditional measures of factor success, such as significant p values and clinically important hazard ratios, specific measures of predictive accuracy at the individual patient level must be added. PCM's success is measured by rates of correct outcome prediction, probabilistic prediction errors, and appropriate predictive scale characteristics.

All along the way PCM relies heavily on traditional prognostic methodology. It uses a modified form of logistic regression analysis to predict the occurrence or nonoccurrence of medical events for a particular patient. It uses a modified form of Cox (proportional hazards) regression to generate individually tailored survival curves. These are just two examples of the many modifications made by PCM to traditional prognostic methodology. All such modifications are designed to operationalize the patient-centered concept and to improve, thereby, individually tailored prognostic accuracy.

The principal impact of adopting PCM is to refocus traditional methodology by extending it. PCM first draws the usual factor-centered conclusions. It then derives an explicit prognostic algorithm to make individually tailored, patient-centered predictions.

2. Selective Focus

PCM focuses on a particular end point. The focal end point is some salient patient outcome (i.e., state, event, or situation related to a targeted patient). Changing the focal end point typically changes the analyses performed and sometimes produces quite different conclusions.

Because of its individual patient orientation PCM does not seek to generate substantive medical conclusions generalizable either across patients or across focal end points. Its purpose is to make an accurate prediction of a focal end point for a targeted patient.

3. Selective Stratification

Refocusing and extending traditional methodology in the PCM manner fundamentally alters what it means for a sample of empirical observations to be representative. It is no longer sufficient just to be population-based. It may even be inappropriate. In the patient-centered context, being population-based may serve the penultimate goal but not necessarily the ultimate goal. To be representative now means to be specifically applicable to supporting accurate predictions relating to a targeted individual patient. This strongly suggests regularly reconceiving the fundamental concept of a patient population in stratified terms. Equally strongly it suggests determining the appropriate principle of stratification, separately, on the basis of whichever particular focal question is being asked. Doing both then requires tailoring all supporting analyses accordingly.

For many cancers there exists a single prognostic factor or a single prognostic index constructed from more than one factor that is widely understood within the medical profession and regularly recorded for most patients. Primary tumor size or thickness is such a single factor. Stage of disease progression is such an index.

PCM selects from among such widely understood and regularly recorded factors and indexes the one that appears to possess the greatest univariate impact. Greatest impact means greatest ability to discriminate reliably among different patients in terms of disease progression—whether or not and when the focal end point occurs.

The selected factor or index is then used to stratify the overall patient population. Separate strata contain distinct subpopulations of patients, where the strata differ significantly in terms of the prevalence of and elapsed time to reach the focal end point.

A sample is drawn from the stratum (subpopulation) regarded as most similar to the targeted patient. Similarity refers to accuracy in predicting the focal end point. A prognostic model is trained on (fitted to data within) the similar-patient sample to produce an explicit prognostic algorithm.

Selective stratification serves to homogenize data relationships within subpopulations. Simultaneously, it introduces heterogeneity across separate strata. Statistical modeling is performed separately within homogenized subpopulations. This tends to improve the fit of prognostic models (e.g., logistic regression and Cox regression) to separately drawn samples of data. Missing observations are also handled separately across heterogeneous strata. The likely consequence of any missing observation related to some particular prognostic factor can then be estimated more accurately by exploiting this heterogeneity.

If no suitable factor or index exists for a given cancer, the patient population is not stratified. When performed, the differentiating consequences of stratification are verified. The differential prevalence of and elapsed time to reach the focal end point across subpopulations are both tested statistically (e.g., via Kaplan-Meier analysis).

Selective stratification is one of the principal devices by which PCM improves individually tailored prognostic accuracy.

4. SPSA Conversion

The Scale Partitioning and Spacing Algorithm (SPSA) is another device to improve prognostic accuracy. Scale partitioning means that the set of possible raw measurement values of a prognostic factor is subdivided into two or more distinct subscales. Scale partitioning is optimized so as to produce the most sensitive and specific prediction of the focal end point. Spacing means ascertaining the apparent "distances" separating partitioned subscales that reveal the "shape" of the univariate relationship linking a prognostic factor to the focal end point. The result is a Univariate Impact-Reflecting Index (UIRI). The raw measurement values of most prognostic factors are automatically converted by SPSA into a corresponding UIRI.

A UIRI indicates the direction, the shape, and the clinical potency of whatever univariate relationship the sample data suggest may exist in the similar-patient population stratum linking each prognostic factor to the focal end point. Direction of impact indicates how more or less of the factor relates to more or less of its impact on the focal end point. Shape of relationship indicates whether the factor's impact is exerted at a constant, accelerating, or decelerating rate at different factor levels. Potency of impact indicates the factor's clinical importance (material influence) relative to the focal end point.

A UIRI is depicted both graphically and algebraically. Its algebraic form is normally incorporated into the prognostic model (explicit algorithm) produced by PCM for a sample of similar patients. Its graphical depiction serves as a visual aid to enhance understanding.

SPSA is a useful tool to the extent that a prognostic factor's impact on some focal end point is genuine, though incompletely understood. A UIRI suggests some form of association or correlation. It may or may not also signal a causal connection linking the prognostic factor to the focal end point in the population stratum containing similar patients. Fortunately, since prediction is the goal of PCM, association or correlation, when genuine, can be useful—as long as it is systematic. The underlying biology need not be understood in detail.

Genuine means that the apparent linkage relationship is more than a statistical artifact resulting from overfitting a prognostic model to inadequate sample data. Quite large samples are required to distinguish genuine relationships (even if only correlational) from spurious correlations. Only large samples can support split-sample reliability testing, whereby the predictive improvements seemingly achieved in an algorithm-fitting sample can be shown to carry over to a completely distinct validation sample drawn from the same population stratum.

On the other hand, if the detailed biological mechanisms mediating a factor's impact were thoroughly understood, data conversion via SPSA would not be helpful. It would not be performed. Yet detailed knowledge of the underlying pathways and connections linking commonly used prognostic factors to popular focal end points is, today, largely nonexistent. Even the shape, as opposed to just the existence and direction, of many linkage relationships remains poorly understood.

PCM, therefore, converts almost all prognostic factor data into corresponding UIRI scores. This does not improve the univariate predictive accuracy of dichotomous prognostic factors such as whether or not a primary tumor has become ulcerated. Such factors possess a directional relationship but without any distinctive shape. In contrast, the predictive accuracy of genuinely quantitative prognostic factors such as tumor size and mitotic rate is sometimes improved substantially. Quantitative factors can display quite distinctive and predictively useful shapes.

5. Dealing with Missing Observations

A sample may contain missing observations on one or more prognostic factors. If not too many observations were missing and if the goal of the analysis were factor-centered, it would be tempting simply to delete patients with missing observations from the analysis.

Becoming patient-centered, however, precludes such a strategy. The goal is to make a specific prediction, even if imprecise, for all patients. SPSA includes detailed procedures to estimate likely end point values for missing observations of all prognostic factors. The efficacy of these procedures is considerably enhanced by selective stratification of the patient population.

SPSA's special handling of missing observations is another device that improves individually tailored prognostic accuracy.

6. Incorporating Additional Factors

The progress of medical science will continue to produce new prognostic factors for various cancers. Incorporating new factors into the analysis via stratification, SPSA, and its special handling of missing observations has been shown to be especially helpful. Substantial increases in the accuracy of individually tailored end point predictions can regularly be achieved by analyzing newly discovered factors in the PCM manner.

A detailed description of PCM can be found in *Patient-Centered Prognosis: A Methodology to Improve Individually Tailored Prognostic Accuracy Illustrated in Two Cancers*, written by the authors of this book and published by iUniverse LLC in April 2013. PCM was first applied to a sample of 1,222 melanoma patients in the United States. PCM was then separately applied to a sample of 1,225 breast cancer patients in Finland. Compared to current prognostic methodology PCM improved substantially the accuracy of individually tailored predictions of disease-specific death within five years of initial diagnosis in both samples. The same results were reported in "A Patient-Centered Methodology That Improves the Accuracy of Prognostic Predictions in Cancer," *PLoS One*, 2013 (8)2:e56435.

1.3   Some of PCM's Principal Benefits

For a number of years the American Joint Committee on Cancer (AJCC) has been focusing on certain prognostic factors useful in predicting the progress of many forms of cancer. We shall designate these traditional or conventional factors. AJCC stage at diagnosis is a prominent example. Patient age at diagnosis and sex of patient are two other examples. So, also, are the size and dimensions of a patient's primary tumor, its histological type, its anatomical location, its degree of ulceration, and its grade or proliferative capacity (e.g., its mitotic rate).

Ongoing medical research continues to identify additional factors that possess prognostic significance. However, unless or until the AJCC "anoints" them, we shall refer to these simply as additional factors. Vascular factors in melanoma and recently discovered, gene-based biomarkers implicated in both the onset and the progression of several cancers constitute additional prognostic factors.

It is common practice to include observations of traditional or conventional factors in the medical records of most patients at the time of their initial diagnosis. Observations of additional factors are less commonly included, and then only at some, typically long-established medical centers.

PCM generates relative predictive potency weights both for traditional or conventional and for additional prognostic factors. These are supplementary to its individually tailored probabilistic predictions of a focal end point.

Potency weights indicate the relative contribution of each factor to making accurate individually tailored probabilistic predictions. Potency weights are both individual-patient-specific and focal-end-point-specific. The weights assigned to (additional) prognostic factors not already included in a patient's initial diagnostic record can suggest which incremental observations would be useful to obtain and in what sequence.

The single most important benefit provided by PCM is greater predictive accuracy. Greater accuracy is useful to patients in making a variety of personal life-planning choices. Greater accuracy is also useful to physicians in making important patient management decisions.

Improving the quality of treatment selection decisions is a striking way to exploit greater predictive accuracy. Using PCM to identify appropriate candidates for the treatment of melanoma via high-dose alpha-2b interferon (IFN) illustrates this application. Substantially better discrimination between appropriate and inappropriate candidates for IFN treatment was documented in both previously cited references to PCM (see "ANNOTATED REFERENCES").

Contemporary guidelines to select melanoma patients for IFN treatment include presenting with a thick primary tumor (exceeding four millimeters) and node-positive disease. Better discrimination was achieved by applying PCM to six traditional and eighteen additional prognostic factors. Facilitating such an improvement is especially welcome in the high-dose IFN context because that treatment normally has a number of seriously unpleasant side effects.

The early portion of this book will illustrate how PCM-generated, individually tailored probabilities that a sentinel lymph node biopsy (SLNB) and that an FDG-PET/CT scan, respectively, will produce a positive test outcome may be used to identify which patients are appropriate candidates to undergo each specific diagnostic procedure. It is the superior predictive accuracy at the individual patient level delivered by PCM that facilitates using it for patient triage.

Specifically, it will be demonstrated that:

1. PCM-generated predictions can be sufficiently accurate to justify their use in the triage of patients both to SLNBs and to PET/CT scans so as to improve the cost-benefit consequences of performing each procedure;
2. PCM-generated predictions can be significantly more accurate than similar predictions produced by contemporary, conventional prognostic procedures, further supporting the adoption of PCM for both purposes;
3. PCM's superior accuracy in predicting SLNB outcomes can be validated as genuine—not a spurious artifact of statistically overfitting a prediction algorithm to inadequate sample data; and
4. cost-benefit trade-offs based on PCM-generated predictions can be tailored specifically both to the cost structure of and to the cultural and other preferences held by any particular medical institution.

1.4 Some of PCM's Limitations

Focusing every predictive analysis on a specific end point experienced by a targeted individual patient; stratifying the patient population, accordingly, into relatively homogeneous subpopulations; preprocessing prognostic factors via SPSA; dealing with missing observations in the SPSA manner; and incorporating additional factors into the analysis via these same analytical devices constitute the means by which PCM achieves its greater predictive accuracy. Unfortunately, the use of these very same devices simultaneously imposes several limitations on the resulting predictions.

Abandoning the comforting assumption that a single, overarching, and reasonably homogeneous patient population exists for every cancer generally requires stratification. Stratification requires significantly larger sample sizes for reliable statistical estimation. It also increases the risk of overfitting the predictive algorithm derived from any prognostic analysis to whatever empirical observations (i.e., training data) are used to produce that algorithm.

SPSA also requires significantly larger sample sizes for reliable statistical estimation. Additional parameters must be estimated to partition the raw measurement scale of each prognostic factor, separately, in each population stratum. This, too, increases the risk of overfitting and for the same reason.

When combined with stratification, dealing with missing observations in the SPSA manner generally does improve predictive accuracy. This is largely because default values assigned to patients with missing observations on some prognostic factor differ systematically according to the separate stratum each patient occupies. The more predictively differentiating the stratification procedure, the more discriminating the assigned, stratum-specific default values become. This improves the accuracy of both logistic and Cox regression. However, estimating numerous default values has a similar overfitting impact.

Adding additional prognostic factors to any analysis increases the number of statistical parameters that must be estimated. When executed in the PCM manner this increase is magnified. Its overfitting impact is likewise magnified.

What does statistical overfitting mean, and when is it a problem?

A prognostic model is fitted via some statistical technique (regression analysis) to some particular collection of empirical observations. Empirical observations are made on selected attributes (prognostic factors) of selected entities (a training sample of patients). The statistical technique produces a prognostic algorithm. Inputs to (independent variables of) the algorithm are values of or indexes constructed from the observed attributes. The output (dependent variable) predicts (probabilistically) the focal end point.

The prognostic algorithm is fitted to a particular collection of empirical observations by choosing a specific set of (numeric) model parameters. The chosen parameters are those that render most plausible (e.g., most likely or prediction-error-minimizing) the observations actually contained in the training data if the assumed underlying model properly characterizes the entities and their related attributes in the population stratum from which that sample was obtained. Hence, training means statistical fitting of the parameters of a particular population model to a specific sample of observations. The prognostic algorithm is trained via the sample observations.

When the number of observations in a training sample becomes "too small" relative to the number of model parameters fitted to the observed data, the resulting prognostic algorithm is said to be overfitted. Its number of observations typically serves as a count of the number of degrees of freedom inherent in a training sample. The number of statistically independent observations in the sample is the dimensionality of (i.e., the number of orthogonal dimensions constituting) its sample space.

Sample sizes are frequently characterized as either "too small" or "large enough" by simple rules of thumb. An example would be that overfitting is avoided so long as the number of sample observations in the training data is at least ten times the number of parameters estimated by the fitted prognostic algorithm. Otherwise, the algorithm may be overfitted. This is because statistical estimation reduces the number of degrees of freedom remaining in the data. The estimation procedure uses them up. Apparent accuracy of estimation is improved at the expense of the degrees of freedom so consumed. We might think of degrees of freedom as the currency we must expend in order to purchase additional accuracy.

PCM consumes many more degrees of freedom inherent within its training data than a typical, factor-centered analysis. Stratification, preprocessing via SPSA, and SPSA's manner of dealing with missing observations all involve the fitting of additional parameters over and above the parameters that are subsequently fitted to training data via multiple regression analysis. That is why special care must be exercised to avoid overfitting.

Some protection against overfitting is provided internally by PCM's admissibility requirements. Virtually any attribute of a patient or aspect of that patient's life situation can serve as a candidate prognostic factor. However, not all candidates are admissible. In order for a candidate attribute or aspect to qualify as an admissible prognostic factor:

1. it must be recorded on a raw measurement scale containing at least two distinguishable, numerically coded values—otherwise, it cannot serve to discriminate among patients in terms of the focal end point;
2. its raw measurement values (if the scale possesses three or more) must indicate increasing or decreasing degrees of whatever attribute or aspect is being measured—otherwise, it cannot be said to constitute

at least an ordinal measure of that raw attribute or aspect;
3. it must be systematically related (either causally or correlationally) to the focal end point—otherwise, it cannot be said to have any genuine prognostic impact;
4. where the systematic relationship must be monotonic throughout the entire scale of values—otherwise, the impact of the prognostic factor on the focal end point cannot be said to be uniformly directional (the SPSA algorithm includes specific steps to verify uniform directionality);
5. where the uniformly directional nature of the relationship must be reasonably well established (e.g., in the relevant scientific literature) in advance of any patient-centered analysis—otherwise, the prognostic methodology cannot be characterized as plausibly predictive (as opposed to just exploratory); and
6. it must be available as raw data in a training sample of similar patients, and at least two distinct scale values must be assigned to patients in that sample—otherwise, it cannot be used to estimate statistically the parameters of a prognostic algorithm applicable to any individual patient, including the targeted patient.

Additional protection against overfitting is provided when the SPSA algorithm partitions the raw measurement scale of a prognostic factor. SPSA possesses a "control knob" to guarantee a minimum partition size (i.e., a minimum count of patients in each subsample associated with each partition of that measurement scale, including the partition associated with missing observations).

Collectively, these admissibility requirements are designed to support reasonably stable statistical estimates of predictive relationships shown by previous research to link selected prognostic factors to the focal end point. They generally necessitate quite large sample sizes.

A reasonable protection against overfitting is also provided by a split-sample reliability test of the prognostic algorithm eventually produced. This serves to verify that whatever improvement in predictive accuracy appears to have been achieved by PCM is genuine. It is not a spurious artifact of statistically overfitting the prediction algorithm to inadequate training data.

Data quality is also essential to PCM. The methodology employs a number of reasonably sophisticated analytical techniques. It does more than just summarize data in terms of means, standard deviations, and cross-tabulations. Noisy patient data, containing many incorrect and inconsistent observations, can neutralize the efficacy of these otherwise useful techniques. Typically, the more sophisticated the analysis, the more easily it can be compromised by even a little noise in the data.

We must acknowledge that the training data used to produce an algorithm that predicts SLNB test results were of distinctly higher-than-average quality. Medical records of the 1,340 patients compiled by the University of California at San Francisco (UCSF) were rechecked and selectively corrected many times. Similar comments apply to the training data used to predict PET/CT scan results for the 269 patients at the California Pacific Medical Center (CPMC). We do not claim that PCM would perform as well on the less clean medical records commonly encountered throughout the world. Much existing medical data would require thorough "precleaning" prior to any useful analysis via PCM.

1.5   Consequences of an Altered and Selective Focus

The ultimate goal of PCM is to make separately tailored predictions about individual patients relative to a focal end point. Assessing the predictive potency of various prognostic factors in stratified patient subpopulations regularly occurs along the way—but only as a repeated penultimate activity.

This changes the fundamental nature of the questions we ask, the hypotheses we formulate and test, and the way we measure success. Such changes are immediate consequences of PCM's altered and selective focus. Can PCM improve prognostic accuracy? That is the overarching question. If so, by how much and compared to what?

When selecting patients to undergo either an SLNB or a PET/CT scan, the test outcome (positive or negative) of actually performing the procedure will be the focal end point to be predicted. Predictions will be stated probabilistically. Each patient's probability of having a positive diagnostic test result will be estimated by a modified form of logistic regression analysis. Our principal measure of predictive accuracy will be the percentage rate of correct outcome predictions enabled by PCM for some set of patients. The relevant hypotheses to formulate and test will be whether or not and the extent to which PCM is successful both in making such predictions accurately and in achieving accuracy improvements compared to similar predictions made by alternative methodologies.

How might one measure the accuracy of a set of probabilistic predictions? We shall do this in three ways.

1. Rank-order the individual probabilistic predictions of a positive SLNB or PET/CT scan generated by logistic regression from largest to smallest. Then test each cut point between adjacent probabilities in the rank order as a possible dichotomous discriminator. Tentatively predict that all patients whose probabilities exceed a given cut point experience a positive outcome, while all patients with lower probabilities experience a negative outcome. Count the number of correct predictions for that cut point. Repeat the process for each possible cut point. Choose the cut point that offers the highest correct count. Designate this the (not necessarily unique) optimum cut point, and designate its corresponding count the maximum possible number of correct predictions. Divide the maximum count by the number of probabilities in the rank order to compute the percentage rate of correct predictions.

   If a receiver operating characteristic (ROC) analysis were performed on the same set of ranked probabilities, an estimated area under the curve (AUC) of 1.00 would correspond to a 100 percent correct prediction rate, and vice versa. ROC/AUC analysis is frequently performed and widely reported in the medical research literature. Our percentage rate of correct predictions is conceptually close to and very highly correlated with an AUC score calculated from the same data set. In many instances throughout this book we shall present both statistics side by side. However, we prefer the percentage rate of correct predictions because it seems to reflect the overarching goal of achieving predictive accuracy in an intuitively more obvious and straightforward manner. Both our SLNB and our PET/CT scan analyses will generate correct prediction rates of approximately 86 percent.

   The United States Weather Bureau faces a similar task in assessing its probabilistic predictions for accuracy and reliability. It makes daily forecasts covering all kinds of weather. Imagine that the chance of rain for a given day at some location is announced to be a number between 20 and 30 percent. As more and more forecasts are made, the mean of all daily probabilistic predictions announcing the chance of rain to fall between 20 and 30 percent should gradually converge toward the actual incidence of rain at that same location during those same days. Also, the actual incidence should fall within the 20-to-30 percent interval. In like manner, mean probabilistic predictions in all other intervals throughout the entire range of forecasts should gradually converge toward their corresponding actual incidences, and the incidences eventually realized should always fall within their respective intervals.

2. We shall divide the set of rank-ordered probabilistic predictions of a positive test result into quartiles. The mean of the probabilities in each quartile will be compared with the actual prevalence of positive outcomes among the patients in that quartile. These two numbers should be about the same in each quartile. The maximum and mean absolute differences between corresponding mean probabilities and actual prevalence will serve as measures of predictive inaccuracy for PCM. They will turn out to be quite small. The pattern of prediction errors observed in different quartiles will also be used to assess predictive reliability at different locations along the probability scale.

When there are only a few distinctly different probability values in a data set, partitioning the scale into a small number of subscales (such as quartiles) may be an appropriate procedure. However, when there are many more distinctly different probabilistic predictions we can investigate their scale characteristics much more thoroughly. The SPSA algorithm will be executed to partition the SLNB probabilistic prediction scale into as many subscales as possible, as long as each subscale encompasses SLNB positivity probabilities for at least enough patients to permit reasonably accurate prevalence estimates. Our SLNB analysis will succeed in generating mean prediction probabilities that converge toward each corresponding actual prevalence in all subscales. When actual prevalence is regressed against mean prediction probability (simple linear regression), an R-squared value (coefficient of determination) in excess of 98 percent will be achieved in both our SLNB and PET/CT scan analyses.

3. Whether or not one methodology produces more accurate predictions than another will be tested, statistically, by matched-sample comparisons. Each sample will contain the set of individually tailored probabilistic predictions of diagnostic test positivity assigned by a particular methodology to each patient. Matching occurs patient-by-patient. Alternative methodologies assign separate test positivity probabilities to each patient.

A Wilcoxon matched-pairs, signed-ranks test will be adopted to compare two methodologies. When more than two are being compared, the Friedman two-way analysis of variance by ranks will be employed.

In all such statistical tests, the uniform null hypothesis will be that no difference in predictive accuracy exists between or among alternative methodologies.

Formal hypothesis tests will generally be nondirectional (i.e., two-tailed tests). It is the existence versus nonexistence of any systematic difference in accuracy that is being tested.

The direction and magnitude of differences in predictive accuracy will be measured by the absolute value of probabilistic prediction errors. A prediction error is the difference between whatever probability some methodology assigns for a positive diagnostic test to a patient and its 0/1 actual occurrence. Zero signifies a negative test result. One signifies a positive test result. The more accurate methodology is the one that generates systematically smaller absolute error differences.

Using probabilistic errors to quantify predictive accuracy can introduce outliers (i.e., extreme values) into the analysis. When a patient actually experiences a rare focal event, the difference between that patient's (typically close to zero) assigned probability and the 1.0 signifying actual occurrence can be much larger than the error differences assigned to the many other patients who do not experience it. Outliers can also arise, although in the reverse manner, with very frequently occurring focal events.

The occurrence of outliers complicates the determination of systematically smaller or larger error differences when means are calculated and compared. It can also undermine the presumption of normally distributed test statistics underlying many parametric procedures (e.g., the analysis of variance and t tests).

Via the magic of the Central Limit Theorem difficulty with outliers is reduced as sample sizes increase. It will sometimes be necessary, however, to assess the direction and magnitude of differences in predictive accuracy by comparing samples of small-to-intermediate size.

The Wilcoxon matched-pairs, signed-ranks test is less sensitive to outliers than the parametric matched-pairs t test. It is based on mean differences in the ranks of matched-pair differences rather than on mean differences between each pair of probabilities, which might include outliers. So also and for the same reason is the Friedman two-way analysis of variance by ranks less sensitive than the parametric analysis of variance (randomized block design). Another possible test, the binomial sign test, is not at all sensitive to outliers when performing a matched-pairs comparison.

Both the Wilcoxon test and the Friedman test have very high relative efficiency (in the neighborhood of 95 percent) in their ability to reject the null hypothesis. Hence, very little needs to be sacrificed to protect effectively against troublesome outliers. These nonparametric tests will be regularly performed throughout the remainder of this book. Occasionally, their slightly more powerful equivalent parametric tests will also be performed and reported, especially when sample sizes are quite adequate.

That the binomial sign test is insensitive to outliers suggests a uniform way to calibrate both the direction and the magnitude of predictive accuracy when comparing different methodologies. Relative predictive accuracy can be encapsulated in an index of error reduction. The index is designed to resemble an ordinary correlation coefficient. It is the signed proportion of net error reductions in any set of matched-pair comparisons calculated as follows.

1. First, select one of two methodologies as more likely to make accurate predictions (e.g., by comparing percentage rates of correct predictions).
2. Then count the number of matched pairs wherein the selected methodology generates the smaller absolute probabilistic prediction error. These

are labeled error reductions.
3. Subtract from this the number of matched pairs wherein the selected methodology generates the larger absolute error. These are labeled error increases.
4. Ignore matched pairs with equal absolute errors.
5. Finally, divide the difference between these two counts by their sum (i.e., the number of matched pairs containing nonidentical absolute errors).

The index ranges in value from -1.0, when all comparisons produce (unanticipated) error increases, to +1.0, when all comparisons produce (anticipated) error reductions. Analogous to a correlation coefficient it has a value of 0.0 when the number of error reductions is exactly offset by an equal number of error increases.

The index of error reduction can be calculated for any set of matched prediction errors. Its sign and magnitude indicate which of any two methodologies generates the more accurate probabilistic predictions. Since it is normalized to fall between -1.0 and +1.0, the relative predictive accuracy of several different methodologies may be determined at a glance. Alternative methodologies may then be ordered according to their relative predictive accuracy.

The distribution of the Wilcoxon test statistic rapidly approaches normality as the number of nontied matched-pair comparisons increases. Whenever the count exceeds twenty-five, this approximation becomes quite satisfactory. Hence, an equivalent standardized Z statistic will generally be computed and referred to the unit normal distribution for statistical significance testing. The Z statistic is the Wilcoxon test statistic divided by its standard deviation. Only for small counts (twenty-five or fewer nontied matched pairs) will an exact probability be computed for Wilcoxon p values.

PCM has been specifically designed to anticipate nontrivial amounts of missing patient data. No patient record is required to possess complete data on all prognostic factors. The SPSA algorithm associates specific probabilistic outcome estimates with every missing observation. This can introduce a substantial number of tied outcome probabilities into the analysis which, in turn, can also skew or otherwise undermine the presumption of normally distributed test statistics.

The Wilcoxon test eliminates within-pair tied observations. The Kruskal-Wallis test, the Mann-Whitney test, and both the Spearman and Kendall rank correlation tests contain explicit procedures that correct for tied observations. Their parametric equivalents lack such procedures and, typically, assume normal distributions.

These considerations constitute a second reason to systematically substitute nonparametric for parametric statistical tests in assessing PCM.

The design of PCM renders it especially vulnerable to overfitting a prognostic algorithm to training data. As previously stated, the same devices that PCM employs to improve predictive accuracy can also produce this unwanted side effect. Unless otherwise indicated, all applications of the SPSA algorithm will be executed with a minimum scale partition size of twenty-five patient observations. This will provide some protection against excessive overfitting. Larger minimum scale partition sizes afford greater protection and will occasionally be adopted.

2.0 ADAPTING PCM TO RENDER SENTINEL LYMPH NODE BIOPSIES MORE COST-EFFECTIVE

The greater predictive accuracy delivered by PCM at the individual patient level can be exploited to identify which patients should and which patients should not undergo some diagnostic test procedure. This is accomplished by adapting PCM to predict the procedure's test outcome. The positive or negative test result becomes PCM's focal event to be predicted.

If PCM's predictions are sufficiently accurate, the possible pain and cost of undergoing a diagnostic procedure may be avoided by some patients who initially appeared to be reasonable candidates but who do not really need the test. PCM may show their likelihood of a positive test outcome to be too low. To take the test would not be worthwhile for them. Other patients, who were initially overlooked as reasonable candidates, might actually undergo the procedure. Surprisingly, PCM may show their likelihood of a positive outcome to be high enough to justify taking the test, after all.

Identifying which patients should and should not undergo a sentinel lymph node biopsy (SLNB) illustrates this eminently actionable application of PCM.

An SLNB is a surgical procedure applied both to melanoma and to breast cancer patients to evaluate their current extent of disease progression. It indicates whether or not an invasive form of the cancer has already penetrated their lymphatic system. The procedure entails the injection of a radiotracer around their primary lesion on the skin or in the breast. The injection is followed by lymphoscintigraphy to ascertain which lymph nodes within a nearby lymphatic basin take up the radioactivity. These are called sentinel lymph nodes. They are said to "light up" under lymphoscintigraphy.

SLNB surgery is expensive. It may also have side effects, such as scarring, infection, lymphedema, and numbness. For both reasons it will be quite useful to compare SLNB's costs and individual patient benefits to identify which patients should and which patients should not undergo the procedure.

The medical records of 1,039 melanoma patients who underwent SLNBs at the University of California at San Francisco (UCSF) between 1987 and 2007 were collected and analyzed. To ensure clean data, their records were checked, rechecked, and selectively corrected many times. Selected attributes of these 1,039 patients are presented in appendix A.

The outcomes of their 1,039 biopsies are tabled below.

VALUE OF ATTRIBUTE SLNSTATE	ABSOLUTE FREQUENCIES (COUNTS)	RELATIVE FREQUENCIES (PROPORTIONS)	CUMULATIVE RELATIVE FREQUENCIES
NEGATIVE	852	.8200	.8200
POSITIVE	187	.1800	1.0000
TOTAL	1039	1.0000	

Note: SLNSTATE designates the outcome of each patient's sentinel lymph node biopsy (SLNB). NEGATIVE indicates that the cancer had not yet involved any regional lymph node(s). POSITIVE indicates that the cancer had involved one or more regional lymph node(s). For these 1,039 patients the SLNB yield (i.e., the generation of positive test outcomes) was 18 percent. There were no missing observations of SLNSTATE.

TABLE OF JOINT ABSOLUTE FREQUENCIES (COUNTS)

VALUE OF ATTRIBUTE SLNSTATE	VALUE OF ATTRIBUTE SLNDUMMY		
	0	1	TOTAL
NEGATIVE	852	0	852
POSITIVE	0	187	187
TOTAL	852	187	1039

Note: SLNDUMMY is a 0/1 dummy attribute created as a numerically coded
       equivalent of the SLNSTATE attribute. A "0" value of SLNDUMMY corresponds
       to a NEGATIVE SLNB outcome, and a "1" value of SLNDUMMY corresponds to a
       POSITIVE SLNB outcome. All logistic regression analyses with SLNB outcome
       as the focal end point to be predicted require this 0/1 dummy attribute
       to be entered as the dependent variable. Since it is merely a recoded
       version of SLNSTATE, SLNDUMMY also possessed no missing observations.

PCM improves the accuracy of predicting as either positive or negative an
individual patient's SLNB outcome by:

1. first stratifying patients according to their risk of experiencing a
   positive SLNB outcome, using both their age at initial diagnosis and
   the thickness (Breslow depth in millimeters) of their primary tumor as
   stratification criteria;
2. then executing the SPSA algorithm, separately, within each risk
   subgroup to transform each traditional (i.e., routinely recorded)
   prognostic factor into a corresponding UIRI;
3. then appending additional, nontraditional prognostic factors
   transformed to corresponding UIRIs by the same SPSA algorithm applied,
   separately, to each risk subgroup;
4. then performing a separate multivariate logistic regression analysis
   within each risk subgroup, using transformed UIRI indexes as
   independent variables and SLNDUMMY as the dependent variable; and
5. merging the results obtained from each risk subgroup's multivariate
   logistic regression analysis into a composite, individually tailored
   prediction algorithm designed to simulate the outcomes of having every
   patient actually undergo an SLNB.

It will be instructive to see how successive steps in this sequence provide
incremental improvements in predictive accuracy.

2.1 Establishing a Base Case for Assessing Accuracy Improvements

For a number of years the American Joint Committee on Cancer (AJCC) has been
focusing on certain widely understood and routinely recorded prognostic factors
useful in predicting the progress of various cancers. In melanoma, prior to
2009, these included:

1. age of patient at the time of initial diagnosis (whole number of years
   as of most recent birthday, where risk increases with increasing age);
2. sex of patient (male or female, with male higher risk);
3. anatomical location of primary tumor (axial, if on head, neck, or
   trunk; peripheral, if on arms or legs, with axial higher risk);
4. thickness of primary tumor (Breslow depth in millimeters, where risk
   increases with increasing thickness);

5. Clark level of primary tumor invasion (I, II, III, IV, or V, where risk increases with increasing Clark level); and
6. ulceration of primary tumor (present or absent, with ulcerated tumors higher risk).

Higher risk was normally interpreted to mean a probably shorter time interval until experiencing successive events indicating further disease progression.

In 2009 the AJCC substituted mitotic rate for Clark level whenever the primary tumor's mitotic rate is ascertainable at initial diagnosis. Mitotic rate counts the number of mitoses observed under the microscope in one square millimeter (a high-powered microscopic field or hpf). Mitotic rate, when ascertainable, was also substituted for Clark level as a way to distinguish between stage 1a and stage 1b patients in the revised AJCC melanoma staging classification recommended for 2010 and beyond. Risk increases with increasing mitotic rate.

We designated these six revised AJCC factors the traditional prognostic factors in melanoma. We designated the specific raw data transformation recommended by the AJCC to measure each traditional factor its corresponding factor index. Appendix A describes how the AJCC constructed each traditional factor index.

We then defined a base case analysis against which to assess improvements in accuracy provided by PCM. The base case analysis was a standard (nonstratified) multivariate logistic regression. SLNB outcome (SLNDUMMY) was its dependent variable. The six traditional AJCC factor indexes (AJCCAGE, AJCCSEX, AJCCSITE, AJCCTHIC, AJCCMITR, AND AJCCULC) served as its independent variables.

These traditional factor indexes have been developed over the years to explain better disease progression in a generic sense. The AJCC seemed to have in mind popular end points such as recurrence, distant metastasis, disease-specific death and overall death.

Their efforts were successful. To the best of our knowledge, however, the traditional factor indexes they constructed were not specifically designed to predict SLNB positivity. Therefore, the first thing to verify in our 1,039-patient sample was that the raw data transformations recommended by the AJCC actually did improve base case predictions of SLNB positivity.

1. The AJCCAGE factor index partitions actual patient age as of most recent birthday prior to initial diagnosis into ten-year intervals.

   A univariate logistic regression of SLNDUMMY on actual patient age at diagnosis generated a highly significant negative regression coefficient with a likelihood ratio chi-square statistic of 10.411 and a corresponding two-tailed p value of 0.0013.

   Substituting AJCCAGE for actual patient age improved these results by a small amount. A slightly more significant negative regression coefficient was generated with a likelihood ratio chi-square statistic of 11.004 and a corresponding two-tailed p value of 0.0009.

   That the regression coefficient was highly significantly negative in both analyses is quite striking. It strongly suggests that being diagnosed with melanoma at an earlier age (not at a later age) is associated with SLNB positivity. Age at diagnosis appears to point in the "wrong" direction (i.e., opposite compared to its impact on other popular indicators of disease progression, such as the occurrence of distant metastasis and disease-specific death).

To confirm that age pointed in the "right" direction with respect to distant metastasis, two additional univariate logistic regressions were executed with this other end point as the dependent variable and with actual age and AJCCAGE, respectively, as independent variables. Both analyses generated positive regression coefficients, as anticipated.

To confirm that age also pointed in the "right" direction with respect to disease-specific death, two additional univariate logistic regressions were executed with this other end point as the dependent variable and with actual age and AJCCAGE, respectively, as independent variables. Both of these analyses also generated positive coefficients.

Other researchers have shown that a patient's age at diagnosis is a significant predictor of SLNB positivity, and also in the reverse direction. One cannot simply dismiss this analysis of the 1,039 patients as some kind of fluke based on an unrepresentative sample.

Rather, the reversal in the direction of impact of patient age on SLNB positivity, compared to its impact on other popular indicators of disease progression, illustrates quite dramatically the importance of tailoring a prognostic analysis separately to separate focal end points. Uncritically adopting the conventional wisdom does not always work. The requirement to verify explicitly with SPSA the directional impact of each prognostic factor is one of PCM's principal virtues. Failing to do so will later be shown to undermine the efficacy of otherwise quite reasonable research efforts.

2. Patient sex is dichotomous. The AJCCSEX factor index assigns zero to being female and one to being male. This indicates that males are at higher risk of disease progression than females. Beside providing this directional guidance in numeric form, however, neither the AJCCSEX factor index nor any other dichotomous index can improve predictive accuracy through logistic regression analysis compared to using its dichotomous raw data input.

The "right" direction of impact was uniformly confirmed by univariate logistic regression analyses for SLNB positivity, distant metastasis, and disease-specific death. The impact of patient sex on SLNB positivity was statistically insignificant, but its impact was significant both on distant metastasis and on disease-specific death, each with a two-tailed p value less than 0.02.

3. The AJCCSITE factor index groups together primary tumors located on the head, neck, and trunk as axial. Primary tumors located on the arms and legs are grouped together as peripheral. An axial location is presumed to be higher risk than a peripheral location, so AJCCSITE scores axial locations as one and peripheral locations as zero.

Surprisingly, a univariate logistic regression of SLNDUMMY on AJCCSITE generated a negative regression coefficient with a likelihood ratio chi-square statistic of 0.482 and a corresponding two-tailed p value of 0.4877. AJCCSITE was similar to AJCCAGE. It, too, pointed (although only weakly) in the "wrong" direction with respect to SLNB positivity.

To confirm that AJCCSITE pointed in the "right" direction with respect to distant metastasis and disease-specific death, two additional univariate logistic regressions were executed with these two other end points, respectively, as dependent variables and with AJCCSITE as the independent variable in each analysis. Both analyses generated positive regression coefficients, as anticipated.

Inspection of anatomical locations revealed a 9.55 percent prevalence of SLNB positivity associated with the upper extremities, a 10.80 percent prevalence associated with the head or neck, a 19.91 percent prevalence associated with the trunk, and a 25.93 percent prevalence associated with the lower extremities. Yes, AJCCSITE's axial versus peripheral grouping was appropriate for predicting distant metastasis and disease-specific death, but not for predicting SLNB positivity.

We experimented with other ways to group anatomical locations of the primary tumor. The best result was achieved by grouping together tumors located on the head, neck, and arms as upper-body and tumors located on the trunk and legs as lower-body. Upper-body tumors seemed to pose a lower risk (10.17 percent prevalence of SLNB positivity) than lower-body tumors (22.04 percent prevalence of SLNB positivity).

A univariate logistic regression of SLNDUMMY on this revised grouping (upper-body scored as zero, lower-body scored as one) generated a significantly positive regression coefficient with a likelihood ratio chi-square statistic of 24.088 and a corresponding two-tailed p value less than 0.00005. These are decidedly more dramatic results.

Note that the grouping of anatomical locations was revised after and on the basis of inferring from the observed sample data the apparently most discriminating relationship linking anatomical location to SLNB positivity. Because of this, the revised regression results cannot be interpreted in the traditional hypothesis testing manner. The existence versus nonexistence of a linking relationship cannot legitimately be tested by means of a measurement (e.g., grouping) procedure specifically designed to maximize its apparent magnitude. That would involve logically circular reasoning.

In contrast, using the revised grouping to test the same linking relationship in a separate sample of patients (e.g., drawn either from an entirely different population or from the same population in the service of a split-sample reliability analysis) would be legitimate. Application to a completely distinct sample would satisfy traditional hypothesis testing logical requirements.

So why did we report the sign of the regression coefficient, the value of the chi-square statistic, and its accompanying p value derived from a logistic regression analysis of the revised grouping? If not legitimately interpretable in traditional hypothesis testing terms then how are these same statistics now to be interpreted? The answer is descriptively rather than in the traditional inferential manner.

Substitution of the revised grouping for the traditional AJCC grouping appears both to clarify the nature of and to strengthen the apparent magnitude of the relationship linking anatomical location to SLNB positivity. The reported statistics indicate an apparent improvement in effective measurement. They suggest that the revised grouping better captures the true underlying relationship reflected in the data.

To the extent that we may have accepted the traditional AJCC way of grouping anatomical locations as universally optimal for predicting all interesting end points including SLNB outcome (not just for the various popular end points for which it was specifically designed) we may be surprised by this suggestion.

The revised grouping just illustrated will later be adopted by PCM. This is because PCM is patient-centered, not factor-centered. PCM does not perform traditional hypothesis tests of the existence, the direction, or the predictive potency of the impact of its prognostic or diagnostic factors on focal end points. It is free to exploit whatever relationships are suggested by the data in its quest to obtain more accurate, individually tailored end point predictions.

However, this additional flexibility does not come without additional cost. It must be purchased by guarding far more diligently than usual against statistical overfitting. These issues and the trade-offs they entail will later be explored in some detail.

4. The AJCCTHIC factor index partitions the raw tumor thickness measurement scale into four intervals (T1, T2, T3, and T4).

   A univariate logistic regression of SLNDUMMY on raw tumor thickness (in millimeters) generated a positive regression coefficient, as anticipated, with a likelihood ratio chi-square statistic of 44.924 and a corresponding two-tailed p value less than 0.00005.

   Substituting AJCCTHIC for raw tumor thickness improved these results by a noticeable amount. A positive regression coefficient was again generated with a likelihood ratio chi-square statistic of 102.585 and a corresponding two-tailed p value less than 0.00005.

   Here is a situation where the AJCC factor index improved the ability of tumor thickness to predict SLNB positivity exactly as anticipated. Substituting AJCCTHIC for raw tumor thickness definitely helped.

   Substituting the AJCC factor index likewise improved the ability of tumor thickness to predict both distant metastasis and disease-specific death as indicated by two more matched pairs of univariate logistic regression analyses.

5. The AJCCMITR factor index partitions the raw mitotic rate measurement scale into two intervals: no mitoses observed versus at least one mitosis observed per one square millimeter high-powered microscopic field.

   A univariate logistic regression of SLNDUMMY on raw mitotic rate generated a highly significant positive regression coefficient with a likelihood ratio chi-square statistic of 23.927 and a corresponding two-tailed p value less than 0.00005. Unfortunately, there were many missing observations. These results were based on only 654 of our 1,039 melanoma patients.

   Substituting AJCCMITR for raw mitotic rate was quite damaging. A much less significant positive regression coefficient was generated with a likelihood ratio chi-square statistic of 6.270 and a corresponding two-tailed p value of 0.0123, based on the same 654 patients.

   The same pattern of results emerged from univariate logistic regressions of distant metastasis and disease-specific death on raw mitotic rate and AJCCMITR. All regressions generated positive coefficients, confirming the uniformly "right" direction of impact, but substituting AJCCMITR for raw mitotic rate diluted substantially its apparent strength of impact on both of these other end points.

It would seem that constructing the AJCCMITR factor index was quite useful in distinguishing between stage 1a and stage 1b patients. This was its original purpose. However, adopting the same index to predict SLNB positivity served to obfuscate rather than to clarify mitotic rate's impact. Yes, its direction of impact was preserved, but at substantially reduced potency. Uncritical acceptance of the conventional wisdom again turned out to be inappropriate.

6. Like patient sex, ulceration of the primary tumor is treated by the AJCC as dichotomous. The AJCCULC factor index assigns zero to being nonulcerated and one to being ulcerated. This indicates that ulcerated tumors produce a higher risk of disease progression than nonulcerated tumors. Beside providing this directional guidance in numeric form, however, the AJCCULC factor index cannot improve predictive accuracy through logistic regression analysis compared to using its dichotomous raw data input.

The "right" direction of impact was uniformly confirmed by univariate logistic regression analyses for SLNB positivity, distant metastasis, and disease-specific death. All impacts were highly significant, with two-tailed p values less than 0.00005.

The next step was to perform a standard multivariate logistic regression of SLNDUMMY on the six traditional AJCC factor indexes. As is common practice, all patients with any missing observations on any prognostic factor were deleted from the analysis. A detailed computer printout is shown below and on the next page enclosed between two horizontal lines.

After removing all undefined values from all expressions, the resulting number of PATIENTs for which each of the 7 expressions possesses a defined value is reduced to 638. This constitutes the effective sample size.

RESULTS OF LOGISTIC REGRESSION ANALYSIS (LINEAR MODEL)

The dependent variable is a binary-coded numeric variable whose values are either 0 or 1. It is embodied in the first expression (parameter) of the LOGREG command, which is just the attribute SLNDUMMY.

The independent variable AJCCAGE is just the attribute AJCCAGE.
The independent variable AJCCSEX is just the attribute AJCCSEX.
The independent variable AJCCSITE is just the attribute AJCCSITE.
The independent variable AJCCTHIC is just the attribute AJCCTHIC.
The independent variable AJCCMITR is just the attribute AJCCMITR.
The independent variable AJCCULC is just the attribute AJCCULC.

Likelihood ratio chi-square statistic: 73.645, 2-tail p value: .0000 (based on 6 degrees of freedom and 638 complete observations).

INDEPENDENT VARIABLE	REGRESSION COEFFICIENT	STANDARD DEVIATION	CHI-SQUARE (DF = 1)	2-TAIL P VALUE	ODDS RATIO MULTIPLIER
intercept	−1.5278	.5805	6.9266	.0085	.2170
AJCCAGE	−.3494	.0685	26.0101	.0000	.7051
AJCCSEX	.2456	.2188	1.2601	.2616	1.2783
AJCCSITE	−.1118	.2138	.2733	.6012	.8943
AJCCTHIC	.6301	.1130	31.1180	.0000	1.8778

AJCCMITR	.0477	.5199	.0084	.9269	1.0489
AJCCULC	.4875	.2270	4.6147	.0317	1.6283

GOODNESS OF STATISTICAL FIT OF LOGISTIC REGRESSION MODEL

Pearson chi-square fit statistic (based on 184 degrees of freedom): 169.936, p value: .7635.

Deviance chi-square fit statistic (based on 184 degrees of freedom): 172.932, p value: .7102.

Several conclusions can be drawn from the printout.

1. The linear model fits the fully defined 638-patient sample data quite satisfactorily.
2. The overall analysis generates a highly significant likelihood ratio chi-square statistic, also suggesting that selecting these six traditional factors to predict SLNB positivity is reasonable.
3. Patient age at diagnosis (AJCCAGE) and primary tumor thickness (AJCCTHIC) are the two most significant prognostic factors. Both are independently highly significant statistically.
4. Ulceration of the primary tumor (AJCCULC) is also an independently significant factor, although less so.
5. Sex of patient (AJCCSEX) and anatomical site of primary tumor (AJCCSITE) are statistically insignificant predictors of SLNB positivity when combined with the other four factors in a multivariate context.
6. Not surprisingly, when measured by AJCCMITR mitotic rate of the primary tumor is also a seemingly insignificant prognostic factor, even though its regression coefficient still points in the "right" direction (i.e., in the positive direction anticipated by the AJCC when the AJCCMITR index was constructed to distinguish between stages 1a and 1b).
7. Of the three independently significant prognostic factors, tumor thickness and ulceration continue to point significantly in the "right" direction, while patient age at diagnosis continues to point quite significantly in the seemingly "wrong" (i.e., unanticipated according to conventional wisdom) direction.

There were missing observations on three of the six traditional AJCC factor indexes: two missing observations of AJCCAGE; 385 missing observations of AJCCMITR; and 149 missing observations of AJCCULC.

To guarantee comparability with the PCM analyses that will follow, missing values of each factor index were replaced by the mean value of that index. Then a multivariate logistic regression of SLNDUMMY was performed on these six augmented traditional AJCC factor indexes. A detailed computer printout is shown below and on the next page enclosed between the two horizontal lines.

```
DEFINE AJCCAGEM: AJCCAGE IF AJCCAGE#UNDEFN ELSE MEAN(AJCCAGE)
DEFINE AJCCMITM: AJCCMITR IF AJCCMITR#UNDEFN ELSE MEAN(AJCCMITR)
DEFINE AJCCULCM: AJCCULC IF AJCCULC#UNDEFN ELSE MEAN(AJCCULC)
```

After removing all undefined values from all expressions, the resulting number of PATIENTs for which each of the 7 expressions possesses a defined value is reduced to 1039. This constitutes the effective sample size.

RESULTS OF LOGISTIC REGRESSION ANALYSIS (LINEAR MODEL)

The dependent variable is a binary-coded numeric variable whose values are either 0 or 1. It is embodied in the first expression (parameter) of the LOGREG command, which is just the attribute SLNDUMMY.

The independent variable AJCCAGEM is just the attribute AJCCAGEM.
The independent variable AJCCSEX is just the attribute AJCCSEX.
The independent variable AJCCSITE is just the attribute AJCCSITE.
The independent variable AJCCTHIC is just the attribute AJCCTHIC.
The independent variable AJCCMITM is just the attribute AJCCMITM.
The independent variable AJCCULCM is just the attribute AJCCULCM.

Likelihood ratio chi-square statistic: 133.542, 2-tail p value: .0000 (based on 6 degrees of freedom and 1039 complete observations).

INDEPENDENT VARIABLE	REGRESSION COEFFICIENT	STANDARD DEVIATION	CHI-SQUARE (DF = 1)	2-TAIL P VALUE	ODDS RATIO MULTIPLIER
intercept	-1.9222	.5479	12.3085	.0005	.1463
AJCCAGEM	-.2922	.0578	25.5540	.0000	.7466
AJCCSEX	.2124	.1871	1.2893	.2562	1.2367
AJCCSITE	-.1177	.1851	.4040	.5251	.8890
AJCCTHIC	.7461	.0858	75.6363	.0000	2.1087
AJCCMITM	-.1178	.5183	.0516	.8203	.8889
AJCCULCM	.4994	.2060	5.8787	.0153	1.6478

GOODNESS OF STATISTICAL FIT OF LOGISTIC REGRESSION MODEL

Pearson chi-square fit statistic (based on 317 degrees of freedom): 310.705, p value: .5891.

Deviance chi-square fit statistic (based on 317 degrees of freedom): 302.086, p value: .7174.

Very little changed by replacing missing values of each traditional factor index with that index's mean value. The effective sample size increased to 1,039. Nevertheless, statistical significance levels failed to improve materially, and the single change in apparent directionality of impact (AJCCMITM) was, therefore, properly ignorable.

The last step was to repeat the same multivariate logistic regression analysis in a stepwise manner. Conventional wisdom was rigorously enforced as if no insights had been gained from any of the preceding univariate analyses. All prognostic factor indexes pointing in the seemingly "wrong" direction and all remaining statistically insignificant factors were purged via backward elimination.

Because just such a procedure is commonly practiced in contemporary prognostic research, this constituted our base case factor-centered analysis against which to calibrate any improvements that PCM might produce. A detailed computer printout is shown on the next page enclosed between the two horizontal lines.

RESULTS OF LOGISTIC REGRESSION ANALYSIS (LINEAR MODEL)

The dependent variable is a binary-coded numeric variable whose values are either 0 or 1. It is embodied in the first expression (parameter) of the LOGREG command, which is just the attribute SLNDUMMY.

The independent variable AJCCTHIC is just the attribute AJCCTHIC.
The independent variable AJCCULCM is just the attribute AJCCULCM.

Likelihood ratio chi-square statistic: 106.481, 2-tail p value: .0000 (based on 2 degrees of freedom and 1039 complete observations).

INDEPENDENT VARIABLE	REGRESSION COEFFICIENT	STANDARD DEVIATION	CHI-SQUARE (DF = 1)	2-TAIL P VALUE	ODDS RATIO MULTIPLIER
intercept	-3.1766	.2080	233.3171	.0000	.0417
AJCCTHIC	.6816	.0792	74.1077	.0000	1.9771
AJCCULCM	.3980	.1999	3.9640	.0465	1.4889

GOODNESS OF STATISTICAL FIT OF LOGISTIC REGRESSION MODEL

Pearson chi-square fit statistic (based on 9 degrees of freedom): 11.989, p value: .2139.

Deviance chi-square fit statistic (based on 9 degrees of freedom): 11.393, p value: .2497.

The base case factor-centered analysis generated respectable results. However, insights gained from the preceding univariate analyses suggest that much has been sacrificed by rigorously enforcing conventional wisdom (i.e., by accepting, uncritically, directional assumptions and measurement procedures that were appropriately developed in other, more "conventional" contexts).

A new attribute (FCSLNPPR) defined by the mathematical model underlying linear logistic regression was then created to encapsulate base case probabilities.

```
DEFINE FCSLNPPR:
EXP(-3.1766+.6816*AJCCTHIC+.3980*AJCCULCM)/[1+
EXP(-3.1766+.6816*AJCCTHIC+.3980*AJCCULCM)]
```

FCSLNPPR stands for factor-centered SLNB positivity probability. This is the factor-centered base case analysis. It assigns an individually tailored base case probability of experiencing a positive SLNB outcome to each of the 1,039 melanoma patients, simulating what would have occurred if an SLNB had actually been undergone. These 1,039 individual probabilities, derived from multiple logistic regression analysis of the six traditional AJCC factor indexes with missing values of each traditional factor index replaced by that index's mean value and with backward elimination, were then subjected to a ROC/AUC analysis.

The area under the complete ROC curve was estimated to be 0.7309.

Several figures have been generated from this base case analysis for visual comparison. They are displayed on the following pages.

The SPSA algorithm was applied to patient age at initial diagnosis to produce a corresponding univariate impact-reflecting index with a minimum subscale size of twenty-five patients. A scattergram of this UIRI is presented in figure 1.

The SPSA algorithm was also applied to primary tumor thickness to produce its corresponding UIRI. In this instance, the minimum subscale size was set at 175 patients to obtain exactly four subscales for easy comparison with the AJCC's traditional demarcation of the T1, T2, T3, and T4 subscales. A scattergram of this UIRI is presented in figure 2.

The shape of figure 2 (consistently increasing at a consistently decreasing rate) reflects quite closely the impact of tumor thickness on melanoma progression repeatedly reported in the literature. Only the three cut points separating the thickness scale into subscales for our sample of 1,039 SLNB patients differed somewhat from the conventional T1, T2, T3, and T4 cut points established by the AJCC for other popular measures of disease progression. Our cut points were 0.85, 1.35, and 2.90 millimeters, respectively, instead of the AJCC's 1.00, 2.00, and 4.00 millimeters.

Figures 1 and 2 showcase rather strikingly the opposite directional impacts of age at diagnosis and tumor thickness on SLNB positivity.

The SPSA algorithm was also applied to the primary tumor's mitotic rate to produce a corresponding UIRI with a minimum subscale size of twenty-five patients. Its scattergram is presented in figure 3.

Figure 3 provides compelling visual evidence that mitotic rate's impact on SLNB positivity is far more complex and interesting than the simple, dichotomous impact envisioned by the construction of the AJCCMITR factor index.

Figure 1

Scattergram of UIRI for Age at Initial Diagnosis

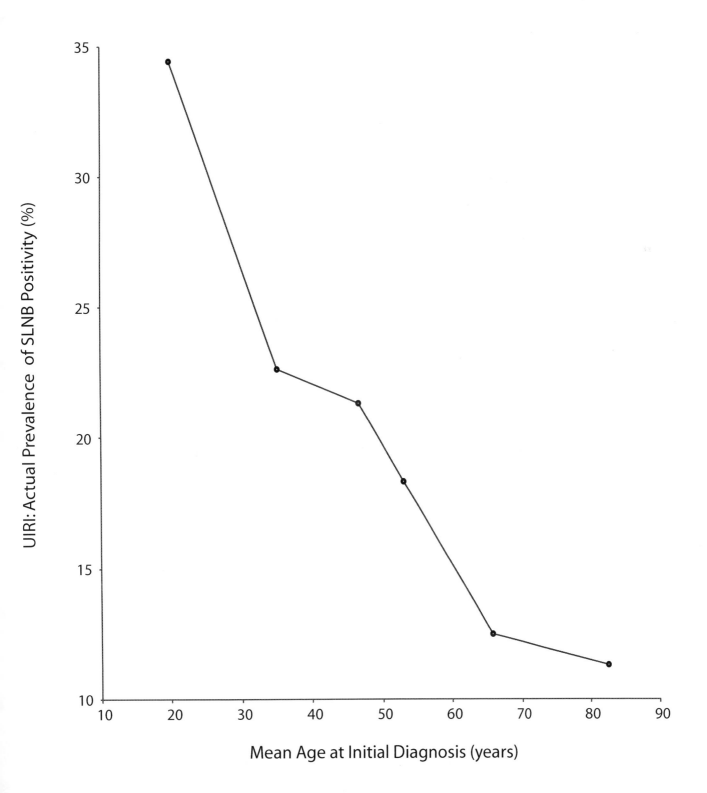

Figure 2

Scattergram of UIRI for Thickness of Primary Tumor

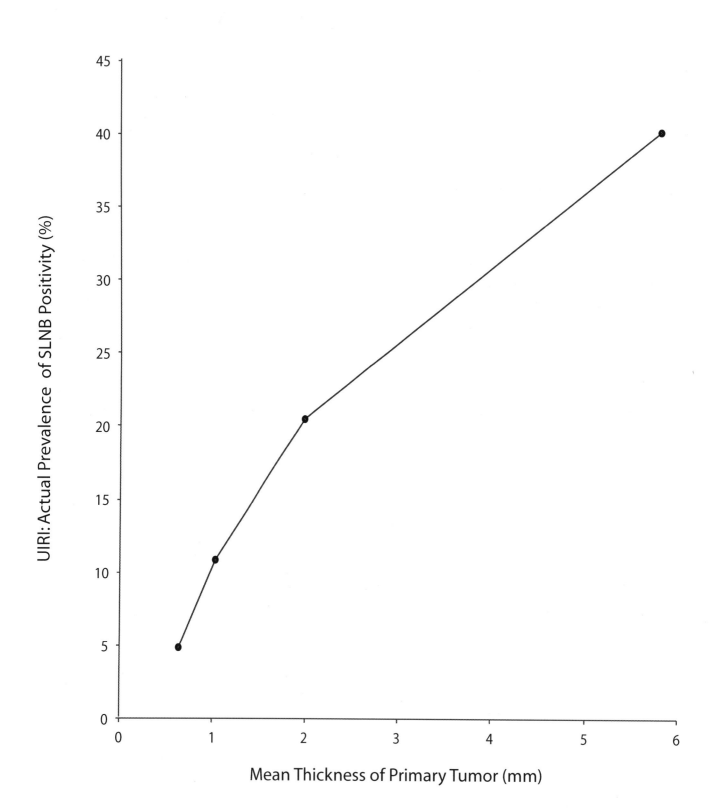

Figure 3

Scattergram of UIRI for Mitotic Rate of Primary Tumor

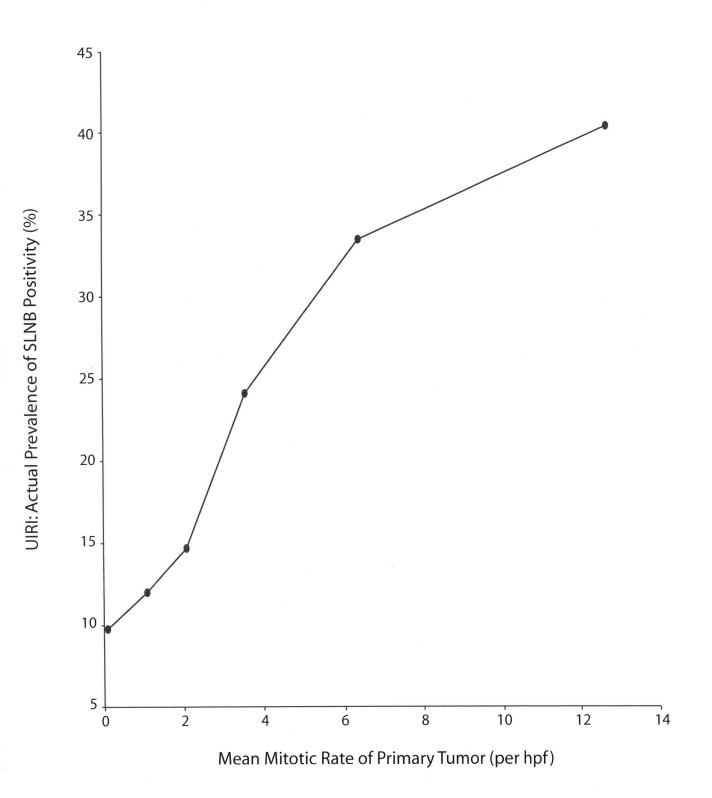

2.2 Stratifying Patients into Low-Risk, Medium-Risk, and High-Risk Subgroups

The next task was to stratify the 1,039 patients into appropriate subgroups.

Among the widely understood and routinely recorded prognostic factors in melanoma AJCC stage is generally regarded as the best single predictor of disease progression. However, the staging index defined by the AJCC includes the patient's nodal status as a major component. In fact, the outcome of an SLNB is frequently used to determine a patient's nodal status. AJCC stage could therefore not be used to stratify patients for the purpose of predicting SLNB outcome. That would have rendered the analysis logically circular.

Instead, we relied on the insights gained from the previous univariate logistic regression analyses. Thickness of the primary tumor and patient age at initial diagnosis were the most potent predictors of SLNB positivity. They were adopted as stratification criteria. The SPSA algorithm was invoked to obtain age fifty-two at initial diagnosis as the best cut point to use for dividing (in the reverse manner) T3 patients between the medium-risk and the high-risk subgroups.

```
DEFINE RISKLEVL:
LOWRISK IF AJCCTHIC=1 ELSE
MEDRISK IF AJCCTHIC=2 OR [AJCCTHIC=3 AND AGE>=52] ELSE
HIGHRISK IF [AJCCTHIC=3 AND AGE<52] OR AJCCTHIC=4
```

TABLE OF JOINT ABSOLUTE FREQUENCIES (COUNTS)

VALUE OF ATTRIBUTE RISKLEVL	VALUE OF ATTRIBUTE SLNSTATE		
	NEGATIVE	POSITIVE	TOTAL
LOWRISK	450	33	483
MEDRISK	265	62	327
HIGHRISK	137	92	229
TOTAL	852	187	1039

The low-risk subgroup included all of the 483 T1 patients (primary tumor thickness no more than one millimeter), with a 33/483 = 6.83 percent actual rate of positive SLNBs.

The medium-risk subgroup included all T2 patients (primary tumor thickness more than one, but no more than two millimeters) and all T3 patients (primary tumor thickness more than two, but no more than four millimeters) who were at least fifty-two years old when initially diagnosed. These 327 patients experienced a 62/327 = 18.96 percent actual rate of positive SLNBs.

The high-risk subgroup included all T4 patients (primary tumor thickness more than four millimeters) and the remaining T3 patients (primary tumor thickness more than two, but no more than four millimeters) initially diagnosed before reaching their fifty-second birthday. These 229 patients experienced a 92/229 = 40.17 percent actual rate of positive SLNBs.

The dramatic between-subgroup differences in the actual rates of positive SLNBs tabled above were highly significant when assessed by a chi-square test (two-tailed p value less than 0.00005) and by a Kruskal-Wallis test corrected for tied observations (two-tailed p value also less than 0.00005).

2.3 Applying the PCM Methodology Separately to the Three Risk Subgroups

After separating patients into risk subgroups, PCM then applied the SPSA algorithm to each of the six traditional AJCC factors. SPSA was uniformly applied to the raw data of each factor to produce its UIRI index. This required executing SPSA three times to produce a UIRI index for each of the six traditional AJCC factors, separately, for each of the three risk subgroups. Each UIRI index was then substituted for its corresponding traditional AJCC factor index as an independent variable for subsequent logistic regression analysis.

When subsample data were used to produce UIRI indexes for all six traditional AJCC factors in all three subgroups according to each factor's univariate relationship to SLNB positivity in that subgroup, any formal hypothesis tests concerning how the factors themselves related to SLNB positivity were thereby compromised. This is because the UIRI index produced to measure each factor was specifically constructed to reflect whatever univariate relationship (especially its shape) the data suggested might exist between that factor and SLNB positivity.

A major advantage of using conventional AJCC factor indexes is that they are not constructed from any particular researcher's data set. Hence, they can be used to test hypotheses concerning the factors employed in almost anybody's research. Nevertheless, because the conventional AJCC factor indexes were not designed for SLNB positivity as a focal end point, because they seemed not to perform very well in this role and because PCM typically does not execute formal hypothesis tests concerning prognostic and diagnostic factors, UIRI indexes were appropriately substituted in this PCM context.

Applying SPSA to the raw data of each factor in each risk subgroup sometimes identified a factor as inadmissible for that subgroup. A factor was deemed inadmissible if the manner in which it indicated the risk of SLNB positivity pointed in the "wrong" direction. From the insights gained in section 2.1 the following indications were deemed directionally correct (judged on a univariate basis).

1. Younger age at initial diagnosis indicates a greater risk of SLNB positivity.
2. A male patient is deemed at greater risk of SLNB positivity than a female patient.
3. Lower-body primary tumor locations (i.e., on the trunk or lower extremities) indicate a greater risk of SLNB positivity than upper-body locations (i.e., on the head, neck, or upper extremities).
4. Thicker primary tumors (measured in millimeters) indicate a greater risk of SLNB positivity than thinner primary tumors.
5. Primary tumors with a higher mitotic rate (measured in mitoses per one square millimeter high-powered field) indicate a greater risk of SLNB positivity than primary tumors with a lower mitotic rate.
6. Ulcerated primary tumors indicate a greater risk of SLNB positivity than nonulcerated primary tumors.

Sex and mitotic rate were identified as directionally incorrect factors in the low-risk subgroup. No traditional AJCC factors were identified as directionally incorrect in either the medium-risk or the high-risk subgroup. Consequently, sex and mitotic rate were eliminated from the subsequent logistic regression analysis of the low-risk subgroup, but no factors were eliminated from further analyses of either the medium-risk or the high-risk subgroup for this reason.

To reduce the possibility of statistical overfitting, only factors achieving a
two-tailed level of statistical significance at or beyond p = 0.05 (after
elimination of directionally incorrect factors) were retained as independent
variables in the multivariate logistic regression analysis associated with each
risk subgroup. Consequently, ulceration was eliminated from the low-risk
analysis; sex, primary tumor location, and ulceration were eliminated from the
medium-risk analysis; and sex and ulceration were eliminated from the high-risk
analysis for this reason.

Again, because observational data were used to construct all UIRI indexes, the
classical concept of statistical significance did not formally apply here,
either. Levels of statistical significance and p values were again construed as
strictly descriptive statistics and were used simply as heuristic guidelines to
help control statistical overfitting.

The three multivariate logistic regression analyses all generated high
likelihood ratio chi-square statistics with p values ranging from p = 0.0001 to
p < 0.00005. All three analyses also demonstrated quite respectable
goodness-of-fit with the linear model underlying logistic regression.
Chi-square p values ranged widely from p = 0.1562 to p = 0.9984.

To distinguish among them, AGELUIRI designated the UIRI for AGE in the low-risk
subgroup, AGEMUIRI designated the UIRI for AGE in the medium-risk subgroup, and
AGEHUIRI designated the UIRI for AGE in the high-risk subgroup. L, M, and H
designators were also used to distinguish UIRI values among subgroups for the
other five traditional AJCC factors.

A composite set of individually tailored probabilities was then obtained from
the outputs of the three multivariate logistic regression subgroup analyses for
the 1,039 patients as follows.

DEFINE PCSLNPPR:
EXP(-6.3401+13.1820*AGELUIRI+18.5508*SITLUIRI+18.4401*THKLUIRI)/[1+
EXP(-6.3401+13.1820*AGELUIRI+18.5508*SITLUIRI+18.4401*THKLUIRI)]
IF RISKLEVL=LOWRISK ELSE
EXP(-6.0511+9.3837*AGEMUIRI+6.9203*THKMUIRI+6.9243*MITMUIRI)/[1+
EXP(-6.0511+9.3837*AGEMUIRI+6.9203*THKMUIRI+6.9243*MITMUIRI)]
IF RISKLEVL=MEDRISK ELSE
EXP(-9.8402+6.3910*AGEHUIRI+4.7685*SITHUIRI+8.7274*THKHUIRI+
3.3915*MITHUIRI)/[1+
EXP(-9.8402+6.3910*AGEHUIRI+4.7685*SITHUIRI+8.7274*THKHUIRI+
3.3915*MITHUIRI)]
IF RISKLEVL=HIGHRISK

PCSLNPPR stands for patient-centered SLNB positivity probability. This is the
patient-centered base case analysis. It assigns an individually tailored
PCM-generated probability of experiencing a positive SLNB outcome to each of
the 1,039 melanoma patients, again simulating what would have occurred if each
patient had actually undergone an SLNB. These 1,039 individual probabilities,
derived via PCM from multiple logistic regression analysis of the same six
traditional AJCC factors, were then subjected to a ROC/AUC analysis.

The area under the complete ROC curve was estimated to be 0.8082.

Stratifying patients into low-risk, medium-risk, and high-risk subgroups;
converting traditional AJCC factors to corresponding UIRI values, separately,
in each subgroup; performing separate logistic regression analyses of SLNB
positivity as predicted by the set of UIRI values in each subgroup; and then
merging the three sets of individually tailored probabilistic outputs to form

the PCM composite PCSLNPPR probabilistic index improved the area under the complete ROC curve (AUC). The composite PCM index's AUC increased by 0.0773 from 0.7309 to 0.8082 compared to the AUC generated by FCSLNPPR in the factor-centered base case analysis.

Referring to the accuracy measures introduced in section 1.5, the corresponding percentage of correct SLNB outcome predictions rose by 2.21 points from 81.81 percent to 84.02 percent. This produced an index of error reduction = 0.340. A Wilcoxon test was performed on the 1,039 matched pairs of probabilistic prediction errors, producing a normalized Z statistic = 8.99, with a two-tailed p value < 0.00005.

2.4 Adding Nontraditional Predictive Factors to Extend the PCM Analysis

Two groups of nontraditional factors were then added to the six traditional AJCC factors in predicting SLNB positivity for the 1,039 melanoma patients.

The first nontraditional group included seven histological factors, all of which were ascertainable at the time of initial diagnosis:

1. TYP - primary tumor's histological subtype (see appendix A for a detailed list of subtypes under the TUMTYPE attribute label);
2. CLR - Clark level of primary tumor invasion (I, II, III, IV, or V, where risk increases with Clark level);
3. TIL - level of primary tumor-infiltrating lymphocytes (risk decreases with higher level);
4. MIC - presence or absence of microsatellites (risk increases, when present);
5. VIN - vascular involvement (impending or actual vascular invasion, where risk increases with greater involvement);
6. ANG - degree of primary tumor vascularity (risk increases with greater degree of vascularization or angiogenesis); and
7. REG - degree of primary tumor regression (risk increases with higher degree of regression).

Higher risk was interpreted here to mean a higher anticipated likelihood of a positive test outcome if an SLNB were undergone.

The second nontraditional group included nine molecular factors, which were also ascertainable at the time of initial diagnosis. These factors were measured aspects of the following nine genes relating to the primary tumor:

1. WNT2;
2. ARPC2;
3. SPP1 (also referred to as osteopontin or OPN);
4. RGS1;
5. FN1;
6. NCOA3;
7. PHIP;
8. POU5; and
9. MITF.

For all genes except PHIP and MITF the measured aspect was degree of gene expression assessed according to the pathologist's four-point scale (absent, slight, moderate, or intense staining intensity derived from immunohistochemical protein analysis). For all seven of these genes a higher degree of gene expression (staining intensity) was uniformly interpreted to mean a higher anticipated likelihood of a positive outcome if an SLNB were undergone.

For PHIP and MITF the measured aspect was mean copy number at the DNA level (i.e., the mean number of copies of the gene per cell in a cluster of at least twenty cells) as determined by Fluorescence In Situ Hybridization (FISH). For both of these genes a higher mean copy number (higher than one copy per chromosome and, therefore, two per cell) was uniformly interpreted to mean a higher anticipated likelihood of a positive outcome if an SLNB were undergone.

Unfortunately, usable tissue was available for only 319 of the 1,039 melanoma patients. For this second nontraditional factor group, therefore, SPSA's ability to deal with missing observations was seriously tested.

One reason why PCM divides predictive factors into separate groups is to accommodate current practice. A complete set of observations is almost never collected. For most patients, complete data are recorded only on traditional factors. This suggests constructing separate predictive algorithms in a cumulative manner for patients with increasing numbers of recorded factors.

Based on the prediction improvements already achieved for the six AJCC traditional factors, the seven factors in the first nontraditional group were converted by SPSA to corresponding UIRI values as previously described. The composite collection of thirteen converted UIRI factors was then subjected to three separate logistic regression analyses, one for each of the three risk subgroups of melanoma patients. The results of the three separate logistic regressions were merged into a composite index called G1SLNPPR, also in the same manner as previously described.

DEFINE G1SLNPPR:

```
EXP(-11.9032+12.4189*AGELUIRI+21.1814*SITLUIRI+19.3000*THKLUIRI+
40.2619*TYPLUIRI+18.5186*CLRLUIRI+15.0647*TILLUIRI)/[1+
EXP(-11.9032+12.4189*AGELUIRI+21.1814*SITLUIRI+19.3000*THKLUIRI+
40.2619*TYPLUIRI+18.5186*CLRLUIRI+15.0647*TILLUIRI)]
IF RISKLEVL=LOWRISK ELSE
EXP(-6.7256+9.8000*AGEMUIRI+6.0145*THKMUIRI+ 5.6725*MITMUIRI+
5.19412*ANGMUIRI)/[1+
EXP(-6.7256+9.8000*AGEMUIRI+6.0145*THKMUIRI+ 5.6725*MITMUIRI+
5.1942*ANGMUIRI)]
IF RISKLEVL=MEDRISK ELSE
EXP(-15.6657+7.1566*AGEHUIRI+4.4576*SITHUIRI+9.3785*THKHUIRI+
4.2331*TYPHUIRI+5.2743*TILHUIRI+3.9013*MICHUIRI+3.2388*VINHUIRI)/[1+
EXP(-15.6657+7.1566*AGEHUIRI+4.4576*SITHUIRI+9.3785*THKHUIRI+
4.2331*TYPHUIRI+5.2743*TILHUIRI+3.9013*MICHUIRI+3.2388*VINHUIRI)]
IF RISKLEVL=HIGHRISK
```

The 1,039 individual probabilities calculated for G1SLNPPR (which account for missing observations of both the six traditional and the seven nontraditional factors in the first group) were then subjected to a ROC/AUC analysis.

The area under the complete ROC curve was estimated to be 0.8352.

Adding the new histological information encapsulated within the seven factors in the first nontraditional group to the six traditional AJCC factors increased the AUC by 0.0270, from 0.8082 achieved by PCSLNPPR to 0.8352 achieved by G1SLNPPR. It increased the comparable percentage of correct SLNB outcome predictions by 1.54 points from 84.02 percent to 85.56 percent. It also produced an index of error reduction = 0.3070. A Wilcoxon test was performed on these 1,039 matched pairs of probabilistic prediction errors, resulting in a normalized Z statistic = 6.41, with a two-tailed p value < 0.00005.

The nine molecular factors in the second nontraditional group were then converted by SPSA to corresponding UIRI values as previously described. Conversion to UIRI values was impossible for all nine genes in the low-risk subgroup due to the large amount of missing data. However, conversion was possible for most genes in both the medium-risk and the high-risk subgroups.

The successfully converted UIRI values from all three factor groups were then subjected to three separate logistic regression analyses, one for each of the three risk subgroups of melanoma patients.

In the medium-risk subgroup only values for OPNMUIRI (the UIRI index for SPP1, also called osteopontin) were sufficiently predictive to be included in that subgroup's logistic regression analysis. The remaining successfully converted UIRIs were combined via a separate logistic regression into a multigene index called GENMUIRI.

In the high-risk subgroup only values for NCOHUIRI (the UIRI index for NCOA3) were sufficiently predictive to be included in the high-risk logistic regression analysis. The remaining successfully converted UIRIs were combined via a separate logistic regression into a multigene index called GENHUIRI.

The results of the three separate logistic regressions were then merged into a composite index called G2SLNPPR, also in the same manner as previously described.

```
DEFINE G2SLNPPR:
EXP(-11.9032+12.4189*AGELUIRI+21.1814*SITLUIRI+19.3000*THKLUIRI+
40.2619*TYPLUIRI+18.5186*CLRLUIRI+15.0647*TILLUIRI)/[1+
EXP(-11.9032+12.4189*AGELUIRI+21.1814*SITLUIRI+19.3000*THKLUIRI+
40.2619*TYPLUIRI+18.5186*CLRLUIRI+15.0647*TILLUIRI)]
IF RISKLEVL=LOWRISK ELSE
EXP(-9.0584+10.1053*AGEMUIRI+5.5269*THKMUIRI+5.0859*MITMUIRI+
5.0375*ANGMUIRI+6.8021*OPNMUIRI+6.0309*GENMUIRI)/[1+
EXP(-9.0584+10.1053*AGEMUIRI+5.5269*THKMUIRI+5.0859*MITMUIRI+
5.0375*ANGMUIRI+6.8021*OPNMUIRI+6.0309*GENMUIRI)]
IF RISKLEVL=MEDRISK ELSE
EXP(-16.7160+7.8949*AGEHUIRI+4.6647*SITHUIRI+9.3925*THKHUIRI+
2.9162*TYPHUIRI+5.8294*TILHUIRI+3.6860*MICHUIRI+3.0240*NCOHUIRI+
2.7716*GENHUIRI)/[1+
EXP(-16.7160+7.8949*AGEHUIRI+4.6647*SITHUIRI+9.3925*THKHUIRI+
2.9162*TYPHUIRI+5.8294*TILHUIRI+3.6860*MICHUIRI+3.0240*NCOHUIRI+
2.7716*GENHUIRI)]
IF RISKLEVL=HIGHRISK
```

The 1,039 individual probabilities calculated for G2SLNPPR (which account for missing observations of the six traditional factors, the seven histological factors in the first nontraditional group and the nine molecular factors in the second nontraditional group) were then subjected to a ROC/AUC analysis.

The area under the complete ROC curve was estimated to be 0.8455.

Adding the new molecular information encapsulated within the nine factors in the second nontraditional group to the six traditional AJCC factors and the seven histological factors in the first nontraditional group increased the AUC by 0.0103, from 0.8352 achieved by G1SLNPPR to 0.8455 achieved by G2SLNPR. It increased the comparable percentage of correct SLNB outcome predictions by 0.10

points from 85.56 percent to 85.66 percent. It also produced an index of error reduction = 0.180. A Wilcoxon test was performed on these 1,039 matched pairs of probabilistic prediction errors, resulting in a normalized Z statistic = 2.93, with a two-tailed p value = 0.0034.

2.5 Improvements in the Accuracy of SLNB Outcome Predictions Achieved by PCM

The addition of sixteen nontraditional predictive factors to the six traditional AJCC factors, when all twenty-two factors were analyzed according to the patient-centered methodology, produced the following improvements in predictive accuracy.

1. Compared to the traditional factor-centered base case (not analyzed via PCM), AUC increased by 11.46 percentage points, from 73.09 percent to 84.55 percent. The percentage of correct predictions increased by 3.85 points, from 81.81 percent to 85.66 percent. The corresponding index of error reduction was 0.3975. These three statistics reflect PCM's overall improvement in accuracy.
2. Compared to the PCM reanalysis of just the same six traditional AJCC factors analyzed by the base case in a conventional manner, AUC increased by 3.73 percentage points, from 80.82 percent to 84.55 percent. The percentage of correct predictions increased by 1.64 points, from 84.02 percent to 85.66 percent. The corresponding index of error reduction was 0.2724. These three statistics reflect the incremental improvement in accuracy provided by the addition of the sixteen nontraditional predictive factors to the six traditional AJCC factors when all twenty-two factors were PCM-analyzed.

Comparing the PCM reanalysis of just the same six AJCC factors analyzed in a conventional manner by the traditional factor-centered base case, AUC increased by 7.73 percentage points, from 73.09 percent to 80.82 percent. The percentage of correct predictions increased by 2.21 points, from 81.81 percent to 84.02 percent. The corresponding index of error reduction was 0.3397. These three statistics reflect PCM's improvement in accuracy when basing predictions solely on the six traditional AJCC factors. From a practical, actionable perspective these may be the most compelling results. The initial diagnosis of most melanoma patients records little more than observations on just these six traditional AJCC factors.

As measured by the index of error reduction and tested by the Wilcoxon matched-pairs, signed-ranks tests, all of the preceding improvements were highly significant. All showed two-tailed p values < 0.00005.

All three of these Wilcoxon tests qualify as legitimate hypothesis tests in the classical (Neyman-Pearson) tradition. The Wilcoxon test is a randomization test whose null hypothesis simply states that no systematic differences exist between the two elements in a set of 1,039 matched pairs of absolute probabilistic prediction errors generated, respectively, by two different prediction methodologies. Pairs of errors are matched patient-by-patient.

Shown on the next page are summary statistics for the individual patient probabilities of experiencing positive SLNB outcomes produced by the four logistic regression analyses generating FCSLNPPR, PCSLNPPR, G1SLNPPR, and G2SLNPPR, respectively.

Notice that the mean probabilities are all identical to each other and equal to the prevalence of SLNB positivity among these 1,039 patients. This is a universally pleasant feature of logistic regression analysis. PCM regularly uses it as an error check to verify that individual patient probabilities of SLNB positivity logistic regression generated by different prediction methodologies have been properly calculated.

Notice also the differences in the minimum-to-maximum ranges and the standard deviations of these individual probabilities. Not only does G2SLNPPR produce the most accurate probabilistic predictions (as just shown in terms of AUC, percentage of correct predictions, and index of error reduction); it also tends to "spread out" its probabilistic predictions more widely than the other three probabilistic logistic regression outputs. Finer discrimination is achieved in combination with, not at the expense of, greater accuracy.

SUMMARY STATISTICS	ATTRIBUTE SLNDUMMY			
n DEFINED	1039			
MINIMUM	0	SLNDUMMY = 0 means negative SLNB outcome.		
MEDIAN	0			
MAXIMUM	1	SLNDUMMY = 1 means positive SLNB outcome.		
MEAN	.1800			
STD. DEV.	.3842			

SUMMARY STATISTICS	ATTRIBUTE FCSLNPPR	ATTRIBUTE PCSLNPPR	ATTRIBUTE G1SLNPPR	ATTRIBUTE G2SLNPPR
n DEFINED	1039	1039	1039	1039
MINIMUM	.0762	.0072	.0007	.0007
MEDIAN	.1402	.1218	.1081	.0973
MAXIMUM	.4870	.8745	.9456	.9483
MEAN	.1800	.1800	.1800	.1800
STD. DEV.	.1286	.1753	.1936	.2021

G2SLNPPR was the most accurate predictor in all of the above senses. Investigation of its scale characteristics throughout its complete logical range from zero to one will reveal other senses in which its probabilistic predictions were also remarkably reliable.

The 1,039 G2SLNPPR individually tailored probabilities were first ranked and divided into quartiles. The mean probability in each quartile was then compared with the actual prevalence of SLNB positivity among patients in that quartile.

These two numbers should converge, statistically, and become approximately equal as the number of patients in each quartile increases. The maximum absolute difference was 0.95 percentage points. The mean absolute difference was 0.58 percentage points. Furthermore, there was no discernible pattern or trend in the succession of quartile probabilities and prevalence.

When there are only a few distinctly different probability values in a data set partitioning the scale into a small number of subscales (such as quartiles) may be both appropriate and sufficient. There were 741 distinctly different values of G2SLNPPR. We can investigate its scale characteristics much more thoroughly.

The SPSA algorithm was executed to partition the scale of G2SLNPPR into as many subscales as possible, as long as each subscale encompassed SLNB positivity probabilities for at least twenty-five patients. Fifteen separate subscales were produced. They are shown as SPSA's printed output on the next page between the two horizontal lines. The corresponding actual prevalence of SLNB positivity is shown as a fraction for each subscale.

The indicator's optimal scale partitioning and numeric rescaling are embodied in the Univariate Impact-Reflecting Index (UIRI) produced by the Scale Partitioning and Spacing Algorithm (SPSA) with a minimum partition (subscale) size set equal to 25. The UIRI's operational definition is shown below.

```
0/60 IF G2SLNPPR<.0082 ELSE
1/66 IF G2SLNPPR>=.0082 AND G2SLNPPR<.0159 ELSE
3/157 IF G2SLNPPR>=.0159 AND G2SLNPPR<.0432 ELSE
1/41 IF G2SLNPPR>=.0432 AND G2SLNPPR<.0489 ELSE
3/105 IF G2SLNPPR>=.0489 AND G2SLNPPR<.071 ELSE
18/169 IF G2SLNPPR>=.071 AND G2SLNPPR<.1339 ELSE
8/56 IF G2SLNPPR>=.1339 AND G2SLNPPR<.1642 ELSE
6/37 IF G2SLNPPR>=.1642 AND G2SLNPPR<.184 ELSE
19/82 IF G2SLNPPR>=.184 AND G2SLNPPR<.2399 ELSE
28/80 IF G2SLNPPR>=.2399 AND G2SLNPPR<.3226 ELSE
17/45 IF G2SLNPPR>=.3226 AND G2SLNPPR<.412 ELSE
24/61 IF G2SLNPPR>=.412 AND G2SLNPPR<.5496 ELSE
17/26 IF G2SLNPPR>=.5496 AND G2SLNPPR<.6391 ELSE
20/29 IF G2SLNPPR>=.6391 AND G2SLNPPR<.78 ELSE
22/25 IF G2SLNPPR>=.78
```

A file named UIRI_SCATTERPLOT.TXT has been created. It contains two columns of data. The first column is labeled UIRI and contains UIRI values calculated for successive scale partitions of the second (indicator) expression in the SPSA command line. The second column is labeled with the operational definition of the second (indicator) expression itself to identify what is being plotted. The means of the indicator expression values in each successive partition are laid out along the horizontal X-axis of the scatterplot, and the corresponding UIRI values are laid out along the vertical Y-axis.

The table below was then constructed. Prediction errors were calculated for each successive subscale as the mean of the G2SLNPPR values falling within that subscale subtracted from the actual prevalence of SLNB positivity among the patients possessing those values of G2SLNPPR.

SUBSCALE	LOWER AND UPPER SUBSCALE BOUNDS		SUBSCALE MEAN	ACTUAL PREVALENCE	PREDICTION ERROR
1	.0000 to	.0082	.0046	.0000	-.0046
2	.0082 to	.0159	.0118	.0152	.0034
3	.0159 to	.0432	.0290	.0191	-.0099
4	.0432 to	.0489	.0463	.0244	-.0219
5	.0489 to	.0710	.0587	.0286	-.0301
6	.0710 to	.1339	.0975	.1065	.0090
7	.1339 to	.1642	.1490	.1429	-.0061
8	.1642 to	.1840	.1729	.1622	-.0107
9	.1840 to	.2399	.2109	.2317	.0208
10	.2399 to	.3226	.2819	.3500	.0681
11	.3226 to	.4120	.3611	.3778	.0167
12	.4120 to	.5496	.4791	.3934	-.0857
13	.5496 to	.6391	.5838	.6538	.0700
14	.6391 to	.7800	.6981	.6897	-.0084
15	.7800 to	1.0000	.8550	.8800	.0250

Since the number of subscales expanded from four (quartiles) to fifteen, subscales contained fewer patient probabilities (between 25 and 169, each). Therefore, the statistical process by which each subscale mean converges toward its corresponding actual prevalence was rendered less complete. The maximum absolute difference between the fifteen subscale means and their corresponding actual prevalence was 8.57 percentage points. The mean absolute difference was 2.60 percentage points.

Taking algebraic signs into account, the mean prediction error should be very close to zero. It was 0.24 percentage points. Both a one-sample t test and a corresponding Wilcoxon test suggested that the population of prediction errors from which this sample of fifteen was drawn differed insignificantly from one with a mean and a median of zero.

When successive subscale means were plotted along the horizontal X-axis and each corresponding actual prevalence was plotted along the vertical Y-axis of a graph, all fifteen points fell close to the straight line through the origin that makes a 45-degree angle with each axis. This line assumes that every actual prevalence exactly equals its corresponding subscale mean. Prediction errors are vertical deviations from the line. The uncorrected R-squared value (coefficient of determination) associated with this line, interpreted as a simple linear regression equation constrained to pass through the origin of the graph, was 0.9819 (equivalent to a 0.9909 linear correlation coefficient).

Inspection of the sequence of prediction errors revealed seven positive and eight negative errors, with relatively large and relatively small errors clustered systematically neither at the extremes of the probability scale nor in its interior. These results were consistent with a random pattern of errors. There was, however, a noticeable and statistically significant tendency for the absolute size of prediction errors to rise with larger probability numbers along the scale.

Based on these observations, it seems appropriate to conclude that individually tailored G2SLNPPR probabilities provide quite accurate predictions of SLNB positivity—especially at low and intermediate probability levels. Figure 4 provides visual evidence of their predictive accuracy.

Conveniently, it will later be shown that accuracy at the low and intermediate probability levels is most important to support our conclusions from the cost-benefit analysis used to justify elimination of excessive SLNBs. Only patients whose PCM-predicted SLNB positivity probabilities are quite small become reasonable candidates to avoid undergoing that expensive surgical procedure with occasional complications.

Figure 4

Scattergram of Predictive Accuracy of
G2SLNPPR Composite Probability

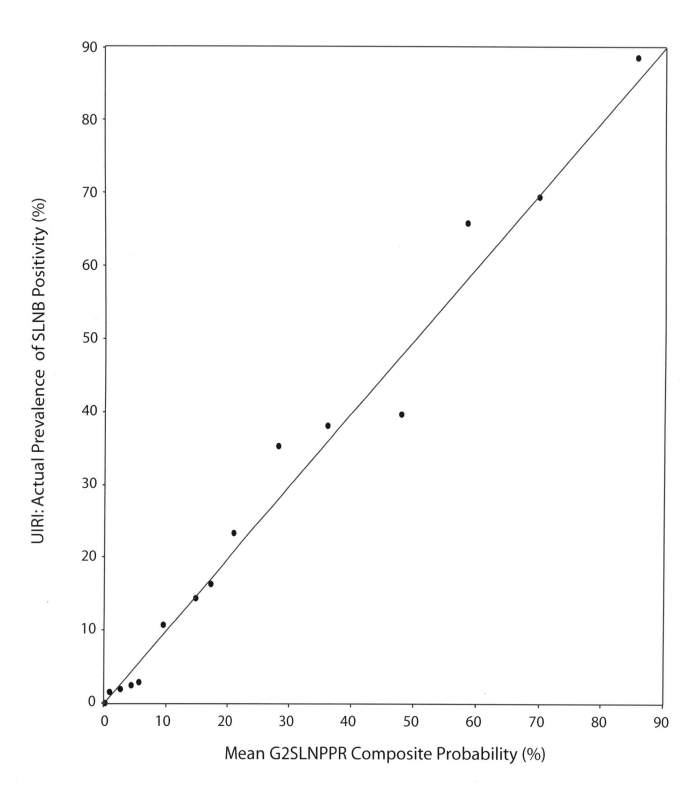

2.6 A Split-Sample Reliability Test for Statistical Overfitting

The apparent predictive accuracy displayed in figure 4 is quite encouraging. If genuine, but only if genuine, practical patient management decisions can be based on these individually tailored probabilities. We need to verify their reliability before proceeding.

It has been demonstrated that PCM generates uniformly better predictions than a typical multivariate logistic regression analysis with backward elimination based on conventional wisdom. All three PCM-generated composite indexes (PCSLNPPR, G1SLNPPR, and G2SLNPPR) delivered significantly more accurate predictions of SLNB positivity than the factor-centered index (FCSLNPPR). Nevertheless, merely achieving statistical significance is not enough.

PCM "uses up" much more sample data than a conventional regression analysis based on a few traditional factor indexes. PCM stratifies the training sample into separate risk subgroups and then performs separate regression analyses in each subgroup. This requires many more regression coefficients to be estimated from the same data. SPSA also identifies cut points to partition the scale of and estimates default missing-data values for each predictive factor separately in each subgroup. These maneuvers consume many more degrees of freedom from the data than conventional analysis. Despite the various protections built into PCM, it is still possible that the increased predictive accuracy is spurious. It may have been purchased at the expense of excessive statistical overfitting.

A split-sample reliability test can shed light on this issue. We shall proceed as follows.

1. First, randomly partition the complete 1,039-patient sample into a training subsample and a validation subsample, each containing approximately the same number of patients.
2. Then recalculate each of the composite indexes embodying individually tailored SLNB positivity probabilities just for patients in the training subsample. This means regenerating a separate prediction algorithm for each separate prediction methodology from just the training data.
3. Apply each of the regenerated prediction algorithms to patients in the validation subsample. This will produce corresponding composite indexes embodying individually tailored SLNB positivity probabilities for patients in the validation subsample.
4. Finally, assess the comparative predictive accuracy achieved by each separate algorithm generated from patients in the training subsample, but then applied to patients in the validation subsample.
5. The training and validation subsamples are completely distinct. They contain neither patients nor any patient data in common. Consequently, whatever accuracy improvements occur in the validation subsample cannot be attributed to overfitting prediction algorithms to data in the training subsample.
6. Yes, one can expect a prediction algorithm initially fitted to patients in a training subsample to lose some accuracy when subsequently applied to a distinct set of patients in a validation subsample. One can anticipate some deterioration in comparable accuracy statistics calculated, first, for patients in the training subsample, then for patients in the validation subsample—but only modest deterioration.
7. The acid test for each separate prediction methodology will therefore be twofold. Is such deterioration only modest, and do statistically significant accuracy improvements in the training subsample persist in the validation subsample (although, perhaps, less strongly)?

8. Failing the acid test would cast doubt on the genuineness of the apparent accuracy improvements reported for the complete, 1,039-patient sample and displayed in figure 4. Passing the acid test comparing each training and validation half-sample would improve our confidence in the genuineness of the accuracy improvements reported for each PCM analysis applied to the twice-as-large complete sample. Individually tailored probabilities generated by each version of the PCM methodology could then be interpreted as reflecting genuine underlying relationships linking its predictive factors to SLNB positivity.

Appendix B documents a split-sample reliability analysis designed to verify PCM's superior predictive accuracy in exactly this manner. Since the incremental improvement in accuracy obtained by adding both groups of sixteen nontraditional factors compared to adding only the first group of seven nontraditional factors was shown to be small (although statistically significant) at the end of section 2.4, appendix B compares only the three predictive methodologies and factor groups used to generate the FCSLNPPR, the PCSLNPPR, and the G2SLNPPR composite indexes.

The 1,039 melanoma patients were randomly partitioned into a training subsample of 521 and a validation subsample of 518. The procedures previously described in sections 2.1 through 2.4 were then applied to the training subsample of 521 patients.

Highlights from appendix B are as follows.

1. The traditional factor-centered base case prediction algorithm (FCSLNPPR) obtained from the 521-patient training subsample via conventional multivariate logistic regression analysis was applied to the 518 patients in the validation subsample. This produced 518 individually tailored SLNB positivity probabilities with a 79.34 percent rate of correct predictions. The comparable rate of correct predictions in the training subsample was 80.23 percent. The difference constituted a 1.11 percent deterioration from the training to the validation subsample.
2. The patient-centered base case prediction algorithm obtained from the same six traditional AJCC factor observations made on the same 521-patient training subsample via the PCM methodology (PCSLNPPR) was also applied to the 518 patients in the validation subsample. This produced a second set of 518 individually tailored SLNB positivity probabilities with a 82.05 percent rate of correct predictions. The comparable rate of correct predictions in the training subsample was 83.69 percent. The difference constituted a 1.96 percent deterioration from the training to the validation subsample.
3. Compared to the factor-centered base case analysis, the PCM improvement in percentage rate of correct predictions in the validation subsample generated an index of error reduction = 0.3514 and a normalized Wilcoxon Z statistic = 4.19, with a two-tailed p value < 0.00005.
4. The prediction algorithm obtained from observations of the same six traditional AJCC factors augmented by sixteen additional nontraditional factors made on the same 521-patient training subsample via the PCM methodology (G2SLNPPR) was also applied to the 518 patients in the validation subsample. This produced a third set of 518 individually tailored SLNB positivity probabilities with a 83.40 percent rate of correct predictions. The comparable rate of correct predictions in the training subsample was 87.14 percent. The difference constituted a 4.29 percent deterioration from the training to the validation subsample.
5. Compared to the PCM analysis of just the six traditional AJCC factors, adding the sixteen nontraditional factors and analyzing all twenty-two

factors via PCM generated in the validation subsample an index of error reduction = 0.2741 and a normalized Wilcoxon Z statistic = 4.07, with a two-tailed p value < 0.00005.

6. Compared to the factor-centered base case analysis of the six traditional AJCC factors, the PCM analysis of all twenty-two factors generated in the validation subsample an index of error reduction = 0.3975 and a normalized Wilcoxon Z statistic = 11.57, with a two-tailed p value < 0.00005.

These results pass both requirements of the acid test. Percentage correct predictions deteriorated only modestly (by less than 5 percent) from training to validation subsamples in all three methodologies. Accuracy improvements produced by both versions of the PCM methodology remained highly significant, statistically, in the validation subsample. Attributing these results to excessive overfitting of prediction algorithms to data in the training subsample is therefore rendered quite implausible.

Notice, however, that the deterioration from training to validation subsamples in percentage of correct predictions increased steadily from 1.11 percent (FCSLNPPR) to 1.96 percent (PCSLNPPR) to 4.29 percent (G2SLNPPR). This is the same sequence in which the three methodologies consumed additional degrees of freedom when fitting their respective prediction algorithms to the same training data. Furthermore, PCM consumed somewhat more degrees of freedom than multivariate logistic regression in order to generate PCSLNPPR compared to FCSLNPPR. PCM consumed dramatically more degrees of freedom in order to generate G2SLNPPR compared to PCSLNPPR.

It is tempting to interpret these two related sequences as evidence of increasing, though still modest overfitting. We may be looking at the beginning of a hockey stick-like increase in deterioration. If true, it would suggest that either reducing the sample size substantially below 1,039 patients or increasing the number of predictive factors substantially above twenty-two or reducing the quality (cleanliness) of the data substantially or any combination thereof might compromise PCM. The current PCM analysis may fall close to the outer limit of only modest deterioration due to statistical overfitting. Data obtained from a different institution describing many melanoma patients who have also undergone SLNBs would be most useful in testing this speculation.

2.7 How PCM's Greater Predictive Accuracy Can Reduce the Cost and Raise the Efficiency of a Diagnostic Test Procedure such as an SLNB

It has just been demonstrated that PCM provides more accurate predictions of the individually tailored outcomes of an SLNB than a conventional, factor-centered methodology:

1. first, by substituting measurement indexes specifically tailored by SPSA to SLNB outcomes realized at a particular medical institution for the conventional factor indexes recommended by the AJCC to predict different, survival-related end points on a generic basis; and
2. then, by implementing the other distinctive PCM devices outlined in section 1.2 that tailor predictions to individual patients; where
3. attributing these improvements in accuracy to nothing more than statistical overfitting has just been ruled out.

So how can PCM's greater predictive accuracy both reduce the cost and, simultaneously, raise the efficiency of a diagnostic test procedure?

Our answer will begin by establishing a historical basis of comparison. That basis will be the experience of the 1,039 patients just analyzed via PCM. All 1,039 patients were diagnosed with melanoma between 1987 and 2007. Each patient then underwent an SLNB. They constituted close to a census of all patients at that institution who underwent SLNBs for melanoma within that time span.

Faculty at the UCSF Melanoma Center adopted a modified version of conventional risk guidelines to make recommendations concerning whether or not a particular patient should undergo an SLN biopsy. The number and severity of high-risk features presented by each patient at initial diagnosis helped to guide these recommendations. Since explicit probabilistic predictions were not generally available between the mid-1990s (when SLNBs were initially offered) and 2007, they could not become the basis for making an appropriate triage of patients.

The actual policy was to recommend an SLNB to any patient:

1. either diagnosed with a primary tumor at least one millimeter in depth (an eligibility criterion established for the Multi-center Selective Lymphadenectomy Trial [MSLT]); or
2. diagnosed with a primary tumor less than one millimeter that underwent an incomplete biopsy (i.e., that possessed a positive deep margin); or
3. diagnosed with a primary tumor less than one millimeter that underwent a complete biopsy but who presented, nonetheless, with one or more high-risk features; where
4. examples of high-risk features included Clark level IV or V, elevated mitotic rate, ulceration, vascular involvement, microsatellite(s), and extensive regression of the primary tumor.

The faculty's goal was to recommend an SLNB to any patient with a sufficiently high likelihood of lymph node positivity. A sufficiently high likelihood was interpreted to mean at least 10 percent. Thus, patients whose risk of lymph node positivity was deemed to approach or exceed 10 percent were recommended to undergo the procedure.

A discussion focusing on the various pros and cons of undergoing an SLNB ensued with those patients deemed to be at lower risk of node positivity. The final faculty recommendation and the patient's decision flowed from this discussion.

Patients typically accepted and acted on whatever the faculty recommended. This was generally but not universally true. For example, no SLNB was recommended for one of these 1,039 patients, but he chose to undergo an SLNB anyway. The details of his rather unusual experience are chronicled in appendix C.

The next step will be to demonstrate how substitution of explicit PCM-generated probabilistic predictions for the policy guidelines listed above could have both reduced the cost and, simultaneously, raised the efficiency of performing SLNBs. This will be accomplished by constructing an alternative recommendation table. The table projects the consequences of relying explicitly on PCM-generated probabilities of SLNB positivity to recommend SLNBs to the 1,039 patients rather than on the modification of conventional guidelines actually adopted, accompanied by a discussion with the patient.

Explicit reliance on PCM-generated positivity probabilities does not mean using them as the sole, firm, and final basis for recommending an SLN biopsy. It does mean using them as the basis for formulating an initial recommendation. Unless discussion with the patient serves to reverse this initial recommendation, it also means using them to establish the default recommendation. Because patients typically accepted and acted on whatever the faculty recommended, it also means that PCM-generated positivity probabilities, therefore, would have largely determined which patients did and which patients did not undergo an SLNB.

The faculty's goal was to achieve an outcome defined in terms of the likelihood of lymph node positivity. So why rely on generic guidelines not painstakingly calculated to achieve this desired result? Why not substitute as both the initial and the default guideline a probabilistic prediction of exactly this desired result, separately tailored by PCM to each individual patient?

There would have been an added bonus to making such a substitution. Discussion with each patient could then have been tailored to PCM's detailed calculation of that patient's likelihood of SLNB positivity. Each of the patient's high-risk features could have been quantified in terms of its separate contribution to a positive SLNB test result. The probabilistic impact of low-risk features could have been similarly quantified. This certainly would have enriched the conversation. In addition, it might have rendered the initial (and default) recommendation more credible, more convincing, and even more likely to be willingly accepted.

The alternative recommendation table first rank-orders all 1,039 patients in ascending sequence according to their G2SLNPPR probabilities. The subset of 187 patients whose actual SLNB outcomes were positive is then identified. The table is constructed on the basis of their probabilities. The consequences of using each SLNB-positive patient's G2SLNPPR probability as an alternative criterion for determining whether each of the 1,039 patients should or should not have been recommended to undergo an SLNB is what the table projects.

Only the first thirty-three (i.e., numerically smallest) of these 187 SLNB-positive G2SLNPPR probabilities appear in the initial column labeled CALCULATED G2SLNPPR CUT POINT. The table is restricted to these thirty-three probabilities because their ascending sequence rose to a level more than high enough to compare their projected alternative consequences with the actual consequences of the intended 10 percent policy.

Using a G2SLNPPR cut point probability as an alternative basis for making SLNB recommendations means that all of the 1,039 patients whose calculated G2SLNPPR probabilities were at least as high as that cut point would have been recommended to undergo an SLNB. All patients with lower G2SLNPPR probabilities would have been recommended to forego the SLNB.

The G2SLNPPR probability-based alternative recommendation table appears below and on the next page.

CALCULATED G2SLNPPR CUT POINT	NUMBER OF ALTERED RECOMMENDATIONS	NUMBER/PERCENT OF PRESCIENT ALTERATIONS		NUMBER OF NONPRESCIENT ALTERATIONS
0.0000	0	0/0	N/A	0
0.0082	60	60/60	100.00%	0
0.0159	126	125/126	99.21%	1
0.0189	145	143/145	98.62%	2
0.0268	194	191/194	98.45%	3
0.0432	283	279/283	98.59%	4
0.0489	324	319/384	98.46%	5
0.0512	339	333/339	98.23%	6
0.0552	357	350/357	98.04%	7
0.0710	429	421/429	98.14%	8
0.0735	438	429/438	97.95%	9
0.0761	451	441/451	97.78%	10

0.0761	451	441/451	97.78%	10
0.0769	458	446/458	97.38%	12
0.0801	468	455/468	97.22%	13
0.0835	480	466/480	97.08%	14
0.0875	490	475/490	96.94%	15
0.0886	493	477/493	96.75%	16
0.0902	497	480/497	96.58%	17
0.0975	520	502/520	96.54%	18
0.0989	523	504/523	96.37%	19
0.1015	531	511/531	96.23%	20
0.1035	538	517/538	96.10%	21
0.1061	541	519/541	95.93%	22
0.1140	548	525/548	95.90%	23
0.1140	548	525/548	95.90%	23
0.1148	561	536/561	95.54%	25
0.1339	598	572/598	95.65%	26
0.1348	600	573/600	95.50%	27
0.1370	602	574/602	95.35%	28
0.1376	605	576/605	95.21%	29
0.1485	621	591/621	95.17%	30
0.1523	625	594/625	95.04%	31
0.1529	632	600/632	94.44%	32
1.0000	1,039	852/1039	82.00%	187

A recommendation not to undergo an SLNB is labeled prescient if the outcome of an SLNB was or would have been negative; otherwise, it is nonprescient. A recommendation to undergo an SLNB is labeled prescient if the outcome of an SLNB was or would have been positive; otherwise, it is nonprescient.

Even though the actual recommendation policy resulted in having all 1,039 patients undergo an SLN biopsy, only 187 patients (18.00 percent) tested positive. These 187 patients were, therefore, treated as if they had received prescient recommendations. The remaining 852 patients (82.00 percent) tested negative. These 852 patients were treated as if they had received nonprescient recommendations.

The number of recommendations treated as nonprescient exceeded the number treated as prescient by more than four to one. This observation suggests an opportunity for substantial improvement.

The top line in the table above (preceding the thirty-three lines reflecting possible alternative cut points) encapsulates the actual results. Alterations are departures from the recommendation policy that produced these results. Since virtually all 1,039 patients were recommended to undergo an SLNB, an altered recommendation constitutes a change from one to undergo an SLNB to a recommendation not to undergo an SLNB. Each alteration relies on the cut point probability tabled in the first column to make such a change.

The bottom line in the table reflects a completely reversed policy. None of the 1,039 patients would have been recommended to undergo an SLNB.

What about patients who did not undergo an SLN biopsy? The table above contains no data on outcomes their SLNBs might have produced. We must deal with these patients separately. The consequences for patients who did not undergo the procedure will be discussed and analyzed in section 2.8.

Referring to the table on this and the previous page, raising the G2SLNPPR cut point to realize an alternative recommendation policy would always increase the number of recommendations not to undergo an SLNB. Each such switch constitutes an altered recommendation. Thus, adopting the first G2SLNPPR cut point (0.0082) would result in sixty altered recommendations. All of these would have been prescient alterations. Sixty of the 1,039 SLNBs would then not have been performed. There were no offsetting medical disbenefits either to patients or to their physicians, so these first sixty altered recommendations would appear to have been noncontroversially appropriate from a medical standpoint.

In contrast, all additional increases in the G2SLNPPR cut point would continue to alter additional recommendations and to reduce, thereby, the number of SLNBs performed—but only by making an ever decreasing percentage of prescient recommendations. Because a decrease in the number of SLNBs performed must be purchased at the expense of an increasingly nonprescient recommendation rate, a trade-off judgment is required. Is there a maximum acceptable rate of nonprescient recommendations?

Consider the following purely hypothetical alternative policy. One might judge that increasing the cutoff probability would be justified as long as the rate of prescient alterations remained at least 95 percent (i.e., as long as deviating from the actual policy would result in prescient recommendation alterations at least 95 percent of the time).

Choosing a cutoff G2SLNPPR probability in the neighborhood of 15.25 percent would serve to implement this hypothetical alternative policy. Looking at the bottom portion of the table, a cutoff G2SLNPPR probability of 15.23 percent would already eliminate 625 (more than half) of the 1,039 SLNBs, while still maintaining a 95.04 percent rate of prescient alterations.

The last column of the alternative recommendation table shows that, except for occasional duplicated values (i.e., ties), relying on each incremental G2SLNPPR cut point probability to recommend an SLNB produces exactly one additional nonprescient recommendation alteration. The table was specifically constructed to showcase this relationship for reasons that will soon become apparent.

However, because the table does not project consequences for any other patients, we must also consider the corresponding impact of relying on each incremental G2SLNPPR cut point probability to make recommendations to patients who did not undergo SLNBs.

2.8 Extending the Analysis to Include Patients Who Did Not Undergo an SLNB

There were many patients who did not undergo an SLNB either by choice or because they did not meet the criteria embodied in the guidelines actually adopted. Based on their attributes, we can now fill out the other side of the picture. We can identify how many and exactly which of these patients would have been recommended to undergo an SLNB instead, if PCM-generated G2SLNPPR probabilities had then been available to facilitate an appropriate triage, and if they had actually been used for this purpose.

Medical records were obtained for 301 patients who were also diagnosed with melanoma at UCSF before or during 2007 but who did not undergo an SLNB. Records for these 301 patients were collected for a variety of prognostic analyses. Many patients were selected for analysis either because they had suffered a relapse or because they had been followed up for at least two years after initial diagnosis without relapse. They constituted a rather high-risk cohort, despite their lower-risk appearance described on the next page. Therefore, they may be viewed as plausible, if not obvious, candidates for an SLNB.

None of the 301 patients showed evidence of nodal involvement at the time of initial diagnosis. None presented with one or more of the following high-risk prognostic features:

1. a thick primary tumor (T4) exceeding four millimeters in Breslow depth;
2. a primary tumor displaying either Clark level IV or V invasion;
3. a primary tumor with a high mitotic rate exceeding 3 mitoses per 1 square millimeter high-powered field (hpf);
4. an ulcerated primary tumor;
5. the presence of one or more microsatellites;
6. vascular involvement (i.e., actual or impending vascular invasion); or
7. prominent vascularity (e.g., angiogenesis) of the primary tumor.

Medical records for these 301 patients were produced by the same pathologist who evaluated the 1,039 patients who did undergo an SLNB. Consequently, these two sets of records were highly comparable. Selected attributes of the 301 patients are presented in appendix D for comparison with the 1,039 patients described in appendix A.

The next step was to partition the 301 patients into low-risk, medium-risk, and high-risk subgroups. The same criteria developed for the 1,039 SLNB patients were applied to the 301 no-SLNB patients.

DESIGNATED RISK GROUP	ABSOLUTE FREQUENCIES (COUNTS)	RELATIVE FREQUENCIES (PROPORTIONS)	CUMULATIVE RELATIVE FREQUENCIES
LOW RISK	204	.6777	.6777
MEDIUM RISK	94	.3123	.9900
HIGH RISK	3	.0100	1.0000
TOTAL	301	1.0000	

As anticipated, the risk of having a positive SLNB was decidedly tilted in the lower direction for these 301 patients compared to the 1,039 SLNB patients.

The same algorithm developed to assign G2SLNPPR positivity probabilities to the 483 low-risk SLNB patients was applied to the 204 low-risk no-SLNB patients. Similarly, the same G2SLNPPR algorithms developed for the 327 medium-risk SLNB patients and for the 229 high-risk SLNB patients were applied, respectively, to the 94 medium-risk no-SLNB patients and to the 3 high-risk no-SLNB patients.

In all three cases a slight modification to the calculation of UIRI values via SPSA was required whenever missing data values were encountered in any of the twenty-two diagnostic factors. Since none of the 301 no-SLNB patients underwent an actual SLNB, no relative frequencies of positive SLNB outcomes appropriate to missing data factor subscales could be used as estimates. Instead, the relative frequencies of positive SLNB outcomes assigned to the 1,039 SLNB patients in the same risk subgroup with missing data on the same diagnostic factor were used for this purpose.

The three separate no-SLNB G2SLNPPR algorithms were then merged into a single, composite G2SLNPPR algorithm in exactly the same manner as was done for the 1,039 SLNB patients. The composite algorithm assigned a probabilistic prediction of SLNB positivity to each of the 301 no-SLNB patients as if each patient were actually to have undergone that diagnostic procedure.

Applying the composite algorithm derived from the 1,039-patient SLNB data to the distinct sample of 301 no-SLNB patients appeared justified in light of the spectacular convergence to actual relative frequencies depicted in figure 4 in conjunction with the split-sample reliability results reported in appendix B.

Now we are ready to apply a common alternative recommendation policy to the combined sample of 1,039 SLNB patients and 301 no-SLNB patients, a total of 1,340 patients. Recommendations to undergo or not to undergo an SLNB will be uniformly based on the G2SLNPPR positivity probability assigned to each patient. Assuming that patients accept their recommendations, the consequences of any such alternative recommendation policy can be assessed and compared with the historical guidelines.

As previously stated, the goal was to implement something close to a 10 percent policy. Therefore, selecting 10 percent as the G2SLNPPR cutoff probability would be an obvious choice for an initial comparison. Only accuracy in implementing the criterion would then change. By retaining a 10 percent cutoff as the recommendation criterion, any reduction in cost and increased efficiency over what actually occurred could then be attributed to substituting the more accurate PCM-generated G2SLNPPR probabilities for the conventional risk guidelines employed, historically, in making actual recommendations.

Applying the 10 percent policy to the 1,039 SLNB patients would have produced the following actual outcomes.

	VALUE OF ATTRIBUTE SLNSTATE		
RECOMMENDATION UNDER THE 10 PERCENT CUTOFF	NEGATIVE	POSITIVE	TOTAL
Eschew SLNB, since G2SLNPPR less than 10%	508	20	528
Perform SLNB, since G2SLNPPR at least 10%	344	167	511
TOTAL	852	187	1039

Of the 1,039 patients who actually underwent SLNBs only 511 (less than half) would have done so under the 10 percent cutoff applied to G2SLNPPR probabilities. The other 528 patients would have been spared. However, while 508 of these 528 altered recommendations (96.21 percent) were prescient, twenty were nonprescient. The twenty nonprescient alterations must be counted as a medical disbenefit produced by the 10 percent G2SLNPPR cutoff relative to actual history.

SUMMARY STATISTICS	SLNB G2SLNPPR	NO-SLNB G2SLNPPR
n DEFINED	511	107
MINIMUM	.1005	.1001
MEDIAN	.2537	.1488
MAXIMUM	.9483	.4017
MEAN	.3229	.1723
STD. DEV.	.2050	.0652

Whereas the mean G2SLNPPR was 0.3229 for the 511 SLNB patients actually and properly recommended for an SLNB under the 10 percent cutoff, the mean G2SLNPPR was only 0.1723 (about half) for the 107 no-SLNB patients actually not recommended for an SLNB but who should have been under the 10 percent cutoff (i.e., because their value of G2SLNPPR was at least 10 percent).

Multiplying 0.1723 by 107 gives 18.44. It is the expected number of positive SLNB outcomes that would have been experienced by no-SLNB patients, assuming the consistent use of G2SLNPPR probabilities with a 10 percent cutoff as the initial basis for recommending to all 1,340 patients that they either undergo or not undergo an SLNB.

Performing an extra 107 SLNBs would certainly have generated an incremental cost compared to performing only the original 1,039 SLNBs. However, the incremental 18.44 prescient positive SLNB outcomes (an expected number) must be counted as a compensating medical benefit purchased by performing these 107 additional SLNBs relative to actual history. Performing the extra 107 SLNBs would have been a direct consequence of applying the same 10 percent G2SLNPPR cutoff probability to the 301 no-SLNB patients.

We now possess sufficient tools to subject many such policies to this type of hypothetical retrospective analysis and to compare the consequences of each with any particular medical institution's actual historical experience. Because the PCM analysis from which these tools are derived is tailored to a particular medical institution, so, also, is any comparative retrospective analysis.

2.9   Identifying the Equilibrating Cutoff Probability that Quantifies Both PCM's Relative Cost Savings and Its Relative Efficiency Improvement

The next step will be to calculate the relative (percentage) cost savings and the corresponding relative (percentage) improvement in triage efficiency enabled by PCM's greater predictive accuracy.

Beginning with the 10 percent cutoff illustrated in the SLNB example, we can accomplish this by simultaneously decreasing the negative impact of the twenty nonprescient altered recommendations made to the 1,039 SLNB patients and increasing the positive impact of the 18.44 prescient altered recommendations made to the 301 no-SLNB patients. Decreases and increases can be continued until these two counts are equalized. Equalizing the counts would alter the total number of SLNBs performed. By doing so, however, it would guarantee that the same number of positive SLNB outcomes realized historically (187 out of 1,039) would also be realized after the selective decreases and increases.

Increasing the cutoff G2SLNPPR probability would always cause more patients originally recommended to undergo an SLNB to eschew it instead. This would cause the number of nonprescient altered recommendations to rise. Decreasing the cutoff G2SLNPPR probability would cause fewer patients originally recommended to undergo an SLNB to eschew it instead, and this would cause the number of nonprescient altered recommendations to fall.

In contrast, increasing the same cutoff G2SLNPPR probability would cause fewer patients originally recommended not to undergo an SLNB to undergo it instead. This would reduce the number of prescient altered recommendations. Decreasing the cutoff G2SLNPPR probability would cause more patients originally recommended not to undergo an SLNB to undergo it instead, and this would cause the number of prescient altered recommendations to rise.

Hence, decreasing the cutoff G2SLNPPR probability below 10 percent by some small amount would serve both to reduce the number of nonprescient altered recommendations among SLNB patients below twenty and to increase the number of prescient altered recommendations among no-SLNB patients above 18.44 so as to balance (i.e., equalize) the negative and positive impacts.

A modified version of the alternative recommendation table has been constructed to illustrate the balancing procedure. The first and third columns of the original table have been retained. They show the consequences of using the G2SLNPPR cutoff probability as the basis for recommending SLNBs to the 1,039 SLNB patients. A column has been added to show the consequences of using the same G2SLNPPR cutoff probability as the basis for recommending SLNBs to the 301 no-SLNB patients. A final column has also been added to show the difference in resulting counts, which the balancing procedure is seeking to reduce to zero.

The modified alternative recommendation table is shown below. It is interpreted below and on the next page.

CALCULATED G2SLNPPR CUT POINT	COUNT OF NONPRESCIENT ALTERED RECOMMENDATIONS FOR 1,039 SLNB PATIENTS	EXPECTED COUNT OF PRESCIENT ALTERED RECOMMENDATIONS FOR 301 NO-SLNB PATIENTS	DIFFERNCE IN COUNTS
0.0000	0	26.71	26.71
0.0082	0	26.64	26.64
0.0159	1	26.48	25.48
0.0189	2	26.45	24.45
0.0268	3	25.82	22.82
0.0432	4	23.85	19.85
0.0489	5	22.75	17.75
0.0512	6	22.65	16.65
0.0552	7	22.39	15.39
0.0710	8	20.91	12.91
0.0735	9	20.62	11.62
0.0761	10	20.61	10.61
0.0761	10	20.61	10.61
0.0769	12	20.32	8.32
0.0801	13	20.32	7.32
0.0835	14	20.23	6.23
0.0875	15	20.15	5.15
0.0886	16	20.15	4.15
0.0902	17	20.15	3.15
0.0975	18	18.64	0.64
0.0989	19	18.64	-0.36
0.1015	20	18.34	-1.66
0.1035	21	18.03	-2.97
0.1061	22	17.82	-4.18
0.1140	23	17.60	-5.40
0.1140	23	17.60	-5.40
0.1148	25	17.48	-7.52
0.1339	26	15.69	-10.31
0.1348	27	15.56	-11.44
0.1370	28	15.56	-12.44
0.1376	29	15.42	-13.58
0.1485	30	12.19	-17.81
0.1523	31	10.70	-20.30
0.1529	32	10.70	-21.30
1.0000	187	0.00	-187.00

Inspection of the table shows that decreasing the cutoff G2SLNPPR probability from 10 percent to an equilibrating value of 9.89 percent would have achieved an almost perfect balance. It would have reduced nonprescient recommendation alterations for the 1,039 SLNB patients from twenty to nineteen. It would have increased the expected count of prescient altered recommendations for the 301 no-SLNB patients from 18.44 to 18.64. The 18.64 - 19 = -0.36 difference was as close to zero as G2SLNPPR probabilities calculated from data describing these 1,340 patients would permit.

So what does it mean to balance the two oppositely directed impacts? Why is it useful to identify an equilibrating G2SLNPPR cutoff probability? What is being equilibrated, and what is gained by doing so?

Under the 9.89 percent equilibrating cutoff probability the nineteen nonprescient recommendation alterations within the 1,039-patient SLNB sample would have caused nineteen patients whose actual SLNB outcomes were known to have been positive to eschew SLNBs. That was a mistake. It would have constituted a medical disbenefit relative to the actual policy.

The expected count of 18.64 prescient positive SLNB outcomes would have resulted from having no-SLNB patients originally recommended to eschew an SLNB actually undergo the procedure. That corrected the mistake. It would have constituted a compensating medical benefit relative to the actual policy.

Adopting as a recommendation policy the equilibrating G2SLNPPR cutoff probability serves to equalize these two impacts as closely as possible. Then, the total (expected) number of positive SLNB outcomes would have remained virtually unchanged. There would have been 186.64 (expected) positive SLNB outcomes for the total of 1,039 + 301 = 1,340 patients. This is almost the same as the 187 positive SLNB outcomes actually experienced by the 1,039 SLNB patients. Hence, compared to the actual history, the differentiating medical disbenefits and compensating medical benefits associated with performing the SLNB diagnostic procedure would have essentially canceled each other out.

We are not claiming that a 9.89 percent policy would have been optimal for any given institution. We are not alleging that it would have been superior in any cost-benefit sense to a 10 percent (or to any other particular recommendation) policy similarly based on G2SLNPPR cutoff probabilities.

Instead, identifying the equilibrating G2SLNPPR cutoff probability is being offered as a way to make a salient comparison. By equalizing the number of positive test outcomes, the smaller number of tests then needed to be performed to achieve the same medical benefit to patients can be compared with the use of conventional guidelines. That is the salient comparison.

A smaller number of required tests constitutes a cost reduction. This is true regardless of the specific dollar cost of performing each test at any given medical institution. Performing fewer tests consumes less of society's valuable resources everywhere.

Looked at from a test yield perspective, the increased ratio of positive test outcomes to the number of tests required to achieve that same positive count constitutes a gain in triage efficiency. A higher test yield does not depend on which specific costs and ways to measure them are deemed locally appropriate. An increased ratio uniformly indicates greater efficiency, regardless of cost.

Relative cost reduction and relative efficiency gain are two sides of exactly the same coin. By designing a uniform metric that is independent of any particular institution's relationships with payers and internal accounting practices both sides of this interesting coin can be illuminated. Useful comparisons are thereby rendered possible both within the same institution at different times (when payer relationships, costs, and accounting practices might change) and across different institutions at the same or different times.

For all of these reasons, calculating an equilibrating cutoff probability facilitates retrospective evaluation. It indicates whether or not and the extent to which substituting PCM-generated probabilities for whatever triage procedure was actually employed could have reduced the relative cost and could have increased the relative efficiency of a particular medical institution's historical experience in performing a particular diagnostic procedure.

Additional consequences of adopting as an alternative recommendation policy the 9.89 percent equilibrating G2SLNPPR cutoff probability would have been as follows.

1. Of the 1,039 SLNB patients, 516 would have been recommended to continue to undergo an SLNB, while the remaining 523 patients would have been recommended to eschew it instead.
2. Of the 301 no-SLNB patients, 109 would have been recommended to undergo an SLNB instead, while the remaining 192 patients would have been recommended to continue to eschew it.
3. Thus, a total of 516 + 109 = 625 SLNBs would have been recommended (and presumably performed).
4. This compared to 1,039 SLNBs actually having been performed.
5. The net cost saving achieved by substituting PCM-generated probabilities for conventional triage methodology and by adopting a 9.89 percent equilibrating cutoff value of G2SLNPPR would have been 1,039 - (516 + 109) = 414 fewer SLNBs performed.
6. Performing 414 fewer SLNBs is equivalent to a 414/1,039 = 39.85 percent cost reduction, regardless of the dollar cost of performing each SLNB.
7. PCM, using the 9.89 percent cutoff probability, would have generated 186.64 positive SLNB outcomes (187 - 19 = 168 actual positive outcomes plus 18.64 expected additional positive outcomes). From the more conventional, guideline-based recommendations actually made virtually the same number (187) of positive SLNB outcomes resulted.
8. PCM would have recommended that only 625 patients actually undergo SLNBs. The guideline-based recommendations required 1,039 SLNBs to produce virtually the same number of positive test outcomes. Therefore, PCM's effective yield was 186.64/625 = 29.86 percent. This compared to the observed 187/1,039 = 18.00 percent yield. The 11.86 yield increase (a 65.89 percent efficiency improvement) was achieved just by changing the triage procedure. No aspects of performing the SLNBs were altered. Only recommendations to undergo or not to undergo an SLNB were based on PCM-generated probabilities rather than on conventional guidelines.

2.10 Possible Problems with the Equilibrating Analysis and Its Conclusions

Of the patients diagnosed with melanoma at UCSF between 1987 and 2007 the number who did not undergo an SLNB far exceeded the number who did. Yet the SLNB sample contained 1,039 patients. The no-SLNB sample contained only 301. The SLNB sample was something close to a census. The no-SLNB sample constituted far less than a census. Do these observations undermine our conclusions?

It is very desirable to obtain as complete as possible a sample of SLNB patients. A census or something close to a census would be ideal. Expending time and energy on a thorough search of a medical institution's patient records is time and energy well spent. The mechanics by which an equilibrating cutoff probability is identified makes this true. In fact, much of the reasoning that underlies the following sensitivity analysis depends on having successfully captured data on (almost) all patients who actually underwent SLN biopsies. We were fortunate to have obtained close to a census of the SLNB patients.

A decidedly more casual approach to no-SLNB patients is permissible. What is important about the no-SLNB sample is that it properly represent the relatively small number of plausible candidates for an SLN biopsy, even though no such candidate actually underwent one. The much larger number of implausible candidates who also did not undergo an SLNB will turn out to be largely irrelevant both to the mechanics of identifying an equilibrating cutoff probability and to the conclusions that may appropriately be drawn therefrom.

An equilibrating cutoff probability sensitivity analysis will demonstrate this.

1. Begin with all patients who did not undergo an SLNB. Partition them into two categories.
2. The first category we shall label plausible candidates. It includes patients who did not undergo an SLNB but who were plausibly close to receiving a positive recommendation for the procedure.
3. An example of a plausible candidate would be a patient who presented at initial diagnosis with none of the particular high-risk features listed in section 2.8 but who subsequently suffered a relapse or recurrence anyway.
4. All 301 no-SLNB patients were treated as plausible candidates. Approximately one-third of them (103) fit the description just given as an example.
5. The second category we shall label implausible candidates. It includes the many more patients who were never seriously considered for an SLNB in terms of the guidelines. None were even close to being considered.
6. An example of an implausible candidate would be a patient whose primary tumor had not yet progressed to its vertical growth phase at initial diagnosis.
7. There were no implausible candidates either among the 1,039 SLNB patients or among the 301 no-SLNB patients. Implausible candidates were completely excluded from our analysis.
8. Now focus on a particular probability of obtaining a positive SLNB which, if used as a cutoff probability in making SLNB recommendations, is believed to have been the equilibrating probability.
9. An equilibrating probability of 9.89 percent was calculated from the analysis of our 1,340-patient cohort.
10. Imagine how including the large number of totally ignored implausible candidates in our analysis might have altered any calculated results and conclusions.
11. Since the SLNB sample was treated as a census, the calculated G2SLNPPR probabilities would not have changed. Neither would the alternative recommendation table presented in section 2.7 have changed for the same reason.
12. Incorporating implausible candidates in our analysis could only change results for no-SLNB patients presented in section 2.8 and included in the modified alternative recommendation table presented in section 2.9.
13. Suppose that all the ignored implausible candidates possessed G2SLNPPR positivity probabilities below the equilibrating cutoff value of 9.89 percent. This is not a preposterous supposition. Most patients who did not undergo an SLNB were judged to possess less than a 10 percent likelihood of being node-positive.
14. Then the calculated value of the equilibrating cutoff probability would not have changed from 9.89 percent. Neither would any of the conclusions based on its calculated value have changed.
15. Only the EXPECTED COUNT OF PRESCIENT ALTERED RECOMMENDATIONS FOR NO-SLNB PATIENTS in the modified alternative recommendation table would have possessed somewhat higher numeric values, and then only with respect to those G2SLNPPR probabilities in the early portion of the table falling below the equilibrating value of 9.89 percent.

16. DIFFERENCE IN COUNTS tabled in the last column of the modified alternative recommendation table would also have changed. Again, however, the only changes would have been related to those G2SLNPPR probabilities falling below the equilibrating value of 9.89 percent.

17. Most importantly, the equilibrating cutoff probability would again have been calculated as 9.89 percent.

18. Now relax the supposition that all implausible candidates possessed G2SLNPPR positivity probabilities below 9.89 percent. Suppose that just the vast majority of such probabilities fell below 9.89 percent. This seems like a very reasonable supposition.

19. Their impact on the EXPECTED COUNT OF PRESCIENT ALTERED RECOMMENDATIONS FOR NO-SLNB PATIENTS would again deteriorate gradually and again evaporate at a G2SLNPPR positivity probability of 9.89 percent.

20. Only the tiny number of implausible candidates and the larger number of ignored plausible candidates possessing G2SLNPPR positivity probabilities above 9.89 percent could alter the numeric value of the equilibrating cutoff probability.

21. We shall continue to ignore the implausible candidates, but we shall consider carefully the ignored plausible candidates.

22. Here is where the representativeness of the 301-patient no-SLNB sample enters the discussion. If we assume that these 301 patients were representative of all plausible candidates for SLN biopsies who did not actually undergo one, we can simulate having included ignored plausible candidates. For example, we can first duplicate and then triplicate the distribution of G2SLNPPR probabilities assigned to the 301 no-SLNB patients in section 2.8. We would then be pretending that we had obtained 602-patient and 903-patient no-SLNB samples whose respective distributions of assigned G2SLNPPR probabilities matched exactly the distribution actually obtained in the 301-patient no-SLNB sample. This constitutes our operational interpretation of representativeness.

23. Analysis of the simulated 602-patient no-SLNB sample would require doubling each EXPECTED COUNT OF PRESCIENT ALTERED RECOMMENDATIONS FOR NO-SLNB PATIENTS in the modified alternative recommendation table and then observing where the altered DIFFERENCE IN COUNTS fell to zero. Since the 1,039-patient SLNB sample was treated as a census, only these last two columns of the table would be affected.

24. A recalculation of the equilibrating cutoff probability for the simulated 602-patient no-SLNB sample would increase its value from 9.89 percent to 13.76 percent. The COUNT OF NONPRESCIENT ALTERED RECOMMENDATIONS FOR 1,039 SLNB PATIENTS would increase from nineteen to twenty-nine as the number of ALTERED RECOMMENDATIONS FOR 1,039 SLNB PATIENTS increased from 523 to 605. The EXPECTED COUNT OF PRESCIENT ALTERED RECOMMENDATIONS FOR 602 NO-SLNB PATIENTS would increase from 18.64 to 30.84 as the number of no-SLNB patients who would now undergo an SLNB increased from 109 to 164. The net result is that 1,039 − (434 + 164) = 441 fewer SLNBs would have been performed.

25. Performing 441 fewer SLNBs is equivalent to a 441/1,039 = 42.44 percent cost reduction and to a [(188.84/598) − (187/1,039)]/(187/1,039) = 75.46 percent higher triage efficiency.

26. Analysis of the simulated 903-patient no-SLNB sample would require tripling each EXPECTED COUNT OF PRESCIENT ALTERED RECOMMENDATIONS FOR NO-SLNB PATIENTS in the modified alternative recommendation table and then observing where the altered DIFFERENCE IN COUNTS fell to zero.

27. A recalculation of the equilibrating cutoff probability for the simulated 903-patient no-SLNB sample would increase its value from 9.89 percent to 15.29 percent. The COUNT OF NONPRESCIENT ALTERED RECOMMENDATIONS FOR 1,039 SLNB PATIENTS would increase from nineteen to thirty-two as the number of ALTERED RECOMMENDATIONS FOR 1,039 SLNB PATIENTS increased from 523 to 632. The EXPECTED COUNT OF PRESCIENT

ALTERED RECOMMENDATIONS FOR 903 NO-SLNB PATIENTS would increase from 18.64 to 32.10 as the number of no-SLNB patients who would now undergo an SLNB increased from 109 to 147. The net result is that 1,039 - (407 + 147) = 554 fewer SLNBs would have been performed.

28. Performing 554 fewer SLNBs is equivalent to a 554/1,039 = 53.32 percent cost reduction and to a [(187.10/485) - (187/1,039)]/(187/1,039) = 114.34 percent higher triage efficiency.

29. A definite pattern emerged from these two analyses. The recalculated equilibrating cutoff probability consistently increased as more ignored plausible candidates were added in simulation to the actual 301-patient no-SLNB sample.

30. This, in turn, caused both the relative cost reduction and its corresponding relative efficiency to become progressively more favorable. Both improvements were achieved simply by substituting PCM-generated G2SLNPPR probabilities for reliance on conventional guidelines as the basis for recommending SLNBs to patients.

Implausible candidates were believed to be far less than 10 percent likely to generate a positive test outcome were they to undergo an SLNB. This means that their likelihood was also far less than 9.89 percent. Therefore, ignoring implausible candidates would seem not to have had an appreciable impact on the calculation of the equilibrating cutoff probability.

Interestingly, ignoring plausible candidates appeared to underestimate the equilibrating probability. Raising that probability would have increased both the resulting cost reduction and the resulting improvement in efficiency. Therefore, to the extent that ignoring plausible candidates biased our two most important conclusions, it was in the conservative direction. If different, the unbiased conclusions would have been even more favorable than those reported.

Closer inspection of the history of the 301 no-SLNB patients also verified that they did represent plausible, if not obvious, candidates for an SLN biopsy. Recall that this sample included many patients who had either suffered a relapse or recurrence following initial diagnosis or who had been followed up for at least two years without experiencing either event. The two-year follow up provided them a reasonable opportunity to experience either event.

Such patients comprised 258/301 = 85.71 percent of the no-SLNB sample. Of them 103/301 = 34.22 percent did subsequently suffer a relapse or recurrence. An even larger portion of the 109 no-SLNB patients who would have been recommended to undergo an SLNB under the 9.89 percent policy (51/109 = 46.79 percent) subsequently suffered a relapse or recurrence.

Assuming that a representative sample of plausible candidates who did not undergo an SLNB can be obtained, is there always an equilibrating cutoff probability such as 9.89 percent? In other words, can a retrospective cost-benefit analysis always be performed to assess and calibrate the room for improvement relative to an institution's historical triage procedure? The answer is yes, excluding certain very unlikely extreme circumstances. However, there is no guarantee that an equilibrating cutoff probability will always indicate the possibility of either lower cost or higher triage efficiency.

Consider the following very unlikely extreme example. If all no-SLNB patients were guaranteed with 100 percent probability to have positive SLNBs, while even the highest positivity probability assigned to SLNB patients fell below 100 percent, and if the number of no-SLNB patients exceeded the number of actual positive test results among the SLNB patients, there would be no equilibrating cutoff probability that could replicate the number of positive test results actually observed.

Alternatively, if the SLNB patient with the lowest positivity probability experienced a positive test result, and if all no-SLNB patients were assigned still lower probabilities, that lowest positivity probability would be a (nonunique) equilibrating cutoff probability. This is not an implausible possibility. It would, however, suggest no room for improvement relative to the institution's historical triage procedure. In the current example it would mean that the conventional guidelines had worked quite satisfactorily.

Whether or not and the extent to which there is room for improvement in a given institution's historical triage procedure relative to a given diagnostic test depends on the circumstances. An institutional audit similar to what has just been presented must actually be performed to find out. An institutional audit is usually possible, but room for substantial improvement is never guaranteed.

2.11 Assessing Cost-Benefit Trade-Offs to Select an SLNB Recommendation
       Policy Appropriate for a Particular Medical Institution

Figure 5 has been produced to illustrate in graphical form the equilibrating analysis just performed algebraically and with tables. Figure 5 relates the resulting yield of positive test results (vertical Y-axis) to the number of SLNBs that were executed in order to generate that yield (horizontal X-axis).

The single point in the northeast portion of figure 5 represents the consequences of the triage policy actually adopted. It resulted in executing 1,039 SLNBs, which generated 187 positive test results.

The policy actually adopted was similar to the triage policy adopted by most melanoma centers during the same historical time period. Patients with primary lesions at least one millimeter thick were typically recommended to undergo an SLNB. In addition, some patients with thin melanomas (no more than one millimeter thick) were also recommended to undergo an SLNB, based on the number and severity of any high-risk features with which they initially presented.

A point on each curve in figure 5 shows the consequences of substituting a particular PCM-generated cutoff probability for the guideline-based triage policy actually adopted. Figure 5 is a downward projection onto two-dimensional cost-benefit space of the three-dimensional relationship whose third dimension records in descending sequence alternative PCM-generated cutoff probabilities.

The upper curve shows the consequences of substituting alternative G2SLNPPR cutoff probabilities. These were generated by the PCM prediction algorithm based on all twenty-two prognostic factors. The result of the detailed equilibrating analysis just performed is represented by the point where the horizontal line at 187 positive SLNB test results intersects this upper curve.

The lower curve shows the alternative consequences of substituting less accurate PCSLNPPR cutoff probabilities generated by the PCM prediction algorithm based on only the six traditional prognostic factors recommended by the AJCC. The result of a comparable equilibrating analysis—applied to PCSLNPPR cutoff probabilities—is represented by the point where the same horizontal line at 187 positive SLNB test results intersects this lower curve.

Substituting a given cutoff probability drawn from either curve means that any patient who is assigned by PCM that or a higher probability of a positive SLNB outcome would have been recommended to undergo an SLNB. Any patient assigned a lower probability would have been recommended not to undergo an SLNB.

Recommendations are assumed to have been accepted and executed. Therefore, substituting each cutoff probability implies both a number of SLNBs that would then necessarily have been executed (horizontal axis, generating an accumulated test cost) and either the number of positive test outcomes that would actually have resulted or the expected number of positive test outcomes that would likely have resulted (vertical axis, generating an accumulated test benefit).

Each curve was produced after first sequencing patients in descending order according to their PCM-generated cutoff probabilities. Thus, the lowest (most southwesterly) point on each curve represents the patient with the highest possible PCM-generated positivity probability. The highest (most northeasterly) point represents the patient with the lowest possible positivity probability.

Each curve is actually a sequence of 488 (not necessarily distinct) points with two logical end points appended. The 187 patients who actually underwent SLNBs with positive outcomes contributed 187 points to each curve. The 301 patients who did not undergo SLNBs contributed the remaining 301 points to each curve. Since tied cutoff probabilities sometimes occurred, the 488 + 2 points that comprise each curve were largely, but not completely distinct.

The 852 patients who underwent SLNBs with negative outcomes are nowhere represented on either curve. This is because each cutoff probability is being viewed as a candidate substitute criterion for the guideline-based triage policy actually adopted. No candidate cutoff probability would ever be selected as an appropriate substitute criterion if there existed at least one other cutoff probability on the same curve that produced the same number of positive test results, but from a smaller number of SLNBs required to achieve them. Because executing any SLNB with a negative outcome always increased the cost of the triage procedure (by one SLNB) but never the benefit (since no additional positive test resulted), such outcomes were uniformly ignored. Plotting points to represent these 852 patients on either curve would only contribute to the clutter, not to the useful information conveyed by figure 5.

Figure 5 is presented on the next page.

Figure 5

SLNB Cost-Benefit Analysis for 1,340 UCSF Patients
(1,039 Patients Underwent SLNBs, while 301 Did Not)

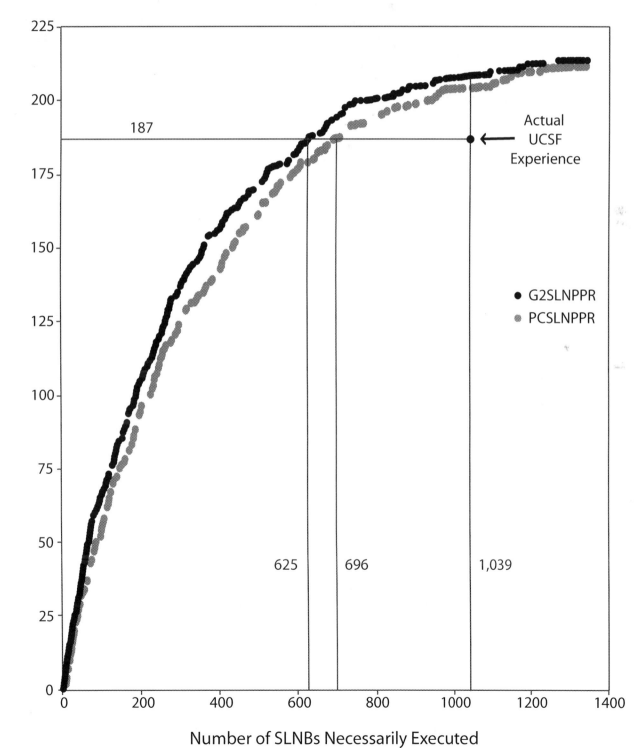

Number of SLNBs Necessarily Executed

Inspection of figure 5 shows that both SLNB positivity yield curves rise consistently but at an ever-decreasing rate, as successively lower cutoff probabilities are considered as substitute candidates for the actual triage policy. Choosing each lower cutoff probability simultaneously requires that an ever-increasing number of SLNBs be executed.

Figure 4 demonstrated that SLNB positivity probabilities converge with great fidelity to the actual frequencies of positive test results. Because of this, consistently rising at an ever-decreasing rate is a direct consequence of the way figure 5 was constructed. This pattern was uniformly reflected in both the upper (G2SLNPPR) and the lower (PCSLNPPR) yield curves. It would also be reflected in any other similarly constructed yield curve based on substantially converging positivity probabilities.

Notice from figure 5 that the upper G2SLNPPR curve is either coincident with or always lies to the northwest of the lower PCSLNPPR curve. There are no crossover points. This has substantial practical implications. Any point in figure 5 that lies due north of or due west of or northwest of another point indicates an unequivocally superior triage consequence compared to that other point. Lying due north means that more positive test results were generated by the same number of SLNBs executed (a benefit enhancement). Lying due west means that the same number of positive test results were generated by executing fewer SLNBs (a cost reduction). Lying northwest means that more positive test results were generated from fewer executed SLNBs (both a benefit enhancement and a cost reduction, simultaneously).

That the G2SLNPPR curve is either coincident with or always to the northwest of the PCSLNPPR curve means that, whenever prognostic factors were analyzed via PCM, using the set of all twenty-two factors to predict SLNB positivity always provided at least an equally good and usually provided a clearly superior candidate cutoff probability compared to relying on just its subset of the traditional six factors recommended by the AJCC. It paid to collect, to record, and to incorporate into a PCM analysis patient data on additional prognostic factors with genuine prognostic significance. Waiting until the AJCC "anoints" a newly discovered, nontraditional factor can preclude a genuine opportunity to save cost and improve efficiency. The wait may last for more than a decade.

We have already demonstrated in sections 2.5 and 2.6 that the additional sixteen nontraditional factors added significantly to prognostic accuracy. Figure 5 demonstrates, in addition, that this increased accuracy can facilitate lower cost and improved triage efficiency in the context of performing a diagnostic test procedure (SLNB). If any medical center can perform a similar historical equilibrating analysis (i.e., conduct an institutional audit) and replicate these pleasant findings, why wait?

Section 2.9 listed the consequences of adopting as an alternative recommendation policy the 9.89 percent equilibrating G2SLNPPR cutoff probability. In figure 5, this 9.89 percent cutoff probability corresponds to the point of intersection of the horizontal line at 187 positive SLNB test results with the upper G2SLNPPR curve.

An equivalent point of intersection between the same horizontal line and the lower PCSLNPPR curve occurs in figure 5 at an equilibrating cutoff probability of 8.94 percent. The consequences of using PCSLNPP probabilities instead of G2SLNPPR probabilities and adopting 8.94 percent as an alternative recommendation policy during the same time period ending in 2007 are listed on the next page.

1. Of the 1,039 SLNB patients, 593 would have been recommended to continue to undergo an SLNB, while the remaining 446 patients would have been recommended to eschew it instead.
2. Of the 301 no-SLNB patients, 103 would have been recommended to undergo an SLNB instead, while the remaining 198 patients would have been recommended to continue to eschew it.
3. Thus, a total of 593 + 103 = 696 SLNBs would have been recommended (and presumably performed).
4. This compared to 1,039 SLNBs actually having been performed.
5. The net cost saving achieved by substituting PCM-generated probabilities for conventional triage methodology and by adopting a 8.94 percent equilibrating cutoff value of PCSLNPPR would have been 1,039 - (593 + 103) = 343 fewer SLNBs performed.
6. Performing 343 fewer SLNBs is equivalent to a 343/1,039 = 33.01 percent cost reduction, regardless of the dollar cost of performing each SLNB.
7. PCM, using the 8.94 percent cutoff probability, would have generated 187.02 positive SLNB outcomes (187 - 17 = 170 actual positive outcomes plus 17.02 expected additional positive outcomes). From the more conventional, guideline-based recommendations actually made virtually the same number (187) of positive SLNB outcomes resulted.
8. PCM would have recommended that only 696 patients actually undergo SLNBs. The guideline-based recommendations resulted in 1,039 SLNBs to produce virtually the same number of positive test outcomes. Therefore, PCM's effective yield was 187.02/696 = 26.87 percent. This compared to the actual 187/1,039 = 18.00 percent yield. The 8.87 yield increase (a 49.28 percent efficiency improvement) was achieved just by changing the triage procedure. No aspects of performing the SLNBs were altered. Only recommendations to undergo or not to undergo an SLNB were based on PCM-generated PCSLNPPR probabilities rather than on conventional guidelines.

Perhaps the most compelling of these results is the suggestion that even a medical center that collects and records only the six traditional AJCC prognostic factors may still be able to obtain cost reductions and triage efficiency improvements close to 33 percent and to 50 percent, respectively. An audit of its historical triage methodology by means of a PCM-generated equilibrating probability analysis could indicate substantial room for improvement.

In 2008 a typical SLN biopsy cost approximately $18,000 at UCSF. Cost, here, was supposed to reflect the total drain on society's valuable resources then required to execute each such biopsy.

This quantity was not intended to reflect the cost to a patient undergoing the SLNB. Neither was it intended to reflect the cost to an insurance company, to a governmental Agency, or to any other entity. Costs to other entities under various circumstances would have differed widely from $18,000.

Taking a drain-on-society's-resources perspective, the total dollar cost savings realizable by substituting PCM-generated G2SLNPPR probabilities for reliance on conventional guidelines as the basis for recommending SLNBs to patients was then estimated to be $18,000 times the reduction in number of SLN biopsies that had to be performed to achieve the same number of positive test outcomes (187) actually achieved.

Using the 9.89 percent equilibrating cutoff value of G2SLNPPR positivity probabilities to recommend SLNBs to patients would have enabled a total dollar cost saving of $18,000 times 414 = $7,452,000.

On a per-patient-considered-for-an-SLNB basis this is equivalent to an average $7,452,000/(1,039+301) = $5,561 cost saving per patient.

On a per-patient-recommended-to-undergo-an-SLNB basis this is equivalent to an average $7,452,000/(516+109) = $11,923 cost saving per patient.

Using the 8.94 percent equilibrating cutoff value of PCSLNPPR positivity probabilities to recommend SLNBs to patients would have enabled a total dollar cost saving of $18,000 times 343 = $6,174,000.

On a per-patient-considered-for-an-SLNB basis this is equivalent to an average $6,174,000/(1,039+301) = $4,608 cost saving per patient.

On a per-patient-recommended-to-undergo-an-SLNB basis this is equivalent to an average $6,174,000/(593+103) = $8,871 cost saving per patient.

Now that we have estimated costs to compare with the benefits of executing a SLN biopsy, how can a particular medical center use G2SLNPPR or PCSLNPPR positivity probabilities and the various tables constructed from them to pick the "best" cutoff probability? We shall illustrate how in terms of the more accurate G2SLNPPR probabilities, although similar conclusions could be drawn from using PCSLNPPR probabilities in their place.

Cost-benefit trade-offs can be made as follows.

1. Pick a G2SLNPPR cutoff probability. That means contemplate revising whatever was the institution's historical recommendation policy by substituting use of the just-picked PCM-generated probability.
2. Compare its tabled and graphed benefits and disbenefits relative to the institution's historical recommendation policy.
3. Judge which contemplated revised recommendation policies (i.e., which contemplated cutoff probabilities) deliver, on balance, a net improvement compared to the institution's historical policy.
4. From among the cutoff probabilities that offer a net improvement pick the one offering the maximum net improvement.
5. Optionally, make judicious interpolations to "round off" the cutoff to a more cosmetically pleasing positive SLNB outcome probability.

Returning to figure 5, there are many points on the G2SLNPPR curve that lie in the northwest quadrant relative to actual historical experience. All of these northwesterly points promise either less cost without giving up any SLNB positivity yield or a greater positivity yield without having to execute more SLNBs or both. In terms of their triage consequences, therefore, substituting any one of the corresponding cutoff probabilities for the conventional, guideline-based triage procedure actually adopted would appear to be unequivocally cost-effective. This clearly indicates room for improvement.

The news gets better. All of these northwesterly points are generated by cutoff probabilities in the neighborhood of 10 percent. Abandoning reliance on conventional guidelines in favor of using any one of them would therefore constitute no break whatsoever from this institution's traditional intentions. It would serve only to reduce cost and to increase SLNB triage efficiency by achieving the intended results more closely.

Not all equilibrating probability analyses would support conclusions as clear as these. The Melanoma Center's triage procedure would have been improved substantially by adopting a cutoff probability had such probabilities been available historically. Going forward, abandoning reliance on conventional guidelines in favor of adopting a cutoff probability would seem eminently wise.

Even after making this decision the question still remains, "Which among the cost-effective cutoff probabilities is optimal for a particular institution?" Picking the optimal cutoff probability means adopting it as the new basis for recommending or not recommending SLNBs to patients. That means altering recommendations compared to historical practice. There may be important qualitative considerations not properly addressed so far in our cost-benefit analysis. How might one judge whether to adjust either upward or downward a seemingly appropriate cutoff probability to reflect these qualitative factors? The following considerations may be useful in making such a judgment.

1. Altering a recommendation from positive to negative is labeled prescient only if the eschewed SLNB would have produced a negative result. Then neither the physician nor the patient is any worse off in terms of making patient management choices and lifestyle choices, respectively. Also, somebody saves $18,000 (at least in an accounting sense).

2. Altering a recommendation from positive to negative is labeled nonprescient if the eschewed SLNB would have tested positive. Yes, somebody still saves the cost of an SLNB, but that somebody may not be the patient, the physician, or the physician's host institution. Far worse, all parties are now deprived of information useful in making patient management and lifestyle choices. If detectable in the legal discovery process, that might even support a claim of malpractice.

3. Altering a recommendation from positive to negative means that one fewer SLNB would be performed, unless the demand for SLNBs exceeds the capacity to perform them. That would reduce somebody's income.

4. Altering a recommendation from negative to positive is labeled prescient only if the previously eschewed, but now performed SLNB would produce a positive result. Both the physician and the patient would then be in possession of information useful in making patient management and lifestyle choices.

5. Whether or not prescient, altering a recommendation from negative to positive would generate an extra cost to somebody. It might also create some complications for the patient. It would likely increase somebody's income. It might decrease the risk of a malpractice suit.

In view of these considerations it is easy to understand why more than an appropriate number of SLNBs might regularly be performed—at least from a drain-on-society's-resources perspective. Our existing legal and health care delivery systems are structured so as to provide numerous and powerful incentives to behave exactly in this manner. Performing an SLNB is the informative, the legally safe, and the financially profitable thing to do. Except for the possibility of complications on the patient's part, incentives not to perform an SLNB are much weaker.

A PCM analysis can be specifically tailored to the patient composition of any particular medical center. Carefully reasoned cost-benefit judgments can also be tailored both to its cost structure and to its distinctive culture.

Tailorability to different patient compositions is facilitated by PCM'S uniform prestratification into separate risk subgroups. This initial procedure serves to attenuate difficulties in achieving representativeness arising from compositional heterogeneity across different medical institutions.

No claim is made that $18,000 is everybody's cost, or even the "right" cost of performing an SLNB. Different institutions face different costs. Everybody's cost will likely change over time. It is easy to substitute for $18,000 whatever cost is appropriate for any particular institution at any given time.

Neither is it claimed that all institutions will elect to balance their costs and benefits in exactly the same manner. Some thrive on innovation, requiring substantial risk taking. Others may prefer to operate more conservatively.

It is even possible to substitute quite different costs and benefits in the analysis to reflect the quite different perspectives of separate entities (different players in the health care delivery arena). This would enable an especially dramatic form of tailoring.

We do, however, make the following claims.

1. The superior accuracy delivered by PCM at the individual patient level can increase prescience.
2. Increased prescience can then be exploited by an institutionally tailored cost-benefit analysis in the manner just illustrated to improve the efficiency of many triage procedures.
3. If the equilibrating cut point portion of a retrospective cost-benefit analysis suggests a substantial opportunity to reduce the cost and to increase the efficiency (based on positive test yield) of a diagnostic procedure compared to whatever triage techniques the institution has employed historically, then the institution might seriously consider altering the way it recommends patients to undergo that procedure.
4. The excessive (i.e., not cost-effective) rate at which such a procedure was being performed could thereby be reduced, along with the unnecessary cost and morbidity.
5. Simultaneously, additional tests could be offered in the future to patients regarded historically as inappropriate candidates but who PCM analysis suggests could benefit from undergoing such a procedure.
6. Our claims are by no means restricted to the SLNB procedure, to melanoma patients, or even to cancer as a malady. These three aspects of our analysis merely served as a convenient illustrative context.

2.12 Concluding Comments

As just stated, our existing legal and health care delivery systems are structured so as to provide numerous and powerful incentives to perform "too many" (rather than "too few") diagnostic and other medical procedures—at least from certain societal perspectives. Performing an SLNB is the medically informative, the legally safe, and the financially profitable thing for health care providers to do. Incentives not to perform an SLNB are much weaker.

Because of this one might expect the overall gain from substituting PCM for conventional, guideline-based triage techniques to be more of a cost saving than an improved medical benefit. Indeed, the analysis we have just performed suggested the possibility of almost a 40 percent cost saving.

The same PCM-based cost-benefit analysis suggested the possibility of an improved medical benefit. By selectively altering the SLNB recommendation policy (i.e., by adopting the 9.89 percent equilibrating cutoff probability), PCM's yield (generation of positive SLNB test results) was improved by 66 percent. The same number of positive SLNB tests (187) was obtained from only 625 instead of the original 1,039 patients.

Were our existing legal and health care delivery systems to become restructured in the future (e.g., by a favorable evolution of Obamacare), the primary virtue of PCM might thereby shift, gradually, from cost reduction to improved medical benefits and to achieving a proper balance between them.

Imagine, for example, a future environment restructured as follows.

First, health care providers are given a fixed financial amount that they are then encouraged to allocate both to preventative procedures and to traditional therapies so as to maximize the overall health and well-being of their patients during their lifetime.

Second, medical malpractice suits are strictly limited to genuine instances of negligence (e.g., to nonexperimental situations where generally accepted standards of medical care are clearly violated).

Unless or until our existing systems are restructured, however, health care providers might be motivated to exploit only that portion of PCM's benefits incrementally beneficial to themselves. In the SLNB context that would mean applying the equilibrating G2SLNPPR probability of 9.89 percent only to the 301 plausible no-SLNB patients to justify performing an additional 109 SLNBs. It would not mean reducing the number of SLNBs actually performed from 1,039 to 516. Why should a health care provider endure a revenue loss to itself and reduced income to its employees; deprive nineteen of its patients and their physicians of valuable medical information; and increase, thereby, the risk of malpractice suits in order to provide cost savings to others (e.g., to insurance companies, to governmental subsidy programs, and, perhaps eventually, to taxpayers)?

An additional 18.64 positive SLNB test outcomes could be expected from performing 109 additional SLNBs. The resulting yield of positive test outcomes of 18.64/109 = 17.10 percent is about the same as the 187/1,039 = 18.00 percent yield realized from the entire group of patients who underwent SLNBs. Everybody seems to win if the additional 109 SLNBs are performed. So why not just do that? It would be consistent with the existing pay-per-procedure-performed manner in which health care costs are currently reimbursed.

Those who believe (as we do) that failing to reduce an excessive number of SLNBs performed would not be in society's best interest should be arguing for an appropriate restructuring of our legal and health care delivery systems. An appropriate restructuring is one that substitutes powerful incentives to health care providers to behave in society's best interest for the distinctly less compelling incentives that currently exist. That means more closely aligning providers' interests with society's interest. Giving health care providers a fixed dollar amount to do the best they can for their patients and allowing them to retain whatever cost savings their more efficient (triage) decisions enable would produce a closer alignment. The closer alignment would result from having providers pocket whatever cost savings they could realize from a more efficient allocation of what would then become viewed as "their own" money.

Allowing patients to obtain their health care from whichever providers actually produce the best outcomes at the lowest cost in a competitive marketplace would force a still closer alignment. Competition really can work when it is allowed to—within appropriate bounds, of course.

Actually (not just nominally) restricting malpractice suits to instances of genuine negligence would also be in society's best interest. Fewer physicians would feel required to abandon their profession rather than pay the ever-increasing cost of malpractice insurance.

Must we wait for a favorable evolution of Obamacare or something like it to obtain PCM's potential benefits? Hopefully not!

Just expanding the triage process to include additional patients PCM suggests are typically overlooked by conventional guidelines could be beneficial both to patients and to health care providers. It might even save lives.

Doing so would also produce solid evidence either to confirm or to disconfirm or to modify PCM's presumption that a predictive algorithm derived from patients who actually underwent some diagnostic procedure also applies to patients who did not. Such evidence, to the extent confirmatory, would serve to allay the suspicion of skeptics who remain unconvinced by results of the type presented in figures 4 and 5 and in the split-sample reliability analysis.

3.0 ADAPTING PCM TO RENDER POSITRON EMISSION TOMOGRAPHY (COMPUTED TOMOGRAPHY)
     SCANS MORE COST-EFFECTIVE: A REPLICATION ANALYSIS

PCM is versatile. Comparable reductions in cost and gains in triage efficiency
can be realized by applying PCM to a different diagnostic procedure
administered to patients at a different medical center.

This section describes how corresponding cost-benefit improvements could have
been obtained by substituting PCM for the conventional, guideline-based method
of triage to positron emission tomography (computed tomography) scans for
melanoma patients at the California Pacific Medical Center (CPMC). A pattern of
cost-benefit improvements similar to what emerged from our previous analysis of
1,340 SLNB patients was realized for these PET/CT scans given at CPMC.

A PET/CT scan is a diagnostic procedure that produces a three-dimensional image
of some functioning bodily process. A radioactive tracer (fluorine-18 labeled
fluorodeoxyglucose, called FDG) is injected into the bloodstream and is taken
up by cells in the target tissue. FDG emits positrons as it decays
radioactively. A pair of gamma rays is produced when a positron encounters a
normal electron and engages in mutual annihilation. A three-dimensional image
of glucose tracer concentration in the target tissue is then constructed from a
computer analysis of the pattern of gamma rays so produced.

Since the overall level of metabolic activity in the target tissue is indicated
by its glucose uptake, PET/CT scans can be administered to various types of
cancer patients in search of tumor metastasis or recurrence after a known
primary tumor has been surgically removed. This is one of the currently most
frequent medical applications of FDG-PET/CT scans.

When used to detect cancer PET/CT scans are not disease-specific. A positive
scan indicates an elevated uptake of glucose. This, in turn, could indicate the
presence of various forms of cancer, as well as some noncancerous condition.
Our interest will be restricted to positivity for melanoma. Throughout the rest
of our discussion, therefore, a positive PET scan will refer exclusively to a
FDG-PET/CT scan outcome specifically positive for the presence of melanoma.

The medical records of eight hundred consecutive patients newly diagnosed with
cutaneous melanoma between 2007 and 2014 by the Center for Melanoma Research
and Treatment at CPMC were collected and reviewed. All patients were seen at
least once both by a dermatological oncologist and by an oncological surgeon
during this time period.

From these eight hundred we selected 173 patients to be in our PET scan sample.
Selection criteria were that each patient must have undergone an FDG-PET/CT
scan as part of the initial staging procedure and that both the patient's
detailed medical record and PET scan report were accessible electronically.
Patients who underwent a nonstaging or a restaging PET scan were excluded.

Outcomes of the scans administered to these 173 patients are tabled below.

VALUE OF ATTRIBUTE PETSTATE	ABSOLUTE FREQUENCIES (COUNTS)	RELATIVE FREQUENCIES (PROPORTIONS)	CUMULATIVE RELATIVE FREQUENCIES
NEGATIVE	137	.7919	.7919
POSITIVE	36	.2081	1.0000
TOTAL	173	1.0000	

Note: PETSTATE designates the outcome of each patient's FDG-PET/CT scan as a specific indicator of melanoma's presence in the target tissue. For these 173 patients the scan's yield (i.e., the generation of scan outcomes specifically positive for melanoma) was 20.81 percent. There were no missing observations of PETSTATE and, therefore, of the PET/CT yield.

VALUE OF ATTRIBUTE PETSTATE	VALUE OF ATTRIBUTE PETDUMMY		
	0	1	TOTAL
NEGATIVE	137	0	137
POSITIVE	0	36	36
TOTAL	137	36	173

Note: PETDUMMY designates a 0/1 dummy attribute created as a numerically coded equivalent of the PETSTATE attribute. A "0" value of PETDUMMY corresponds to a NEGATIVE PET/CT scan, and a "1" value of PETDUMMY corresponds to a POSITIVE PET/CT scan. All logistic regression analyses with PET/CT scan outcome as the focal end point to be predicted require this 0/1 dummy attribute to be entered as the dependent variable. Since it is merely a recoded version of PETSTATE, PETDUMMY also possessed no missing values.

Most of the 173 melanoma patients were diagnosed with known primary tumors. For six patients, however, no primary tumor was detected at the time of their initial diagnosis. The absence of a known primary tumor produced a number of missing observations in the patient's medical record. Interestingly, the absence of a known primary tumor turned out to be predictive of PET/CT scan positivity for reasons that will be explained later.

Selected attributes of all 173 patients included in our PET scan sample appear in appendix E. Also recorded are the transformations into corresponding factor indexes recommended by the AJCC for prognostic purposes. These transformations relate to the AJCC's six traditional prognostic factors in predicting melanoma progression and to Clark level of primary tumor invasion. Appendix E shows that our PET scan sample encompassed mostly higher-risk (e.g., T3 and T4) patients.

PCM could be expected to improve the accuracy of predicting as either positive or negative an individual patient's PET/CT scan outcome by:

1. first stratifying patients according to their risk of generating a positive scan, using as a stratification criterion the single most discriminating prognostic factor selected from among those widely understood within the medical profession and routinely recorded for most patients (e.g., primary tumor thickness);
2. then executing the SPSA algorithm (separately within each risk subgroup) to transform each traditional (i.e., routinely recorded) prognostic factor into a corresponding UIRI;
3. then adding additional, nontraditional prognostic factors—transformed to corresponding UIRIs by the same SPSA algorithm applied, separately, to each risk subgroup;
4. then performing a separate multivariate logistic regression analysis within each risk subgroup, using transformed UIRI indexes as independent variables and PETDUMMY as the dependent variable; and
5. merging the results obtained from each risk subgroup's multivariate logistic regression analysis into a composite, individually tailored prediction algorithm designed to simulate the outcomes of having every patient actually undergo a PET/CT scan.

That is exactly what was done in the forgoing SLNB analysis. This time, however, our PET scan sample of 173 patients was too small to stratify initially according to a patient's risk of generating a scan positive for melanoma. The stratified subsamples would have been too small to support reliable statistical estimates. We must omit PCM's normal first step. Instead, we shall perform each of the subsequent steps listed on the previous page, but only once and applied to the entire unstratified sample of 173 patients.

3.1 Establishing a Base Case for Assessing Accuracy Improvements

As before, we designated the six AJCC factors described in appendix E the traditional prognostic factors in melanoma. We also designated the specific raw data transformation recommended by the AJCC to measure each traditional factor its corresponding factor index.

Univariate logistic regressions of PET/CT outcome (PETDUMMY) on each factor and factor index generated the following results.

1. The AJCCAGE factor index partitions actual patient age as of most recent birthday prior to initial diagnosis into ten-year intervals.

   A univariate logistic regression of PETDUMMY on actual patient age at diagnosis (AGEDIAG) generated a statistically insignificant positive regression coefficient with a likelihood ratio chi-square statistic of 0.499 and a corresponding two-tailed p value of 0.4801. There were no missing observations in this analysis.

   Substituting AJCCAGE for actual patient age rendered the impact even weaker. A slightly less significant positive regression coefficient was generated with a likelihood ratio chi-square statistic of 0.078 and a corresponding two-tailed p value of 0.7803. This result was also based on all 173 observations.

   That the regression coefficient was positive (though insignificantly so) in both analyses stands in sharp contrast to the previously reported significantly negative impact of age at diagnosis on SLNB positivity. This time, the conventional wisdom was correct. Age at diagnosis appeared to point weakly in the "right" direction.

2. Patient sex is dichotomous. The AJCCSEX factor index assigns zero to being female and one to being male. By so doing it reflects the conventional wisdom that males are at higher risk of melanoma progression than females. Beside providing this directional guidance in numeric form, however, neither the AJCCSEX factor index nor any other dichotomous index can improve predictive accuracy through logistic regression analysis compared to using its dichotomous raw data input.

   The "right" direction was confirmed. The impact of patient sex on PET/CT positivity was statistically significantly positive with a likelihood ratio chi-square statistic of 5.027 and a corresponding two-tailed p value of 0.0250 based on all 173 observations.

3. The AJCCSITE factor index groups together primary tumors located on the head, neck, and trunk as axial. Primary tumors located on the upper and lower extremities are grouped together as peripheral. An axial location is presumed to be higher risk than a peripheral location, so AJCCSITE scores axial locations as one and peripheral locations as zero.

A detailed inspection of anatomical locations revealed a 15.09 percent prevalence of PET/CT positivity associated with the trunk, a 18.64 percent prevalence associated with the head or neck, a 20.00 percent prevalence associated with the upper extremities, and a 26.67 percent prevalence associated with the lower extremities.

We experimented with various ways to group these four anatomical locations. We also found that among dichotomous groupings, the best discrimination was achieved by grouping tumors as axial versus peripheral. This was in line with conventional wisdom.

Although AJCCSITE's axial versus peripheral grouping seemed appropriate, it pointed weakly in the "wrong" direction. Axial primary tumors were less likely, not more likely to produce a positive PET/CT result. The univariate logistic regression of PET/CT positivity on AJCCSITE generated a negative regression coefficient with a likelihood ratio chi-square statistic of 1.033 and a corresponding two-tailed p value of 0.3094.

Six of the 173 patients presented with unknown primary tumors at initial diagnosis. Four of these six patients (66.67 percent) generated positive PET/CT scans. This was a significantly higher prevalence of PET positivity than the 19.16 percent generated by the other 167 patients (chi square two-tailed p value = 0.0212).

A possible explanation of this higher prevalence of PET positivity is a delay in diagnosis. If no primary tumor is identified an initial melanoma diagnosis is likely to occur at a later stage in disease progression. Later-stage progression is likely to increase the chances of PET positivity for any target tissue suspected to have become melanoma-involved.

It turned out that three of the six patients diagnosed with unknown primaries were initially staged 3b, two were initially staged 3c, and the sixth could not be properly staged. Of the 152 patients with known primaries who could be properly staged at initial diagnosis 120 (78.95 percent) were staged either as somewhere in stage 1 or stage 2 or as stage 3a (chi square two-tailed p value = 0.0004). This highly significant difference in stage at initial diagnosis was consistent with our explanation.

Note that missing data on primary tumor location was directionally informative. PCM's unusual way of handling missing observations will later exploit this directional difference to improve the accuracy of PET positivity predictions.

4. The AJCCTHIC factor index partitions the raw tumor thickness measurement scale into four intervals (T1, T2, T3, and T4).

A univariate logistic regression of PETDUMMY on raw tumor thickness (in millimeters) generated a positive regression coefficient, as anticipated, with a likelihood ratio chi-square statistic of 3.973 and a corresponding two-tailed p value of 0.0462. This result was based on 154 observations.

Substituting AJCCTHIC for raw tumor thickness improved these results. A positive regression coefficient was again generated with a likelihood ratio chi-square statistic of 4.818 and a corresponding two-tailed p value of 0.0282. This result was based on the same 154 observations.

Here is a situation where the AJCC factor index improved the ability of tumor thickness to predict PET positivity, also as anticipated by conventional wisdom. Substituting AJCCTHIC for raw tumor thickness did help a bit, just as it did in the SLNB analysis.

5. The AJCCMITR factor index partitions the raw mitotic rate measurement scale into two intervals: no mitoses versus at least one mitosis observed per one square millimeter high-powered microscopic field.

   A univariate logistic regression of PETDUMMY on raw mitotic rate generated a very insignificant positive regression coefficient with a likelihood ratio chi-square statistic of 0.581 and a corresponding two-tailed p value of 0.4458. Conventional wisdom was "right" about the direction of impact. These results were based on 134 observations.

   Substituting AJCCMITR for raw mitotic rate produced a modest improvement. A positive regression coefficient was generated with a likelihood ratio chi-square statistic of 2.097 and a corresponding two-tailed p value of 0.1476 based on the same 134 observations.

6. Like patient sex, ulceration of the primary tumor is treated by the AJCC as dichotomous. The AJCCULC factor index assigns zero to being nonulcerated and one to being ulcerated. Ulcerated tumors are presumed to pose a higher risk of disease progression. Beside providing this directional guidance in numeric form, however, the AJCCULC factor index cannot improve predictive accuracy through logistic regression analysis compared to using its dichotomous raw data input.

   The "right" direction of impact was confirmed, though insignificantly, by univariate logistic regression of PETDUMMY on AJCCULC. A positive regression coefficient was generated with a likelihood ratio chi-square statistic of 1.635 and a corresponding two-tailed p value of 0.2010. This result was based on 145 observations.

The next step was to perform a standard multivariate logistic regression of PETDUMMY on the six traditional AJCC factor indexes. As is common practice, all patients with any missing observations on any prognostic factor were deleted from the analysis. A detailed computer printout is shown below and on the next page enclosed between two horizontal lines.

After removing all undefined values from all expressions, the resulting number of PATIENTs for which each of the 7 expressions possesses a defined value is reduced to 131. This constitutes the effective sample size.

RESULTS OF LOGISTIC REGRESSION ANALYSIS (LINEAR MODEL)

The dependent variable is a binary-coded numeric variable whose values are either 0 or 1. It is embodied in the first expression (parameter) of the LOGREG command, which is just the attribute PETDUMMY.

The independent variable AJCCAGE is just the attribute AJCCAGE.
The independent variable AJCCSEX is just the attribute AJCCSEX.
The independent variable AJCCSITE is just the attribute AJCCSITE.
The independent variable AJCCTHIC is just the attribute AJCCTHIC.
The independent variable AJCCMITR is just the attribute AJCCMITR.
The independent variable AJCCULC is just the attribute AJCCULC.

Likelihood ratio chi-square statistic: 14.003, 2-tail p value: .0296 (based on 6 degrees of freedom and 131 complete observations).

INDEPENDENT VARIABLE	REGRESSION COEFFICIENT	STANDARD DEVIATION	CHI-SQUARE (DF = 1)	2-TAIL P VALUE	ODDS RATIO MULTIPLIER
intercept	-16.4757	713.9434	.0005	.9816	.0000
AJCCAGE	-.1187	.2035	.3400	.5598	.8881
AJCCSEX	1.9817	1.0969	3.2640	.0708	7.2553
AJCCSITE	-.7253	.5521	1.7258	.1890	.4842
AJCCTHIC	.7972	.3749	4.5227	.0334	2.2194
AJCCMITR	11.5381	713.9424	.0003	.9871	102551.3079
AJCCULC	.1232	.5483	.0505	.8222	1.1311

GOODNESS OF STATISTICAL FIT OF LOGISTIC REGRESSION MODEL

Pearson chi-square fit statistic (based on 71 degrees of freedom): 112.960, p value: .0011.

Deviance chi-square fit statistic (based on 71 degrees of freedom): 53.557, p value: .9391.

This analysis is not entirely satisfactory. Two prominent problems are:

1. the statistical instability of the regression coefficient estimated for AJCCMITR (it has an excessive standard deviation, producing an even more excessive odds ratio); and
2. its Pearson chi-square fit statistic, which suggests a statistically significantly poor fit of the logistic regression model to the data (although its deviance chi-square fit statistic suggests a plausible fit).

SUMMARY STATISTICS	ATTRIBUTE AJCCAGE	ATTRIBUTE AJCCSEX	ATTRIBUTE AJCCSITE	ATTRIBUTE AJCCTHIC	ATTRIBUTE AJCCMITR	ATTRIBUTE AJCCULC
n DEFINED	173	173	167	154	134	145
MINIMUM	1	0	0	1	0	0
MEDIAN	6	1	1	3	1	0
MAXIMUM	8	1	1	4	1	1
MEAN	5.7168	.7919	.6707	2.9545	.9552	.4207
STD. DEV.	1.4804	.4059	.4700	.9352	.2068	.4937

There were missing values of four of the six traditional AJCC factor indexes:

1. the six missing values of AJCCSITE associated with the six patients who presented with unknown primary tumors;
2. the six missing values of AJCCTHIC associated with these same six patients, plus thirteen missing values associated with patients who presented with known primaries;
3. the six missing values of AJCCMITR associated with these same six patients, plus thirty-three missing values associated with patients who presented with known primaries; and
4. the six missing values of AJCCULC associated with these same six patients, plus twenty-two missing values associated with patients who presented with known primaries.

Both to ameliorate the problems with the initial analysis and, more importantly, to guarantee comparability with the PCM analyses that will follow missing values of each factor index were replaced by the mean value of that index.

```
DEFINE AJCCSITM: AJCCSITE IF AJCCSITE#UNDEFN ELSE MEAN(AJCCSITE)
DEFINE AJCCTHCM: AJCCTHIC IF AJCCTHIC#UNDEFN ELSE MEAN(AJCCTHIC)
DEFINE AJCCMITM: AJCCMITR IF AJCCMITR#UNDEFN ELSE MEAN(AJCCMITR)
DEFINE AJCCULCM: AJCCULC IF AJCCULC#UNDEFN ELSE MEAN(AJCCULC)
```

SUMMARY STATISTICS	ATTRIBUTE AJCCAGE	ATTRIBUTE AJCCSEX	ATTRIBUTE AJCCSITM	ATTRIBUTE AJCCTHCM	ATTRIBUTE AJCCMITM	ATTRIBUTE AJCCULCM
n DEFINED	173	173	173	173	173	173
MINIMUM	1	0	.0000	1.0000	.0000	.0000
MEDIAN	6	1	1.0000	3.0000	1.0000	.4207
MAXIMUM	8	1	1.0000	4.0000	1.0000	1.0000
MEAN	5.7168	.7919	.6707	2.9545	.9552	.4207
STD. DEV.	1.4804	.4059	.4618	.8823	.1820	.4520

Then a multivariate logistic regression of PETDUMMY was performed on these six augmented traditional AJCC factor indexes. A detailed computer printout is shown below and on the next page enclosed between the two horizontal lines.

After removing all undefined values from all expressions, the resulting number of PATIENTs for which each of the 7 expressions possesses a defined value is reduced to 173. This constitutes the effective sample size.

RESULTS OF LOGISTIC REGRESSION ANALYSIS (LINEAR MODEL)

The dependent variable is a binary-coded numeric variable whose values are either 0 or 1. It is embodied in the first expression (parameter) of the LOGREG command, which is just the attribute PETDUMMY.

The independent variable AJCCAGE is just the attribute AJCCAGE.
The independent variable AJCCSEX is just the attribute AJCCSEX.
The independent variable AJCCSITM is just the attribute AJCCSITM.
The independent variable AJCCTHCM is just the attribute AJCCTHCM.
The independent variable AJCCMITM is just the attribute AJCCMITM.
The independent variable AJCCULCM is just the attribute AJCCULCM.

Likelihood ratio chi-square statistic: 11.588, 2-tail p value: .0718 (based on 6 degrees of freedom and 173 complete observations).

INDEPENDENT VARIABLE	REGRESSION COEFFICIENT	STANDARD DEVIATION	CHI-SQUARE (DF = 1)	2-TAIL P VALUE	ODDS RATIO MULTIPLIER
intercept	-3.7375	2.0408	3.3540	.0670	.0238
AJCCAGE	-.0720	.1417	.2583	.6113	.9305
AJCCSEX	1.4407	.6701	4.6223	.0316	4.2235
AJCCSITM	-.6822	.4240	2.5892	.1076	.5055
AJCCTHCM	.4209	.2633	2.5559	.1099	1.5233
AJCCMITM	.7540	1.9066	.1564	.6925	2.1254
AJCCULCM	.0408	.4526	.0081	.9282	1.0416

GOODNESS OF STATISTICAL FIT OF LOGISTIC REGRESSION MODEL

Pearson chi-square fit statistic (based on 103 degrees of freedom): 119.687, p value: .1249.

Deviance chi-square fit statistic (based on 103 degrees of freedom): 108.497, p value: .3363.

This is a distinctly improved analysis. Instability in the estimate of the regression coefficient for AJCCMITM has been eliminated. Both chi-square fit statistics have been rendered respectable.

Notice, however, that the overall two-tailed p value associated with the likelihood ratio chi-square statistic has changed from 0.0296 to 0.0718, suggesting some deterioration in statistical significance. This occurred despite the forty-two-patient increase in effective sample size from 131 to 173.

The unexpected deterioration may have resulted, at least in part, from excluding the six patients who presented with unknown primaries from the initial analysis, but then including them in the augmented analysis.

We know that these six patients were initially diagnosed at systematically later stages of melanoma progression. Had their primaries then been identified, it is plausible to guess that they would have been thicker than average, that they would have displayed a higher-than-average mitotic rate, and that they would have been ulcerated with higher-than-average likelihood.

To incorporate all 173 patients into the augmented analysis mean (not higher-than-mean) values were uniformly substituted for their missing values. This may have introduced a systematic bias into the data. The impact of tumor thickness, mitotic rate, and ulceration may have been inadvertently attenuated for the six patients presenting with unknown primaries. That would have counteracted the normally favorable impact of increased sample size on the overall statistical significance of the augmented analysis.

Our subsequent PCM analysis will avoid this problem. PCM does not uniformly assume that being missing or otherwise undefined signifies a value that is "typical" of (e.g., average among) nonmissing values. One of PCM's principal virtues is that it regularly inspects the data. Instead of making a conventional assumption, it calculates and substitutes a "most likely" value, specifically tailored to what the data appear to show.

In the case of all six patients presenting with unknown primaries PCM will later substitute riskier-than-average values of AJCCSITE, AJCCTHC, AJCCMITR, and AJCCULC for their missing values. This will improve the accuracy of individually tailored predictions of PET/CT positivity.

The next step was to repeat the same multivariate logistic regression analysis in a stepwise manner. Conventional wisdom was rigorously enforced. Prognostic factor indexes pointing in the seemingly "wrong" direction and statistically insignificant factors were purged via backward elimination.

Because just such a procedure is commonly practiced, this will constitute our base case factor-centered analysis against which to calibrate any improvements that PCM might produce. A detailed computer printout is shown on the next page enclosed between the two horizontal lines.

After removing all undefined values from all expressions, the resulting number of PATIENTs for which each of the 3 expressions possesses a defined value is reduced to 173. This constitutes the effective sample size.

RESULTS OF LOGISTIC REGRESSION ANALYSIS (LINEAR MODEL)

The dependent variable is a binary-coded numeric variable whose values are either 0 or 1. It is embodied in the first expression (parameter) of the LOGREG command, which is just the attribute PETDUMMY.

The independent variable AJCCSEX is just the attribute AJCCSEX.
The independent variable AJCCTHCM is just the attribute AJCCTHCM.

Likelihood ratio chi-square statistic: 8.437, 2-tail p value: .0147 (based on 2 degrees of freedom and 173 complete observations).

INDEPENDENT VARIABLE	REGRESSION COEFFICIENT	STANDARD DEVIATION	CHI-SQUARE (DF = 1)	2-TAIL P VALUE	ODDS RATIO MULTIPLIER
intercept	-3.6409	.9473	14.7731	.0001	.0262
AJCCSEX	1.1916	.6391	3.4767	.0622	3.2924
AJCCTHCM	.4229	.2373	3.1759	.0747	1.5264

GOODNESS OF STATISTICAL FIT OF LOGISTIC REGRESSION MODEL

Pearson chi-square fit statistic (based on 7 degrees of freedom): 16.810, p value: .0187.

Deviance chi-square fit statistic (based on 7 degrees of freedom): 16.656, p value: .0198.

Several conclusions can be drawn from the printout.

1. The linear model does not appear to fit the 173-patient sample data very well. Both the Pearson and the deviance fit statistics suggest that the null hypothesis specifying a good fit may be rejected.
2. Nevertheless, the overall analysis generates a significant likelihood ratio chi-square statistic, suggesting that these two traditional factor indexes may be useful in predicting PET/CT positivity.
3. Sex of patient (AJCCSEX), with no missing observations, and primary tumor thickness transformed by the AJCC into the conventional T1 vs. T2 vs. T3 vs. T4 index (AJCCTHCM), with mean index values substituted for missing data, appear to be independently predictive of PET/CT positivity.
4. Both factor indexes point in the "right" direction, and both are statistically significant predictors, albeit only on a one-tailed, but not on a two-tailed basis.

A new attribute (FCPETPPR) defined by the mathematical model underlying linear logistic regression was then created to encapsulate base case probabilities.

```
DEFINE FCPETPPR:
EXP(-3.6409+1.1916*AJCCSEX+.4229*AJCCTHCM)/[1+
EXP(-3.6409+1.1916*AJCCSEX+.4229*AJCCTHCM)]
```

FCPETPPR stands for factor-centered PET/CT positivity probability. It assigns an individually tailored base case probability of producing a positive PET/CT scan to each of the 173 melanoma patients. These 173 individual probabilities, derived from multivariate logistic regression analysis of the six traditional AJCC factor indexes with missing values of each index replaced by that index's mean value and with backward elimination, were then subjected to a ROC/AUC analysis.

The area under the complete ROC curve was estimated to be 0.6124.

Several figures have been generated from this base case analysis for visual comparison. They are displayed on the following pages.

The SPSA algorithm was applied to patient age at initial diagnosis to produce a corresponding univariate impact-reflecting index with a minimum subscale size of twenty-five patients. A scattergram of this UIRI is presented in figure 6. The opposite directions of impact of age on PET/CT scan result versus SLNB result is obvious from a visual comparison of figure 6 with figure 1.

The SPSA algorithm was also applied to primary tumor thickness to produce its corresponding UIRI. The minimum subscale size was again twenty-five patients. Fortuitously, four subscales emerged, rendering it easy to compare the UIRI with the AJCC's traditional demarcation of the T1, T2, T3, and T4 subscales. A scattergram of this UIRI is presented in figure 7.

The shape of figure 7 (consistently increasing at a consistently decreasing rate) once again reflects quite closely the impact of tumor thickness repeatedly reported in the literature and shown in figure 2.

The SPSA algorithm was also applied to the primary tumor's mitotic rate to produce a corresponding UIRI with a minimum subscale size of twenty-five patients. Its scattergram is presented in figure 8.

The same "S-shaped" UIRI presented in figure 3 is reproduced in figure 8. Mitotic rate's impact on PET/CT positivity, just like its impact on SLNB positivity, appears to be far more complex and interesting than the simple, dichotomous impact envisioned by the construction of the AJCCMITR factor index.

Figure 6

Scattergram of UIRI for Age at Initial Diagnosis

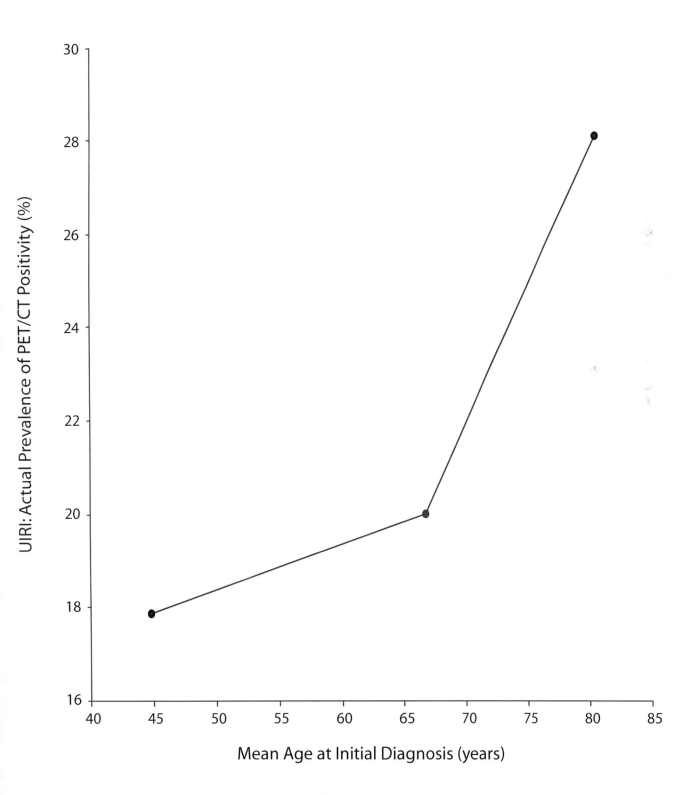

Figure 7

Scattergram of UIRI for Thickness of Primary Tumor

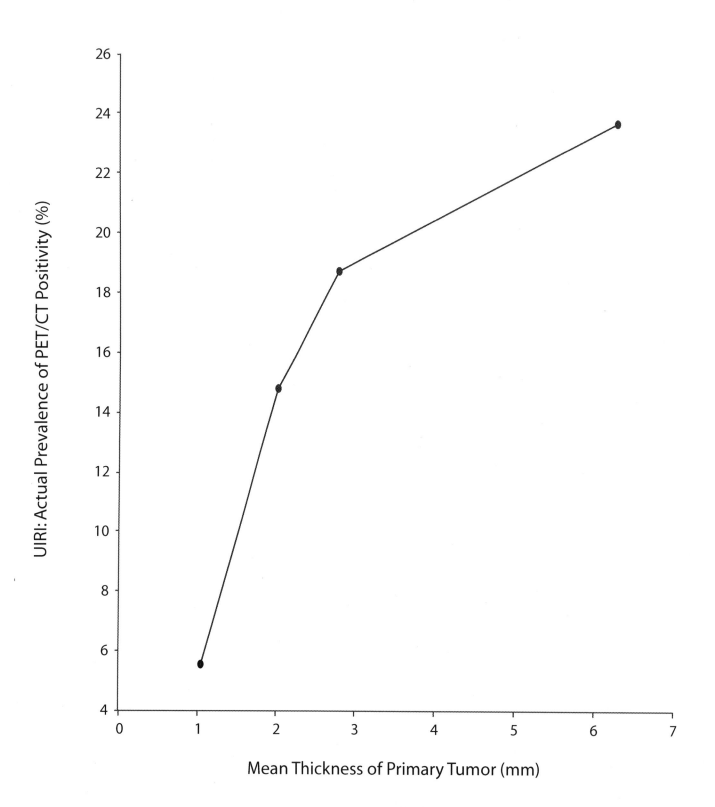

Figure 8

Scattergram of UIRI for Mitotic Rate of Primary Tumor

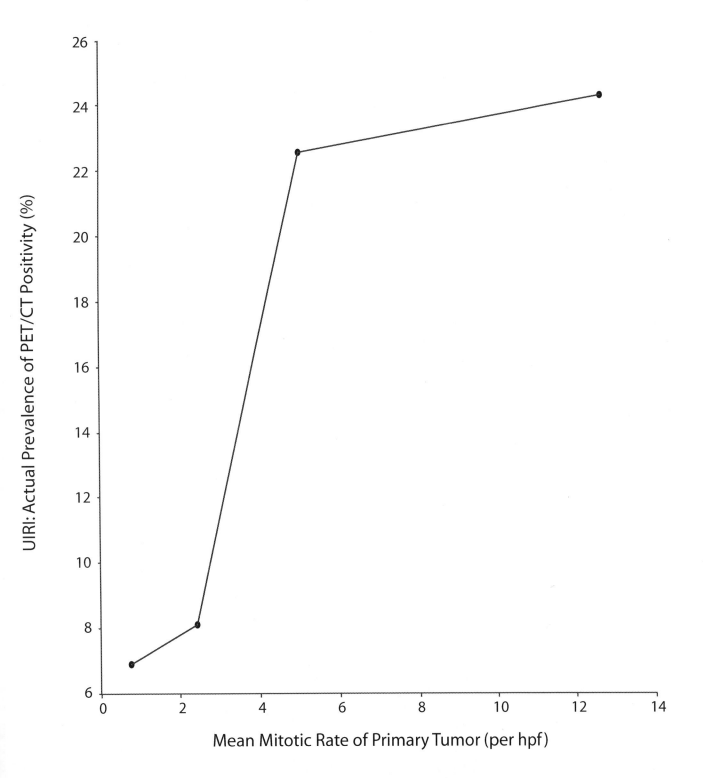

3.2 Applying the PCM Methodology to the Six Traditional AJCC Factors

The SPSA algorithm was similarly applied to the raw data of the other three traditional AJCC prognostic factors to produce their corresponding UIRI indexes. Visual inspection of figures 6, 7, and 8 and the conclusions drawn in section 3.1 suggested the following directions of univariate impact.

1. Later age at initial diagnosis indicates a greater risk of PET/CT positivity than earlier age.
2. A male patient is deemed at greater risk of PET/CT positivity than a female patient.
3. Peripheral primary tumor locations (i.e., on the upper or lower extremities) indicate a greater risk of PET/CT positivity than axial locations (i.e., on the head, neck, or trunk).
4. Thicker primary tumors indicate a greater risk of PET/CT positivity than thinner primary tumors.
5. Primary tumors with a higher mitotic rate indicate a greater risk of PET/CT positivity than primary tumors with a lower mitotic rate.
6. Ulcerated primary tumors indicate a greater risk of PET/CT positivity than nonulcerated primary tumors.

The next step was to perform the procedural equivalent of a multivariate logistic regression analysis of PETDUMMY on the six UIRI indexes calculated, respectively, from the six traditional AJCC prognostic factors.

The procedure was executed with backward elimination. To reduce the possibility of statistical overfitting only UIRIs pointing in the "right" direction and achieving a one-tailed level of statistical significance at or beyond $p = 0.05$ were retained as independent variables.

Recall that because observational data were used to construct all UIRI indexes, the classical concept of statistical significance did not formally apply here. P values were interpreted as purely descriptive statistics. Just as in the previously reported SLNB analysis, they were used only as heuristic guidelines to help control statistical overfitting.

The result was to eliminate UIRI indexes computed for age at diagnosis and mitotic rate as predictors. Although interpretable only heuristically, the four remaining UIRIs (SEXUIRI, SITUIRI, THKUIRI, and ULCUIRI) produced respectable goodness-of-fit statistics, a high overall likelihood ratio chi-square statistic with $p < 0.00005$, and chi-square one-tailed p values associated with the individual indexes ranging from $p = 0.010$ to $p = 0.026$.

Individually tailored probabilities of PET/CT positivity were then obtained as follows.

DEFINE PCPETPPR:
EXP(-6.7407+8.4926*SEXUIRI+7.5075*SITUIRI+4.9390*THKUIRI+3.6370*ULCUIRI)/
[1+EXP(-6.7407+8.4926*SEXUIRI+7.5075*SITUIRI+4.9390*THKUIRI+3.6370*ULCUIRI)]

PCPETPPR stands for patient-centered PET/CT positivity probability. It assigns an individually tailored PCM-generated probability of producing a positive PET/CT test result to each of the 173 melanoma patients. PCPETPPR predicts what would have occurred if each patient had actually undergone an FDG-PET/CT scan. These 173 individual probabilities were then subjected to a ROC/AUC analysis.

The area under the complete ROC curve was estimated to be 0.7636.

The PCM probability's AUC increased dramatically by 0.1512 from 0.6124 to 0.7636 compared to the AUC generated by FCPETPPR in the factor-centered base case analysis. Referring to the accuracy measures introduced in section 1.5, the corresponding maximum percentage of correct PET/CT outcome predictions rose equally dramatically by 13.87 points from 68.21 percent to 82.08 percent. This produced an index of error reduction of 0.4798. A Wilcoxon test was performed on the 173 matched pairs of probabilistic prediction errors, producing a normalized Z statistic = 5.23 with a two-tailed p value < 0.00005.

That the patient-centered base case predictive accuracy results exceeded the factor-centered base case results is no surprise. What is surprising is the magnitude of the improvement. One of PCM's principal devices mediating accuracy improvement is the initial stratification of patients into relatively homogeneous risk subgroups. This was impossible because of the small sample size (only 173 PET/CT patients versus 1,039 SLNB patients). Yet the improvement was unusually high and highly significant. How can this be?

Part of the explanation lies with PCM's initial attempt to verify conventional wisdom. PCM always inspects the data presented to it. UIRI indexes tailored by SPSA to such data are uniformly substituted for traditional AJCC factor indexes. This sometimes confirms the conventional wisdom, as in the case of age at initial diagnosis and tumor thickness. It sometimes corrects or modifies the conventional wisdom, as in the case of anatomical location and mitotic rate of the primary tumor.

Part of the explanation lies with the six patients who presented with unknown primary tumors at initial diagnosis. PCM's unusual way of handling missing observations assigned to all six of them substantially higher-than-average PET/CT positivity probabilities for the reasons previously explained. Four of these six patients actually produced positive PET/CT scans.

Part of the explanation lies with missing observations on the thickness, the mitotic rate, and the presence or absence of ulceration of primary tumors. PCM detected that seventeen out of the forty-two patients with missing observations on at least one of these three predictors had positive PET/CT scans. That was almost half of the thirty-six positive scans generated by all 173 patients. PCM's way of handling undefined data values also exploited this observation to improve its predictive accuracy and to guarantee that every one of the 173 patients received an explicit probabilistic prediction.

3.3 Adding Nontraditional Predictive Factors to Extend the PCM Analysis

Data on more than fifteen additional factors were included in patient records at the time of initial diagnosis. Lymphadenopathy, skin type, eye and hair color, and both itching and bleeding of the primary tumor were among the additionally recorded clinical factors. AJCC stage of melanoma progression, Clark's level of primary tumor invasion, vascular invasion, the presence of microsatellites, and the prevalence of tumor-infiltrating lymphocytes were among the additionally recorded pathological factors. Familial and personal history factors were also recorded, such as relatives with melanoma or other cancers, excessive sun exposure, and repeated blistering of the skin.

Univariate logistic regression analyses were performed to ascertain the impact of each additional factor on PET/CT positivity. Appendix E reports the composition of the 173 patients in the PET scan sample in terms of the six AJCC traditional prognostic factors and the subset of additional factors demonstrating a significant univariate impact. That is how appendix E was constructed. Additional factors not described in appendix E were eliminated from further consideration because they appeared to lack any appreciable predictive value.

The equivalent of a multivariate logistic regression analysis of PETDUMMY on the six UIRI indexes calculated from the six traditional AJCC prognostic factors and on UIRI indexes calculated from the subset of additional nontraditional factors demonstrating a significant univariate impact was performed. Once again, the procedure was executed with backward elimination to reduce the possibility of statistical overfitting. Only UIRIs pointing in the "right" direction and achieving a one-tailed level of statistical significance at or beyond $p = 0.05$ were retained as independent variables.

The result was to eliminate all UIRI indexes except those calculated from patient sex, primary tumor thickness, lymphadenopathy, bleeding of the primary tumor, eye color (blue eyes were higher risk), and skin blistering due to sun exposure. The first four of these were the most predictive of PET/CT positivity. Adding UIRI indexes calculated from eye color and skin blistering helped somewhat, but the accuracy of predictions did not improve significantly. Therefore, only the first four predictors were retained.

These four UIRIs (SEXUIRI, THKUIRI, LYMUIRI, and BLEUIRI) produced respectable goodness-of-fit statistics, a high overall likelihood ratio chi-square statistic with $p < 0.00005$, and chi-square one-tailed p values associated with the individual indexes ranging from $p = 0.00004$ to $p = 0.046$.

Individually tailored probabilities of PET/CT positivity were then obtained as follows.

DEFINE G1PETPPR:
EXP(-6.8466+9.4357*SEXUIRI+4.4498*THKUIRI+4.1346*LYMUIRI+5.7913*BLEUIRI)/
[1+EXP(-6.8466+9.4357*SEXUIRI+4.4498*THKUIRI+4.1346*LYMUIRI+5.7913*BLEUIRI)]

G1PETPPR stands for PET/CT positivity probability assigned by the diagnostic algorithm shown above. The algorithm was generated from the best set of extended prognostic factors selected by and processed by PCM. Separate values of G1PETPPR are individually tailored PCM-generated probabilities of producing a positive PET/CT test result. They are assigned by the diagnostic algorithm to each of the 173 melanoma patients. G1PETPPR predicts what would have occurred if each patient had actually undergone an FDG-PET/CT scan. These 173 individual probabilities were then subjected to a ROC/AUC analysis.

The area under the complete ROC curve was estimated to be 0.8651.

The extended PCM probability's AUC increased substantially by 0.1015 from 0.7636 to 0.8651 compared to the AUC generated by PCPETPPR. Referring to the accuracy measures introduced in section 1.5, the corresponding maximum percentage of correct PET/CT outcome predictions rose by 4.03 points from 82.08 percent to 86.11 percent. This produced an index of error reduction of 0.3988. A Wilcoxon test was performed on the 173 matched pairs of probabilistic prediction errors, producing a normalized Z statistic = 5.24 with a two-tailed p value < 0.00005.

For easy comparison, the table on the next page summarizes the relative predictive accuracy of the probabilities produced, respectively, by the three diagnostic algorithms, FCPETPPR, PCPETPPR, and G1PETPPR.

Table P. Comparison of Accuracy Achieved in Predicting the
Outcome of an FDG-PET/CT Scan Through Differing Predictive
Methodologies and Differing Collections of Predictive Factors
(Complete Sample: N=173)

Pedictive Methodology	Correct Predictions	Index of Error Reduction	Wilcoxon Z Value	2-Tail P Value
Factor-Centered Base Case (six traditional AJCC factors)	68.21%	N/A	N/A	N/A
Patient-Centered Base Case (same six AJCC factors)	82.08%	0.4798	5.23	< 0.00005
Patient-Centered Methodology (same six AJCC + added factors)	86.11%	0.3988	5.24	< 0.00005

Notes:

1. Results in the first row were produced by executing a multivariate
   logistic regression analysis of the six traditional factor indexes
   exactly as defined by and measured by the AJCC, except that missing
   observations of each index were uniformly replaced by the mean value
   of that index in the complete 173-patient sample. Factor indexes
   pointing in the "wrong" direction (i.e., possessing a negative
   regression coefficient) were first removed from the analysis. Then
   stepwise multiple logistic regression was performed with backward
   elimination.
2. Results in the second and third rows were produced by applying the
   Patient-Centered Methodology (PCM) to the same raw data observations
   (e.g., not transformed by the AJCC into factor indexes) of the same
   predictive factors gathered from the same 173 patients. The second
   row reanalyzed the same six traditional AJCC factors, but via PCM.
   The third row added more than fifteen clinical and pathological
   predictive factors and analyzed via PCM the subset of these many
   factors that were significantly predictive of PET/CT positivity on
   a univariate basis.
3. All three tabled predictive algorithms assigned an individually
   tailored probability of having a positive PET/CT outcome to each of
   the 173 patients.
4. Correct Predictions in the table stands for the maximum percentage
   of correct predictions of PET/CT outcomes enabled by the particular
   predictive methodology and factor collection tabled in each
   successive row.
5. Index of Error Reduction, Wilcoxon Z Value, and accompanying 2-Tail
   P Value refer to the results of Wilcoxon matched-pair, signed-rank
   tests performed on the accuracy of individually tailored
   probabilistic predictions made by the particular predictive
   methodology and factor collection tabled in each successive row,
   compared to comparable predictions made by the methodology and
   factor collection tabled in the row immediately above. Each Wilcoxon
   test was applied to 173 matched pairs of differences (usually
   reductions) in absolute-value probabilistic prediction errors. An
   individual patient's probabilistic prediction error is the
   difference between the predicted probability of a positive PET/CT
   scan assigned to that patient and the actual PET/CT outcome (zero
   for negative scan, one for positive scan).

6. The Index of Error Reduction is designed to mirror a correlation coefficient. It is calculated as the number of net error reductions (i.e., the number of reductions minus the number of increases) as a signed proportion of the total number of nonidentical matched-pair comparisons. The index ranges in value from -1.0, if all comparisons generate error increases, to +1.0, if all comparisons generate error reductions. Analogous to a correlation coefficient the index has a value of 0.0 if the number of error reductions is exactly counterbalanced by the number of error increases.

7. The distribution of differences between absolute probabilistic prediction errors can be quite skewed. It can also possess occasional outliers (extreme values). Because of this, matched pairs of error differences were tested by the Wilcoxon matched-pairs, signed-ranks test instead of by the more traditional matched-pairs t test. The t test assumes normally distributed data, while the Wilcoxon test makes no distributional assumptions. The Wilcoxon test is also less sensitive to outliers. Compared to the t test, the Wilcoxon test has a relative efficiency near 95 percent for small samples and slightly better than 95 percent for large samples. The Wilcoxon test produces exact one-tailed and two-tailed p values for sample sizes up to twenty-five. A normalized Z statistic corresponding to the Wilcoxon T statistic is calculated for sample sizes greater than twenty-five. The Z value is then referred to the unit normal distribution to obtain appropriate p values.

8. As measured by the index of error reduction and tested by the Wilcoxon matched-pairs, signed-ranks tests, both of the tabled improvements were highly significant. Both showed two-tailed p values less than 0.00005.

9. Both of these Wilcoxon tests qualify as legitimate hypothesis tests in the classical (Neyman-Pearson) tradition. The Wilcoxon test is a randomization test whose null hypothesis simply states that no systematic differences exist between the two elements in a set of 173 matched pairs of absolute probabilistic prediction errors generated, respectively, by two different prediction methodologies. Pairs of errors are uniformly matched patient-by-patient.

Shown on the next page are summary statistics for the individual patient probabilities of generating positive PET/CT scans produced by the three predictive algorithms. Notice, once again, that the mean probabilities are all identical to each other and equal to the prevalence of PET/CT positivity among the 173 patients. Notice, also, the differences in the minimum-to-maximum ranges and the standard deviations of these individual probabilities. Not only does G1PETPPR produce the most accurate probabilistic predictions (as just shown in terms of AUC, percentage of correct predictions, and index of error reduction); it also tends to "spread out" its probabilistic predictions more widely than the other two probabilistic logistic regression outputs. Finer discrimination is once again achieved in combination with greater accuracy, not at the expense of greater accuracy.

SUMMARY STATISTICS	ATTRIBUTE PETDUMMY
n DEFINED	173
MINIMUM	0
MEDIAN	0
MAXIMUM	1
MEAN	.2081
STD. DEV.	.4059

SUMMARY STATISTICS	ATTRIBUTE FCPETPPR	ATTRIBUTE PCPETPPR	ATTRIBUTE G1PETPPR
n DEFINED	173	173	173
MINIMUM	.0385	.0149	.0071
MEDIAN	.2349	.1606	.0904
MAXIMUM	.3191	.6760	.9055
MEAN	.2081	.2081	.2081
STD. DEV.	.0858	.1672	.2421

G1PETPPR was the most accurate predictor in all of the above senses. Investigation of its scale characteristics throughout its complete logical range from zero to one will reveal other senses in which its probabilistic predictions were also remarkably reliable.

The 173 G1PETPPR individually tailored probabilities were first ranked and divided into quartiles. The mean probability in each quartile was then compared with the actual prevalence of PET/CT positivity among patients in that quartile.

These two numbers should converge, statistically, and become approximately equal as the number of patients in each quartile increases. The maximum absolute difference was 2.63 percentage points. The mean absolute difference was 1.75 percentage points. Furthermore, there was no discernible pattern or trend in the succession of quartile probabilities and prevalence.

When there are only a few distinctly different probability values in a data set, partitioning the scale into a small number of subscales, such as quartiles, may be an appropriate procedure. There were thirty-three distinctly different values of G1PETPPR. Consequently, we can investigate its scale characteristics somewhat more thoroughly.

The SPSA algorithm was executed to partition the scale of G1PETPPR into as many subscales as possible, as long as each subscale encompassed PET/CT positivity probabilities for at least twenty-five patients. Five separate subscales were produced. They are shown as SPSA's printed output below and on the next page between the two horizontal lines. The corresponding actual prevalence of PET/CT positivity is shown as a fraction for each subscale.

The indicator's optimal scale partitioning and numeric rescaling are embodied in the Univariate Impact-Reflecting Index (UIRI) produced by the Scale Partitioning and Spacing Algorithm (SPSA) with a minimum partition (subscale) size set to twenty-five. The UIRI's operational definition is shown on the next page.

```
1/38 IF G1PETPPR<.0457 ELSE
1/27 IF G1PETPPR>=.0457 AND G1PETPPR<.0888 ELSE
3/43 IF G1PETPPR>=.0888 AND G1PETPPR<.2024 ELSE
8/31 IF G1PETPPR>=.2024 AND G1PETPPR<.3051 ELSE
23/34 IF G1PETPPR>=.3051
```

A file named UIRI_SCATTERPLOT.TXT has been created. It contains two columns of data. The first column is labeled UIRI and contains UIRI values calculated for successive scale partitions of the second (indicator) expression in the SPSA command line. The second column is labeled with the operational definition of the second (indicator) expression itself to identify what is being plotted. The means of the indicator expression values in each successive partition are laid out along the horizontal X-axis of the scatterplot, and the corresponding UIRI values are laid out along the vertical Y-axis.

The table below was then constructed. Prediction errors were calculated for each successive subscale as the mean of the G1PETPPR values falling within that subscale subtracted from the actual prevalence of PET/CT positivity among the patients possessing those values of G1PETPPR.

SUBSCALE	LOWER AND UPPER SUBSCALE BOUNDS	SUBSCALE MEAN	ACTUAL PREVALENCE	PREDICTION ERROR
1	.0000 to .0457	.0227	.0263	.0036
2	.0457 to .0888	.0563	.0370	-.0193
3	.0888 to .2024	.1094	.0698	-.0396
4	.2024 to .3051	.2269	.2581	.0312
5	.3051 to 1.0000	.6435	.6765	.0330

Since the number of subscales expanded from four (quartiles) to five, subscales contained fewer patient probabilities (between 27 and 43 each). Therefore, the statistical process by which each subscale mean converges toward its corresponding actual prevalence was rendered less complete. The maximum absolute difference between the five subscale means and their corresponding actual prevalence was 3.96 percentage points. The mean absolute difference was 2.53 percentage points.

Taking algebraic signs into account, the mean prediction error should be very close to zero. It was 0.18 percentage points. Both a one-sample t test and a corresponding Wilcoxon test suggested that the population of prediction errors from which this sample of five was drawn differed insignificantly from one with a mean and a median of zero.

When successive subscale means were plotted along the horizontal X-axis and each corresponding actual prevalence was plotted along the vertical Y-axis of a graph, all five points fell close to the straight line through the origin that makes a 45-degree angle with each axis. This line assumes that every actual prevalence exactly equals its corresponding subscale mean. Prediction errors are vertical deviations from the line. The uncorrected R-squared value (coefficient of determination) associated with this line, interpreted as a simple linear regression equation constrained to pass through the origin of the graph, was 0.9868 (equivalent to a 0.9934 linear correlation coefficient).

Inspection of the sequence of prediction errors revealed three positive and two negative errors, with relatively large and relatively small errors clustered systematically neither at the extremes of the probability scale nor in its interior. These results were consistent with a random pattern of errors. There

was, however, a slight but statistically insignificant tendency for the
absolute size of prediction errors to rise with larger probability numbers
along the scale.

Based on these observations, it seems appropriate to conclude that individually
tailored G1PETPPR probabilities provide quite accurate predictions of PET/CT
positivity. Figure 9 provides visual evidence of their predictive accuracy.

Figure 9

Scattergram of Predictive Accuracy of G1PETPPR Probability

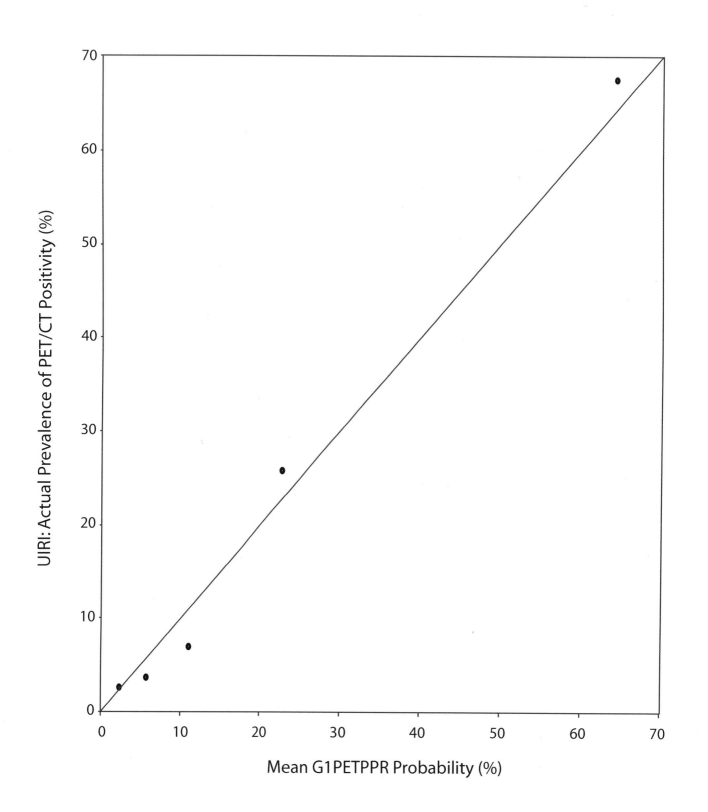

3.4 How PCM's Greater Predictive Accuracy Can Reduce the Cost and Raise the Efficiency of FDG-PET/CT Scans

It has just been demonstrated that PCM provides more accurate predictions of the individually tailored outcomes of a PET/CT scan than a conventional, factor-centered methodology:

1. first, by substituting measurement indexes specifically tailored by SPSA to PET/CT outcomes realized at a particular medical center for the conventional factor indexes recommended by the AJCC to predict different, survival-related end points on a generic basis; and
2. then by implementing the other distinctive PCM devices outlined in section 1.2 that tailor predictions to individual patients, excluding the initial stratification of patients into separate risk subgroups.

So how can PCM's greater predictive accuracy both reduce the cost and, simultaneously, raise the triage efficiency of a PET scan?

Our answer will begin by establishing a historical basis of comparison. That basis will be the experience of the 173 patients just analyzed via PCM. All of these patients were diagnosed with melanoma between 2007 and 2014. Each of them subsequently underwent a PET/CT scan. They constituted close to a census of the patients who received PET/CT scans for melanoma at CPMC during that time period.

Conventional risk guidelines were used to make recommendations concerning whether or not a particular patient should have a PET scan. Typically, a higher-risk patient presenting with a primary tumor that was of at least intermediate thickness (greater than two millimeters in depth) was recommended to do so.

For patients with thinner tumors, the number and severity of other high-risk features presented at initial diagnosis could also trigger a recommendation to undergo the procedure. Examples of high-risk features included presenting with a primary tumor that displayed either a Clark level IV or V of invasion or that possessed an elevated mitotic rate (greater than three mitoses per square millimeter hpf).

Patients satisfying none of the above criteria were generally not recommended to have a PET/CT scan.

Since no explicit probabilistic predictions were available between 2007 and 2014 they could not be used to facilitate an appropriate triage of patients. The conventional risk guidelines were presumed to indicate a sufficient likelihood of PET/CT scan positivity to warrant undergoing the procedure.

Patients typically accepted and acted on whatever was recommended.

The next step will be to demonstrate how substitution of explicit PCM-generated probabilistic predictions for the conventional guidelines could have both reduced the cost and, simultaneously, raised the triage efficiency of performing PET/CT scans. This will be accomplished by replicating our analysis of SLNBs. We shall extend the analysis to include patients who did not undergo a PET/CT scan. Then we shall identify the equilibrating cutoff probability that quantifies both PCM's relative cost savings and its triage efficiency improvement.

3.5 Analysis of Patients Who Did Not Undergo an FDG-PET/CT Scan

Medical records were obtained for ninety-six patients who were also diagnosed
with melanoma at CPMC between 2007 and 2014 but who did not undergo a PET/CT
scan. The criteria for selecting these ninety-six no-PET scan patients were:

   1. each was judged to be a plausible candidate for a PET/CT scan; but
   2. none was an obvious candidate because none was judged to possess a
      sufficiently high likelihood of producing a scan result positive for
      melanoma to warrant undergoing the procedure.

Selected attributes of these ninety-six patients appear in appendix F.
Collectively, they also represented close to a census of no-PET scan patients
satisfying both criteria during the designated time period. Appendix F shows
that slightly more than half were lower-risk patients (i.e., T1 and T2 patients
with a primary tumor thickness no greater than two millimeters).

3.6 Identifying the Equilibrating Cutoff Probability that Quantifies Both
     PCM's Relative Cost Savings and Its Relative Efficiency Improvement

The next step will be to calculate the relative (percentage) cost savings and
the corresponding relative (percentage) improvement in triage efficiency
enabled by PCM's greater predictive accuracy.

The equilibrating procedure presented in section 2.9 for SLNBs was replicated
for PET/CT scans. Similar calculations generated an equilibrating cutoff
probability of 12.08 percent. This compared to 9.89 percent in the case of
SLNBs. It suggested that only patients in the PET sample of 173 with G1PETPPR
probabilities at least 0.1208 plus all patients in the no-PET sample of
ninety-six with G1PETPPR probabilities at least 0.1208 should have been
recommended to undergo a PET/CT scan. The remainder of the 269 patients should
have been recommended not to undergo a PET/CT scan.

Consequences of adopting as an alternative recommendation policy the 12.08
percent equilibrating G1PETPPR cutoff probability would have been as follows.

   1. Of the 173 PET patients, seventy-nine would have been recommended to
      continue to undergo a PET/CT scan, while the remaining ninety-four
      patients would have been recommended to eschew it instead.
   2. Of these ninety-four patients recommended not to undergo a PET/CT scan
      four actually produced positive test results for melanoma.
   3. Of the ninety-six no-PET patients, fifteen would have been recommended
      to undergo a PET/CT scan instead, while the remaining eighty-one
      patients would have been recommended to continue to eschew it.
   4. From these fifteen no-PET patients recommended to undergo a PET/CT scan
      the expected number of positive test results would have been 4.44.
   5. Thus, a total of 79 + 15 = 94 PET/CT scans would have been recommended
      (and presumably performed).
   6. This compared to 173 scans actually having been performed.
   7. The net cost savings achieved by substituting PCM-generated
      probabilities for conventional triage methodology and by adopting a
      12.08 percent equilibrating cutoff value of G1PETPPR would have been
      173 - (79 + 15) = 79 fewer PET/CT scans performed.
   8. Performing seventy-nine fewer scans is equivalent to a 79/173 = 45.66
      percent cost reduction, regardless of the dollar cost of each scan.
   9. PCM, using the 12.08 percent cutoff probability, would have generated

36.44 positive scan outcomes (36 - 4 = 32 actual positive outcomes plus
4.44 expected additional positive outcomes). From the more
conventional, guideline-based recommendations actually made virtually
the same number (36) of positive PET/CT outcomes resulted.

10. PCM would have recommended that only ninety-four patients actually
undergo PET/CT scans. The guideline-based recommendations required 173
scans to produce virtually the same number of positive test outcomes.
Therefore, PCM's effective yield was 36.44/94 = 38.77 percent. This
compared to the actual 36/173 = 20.81 percent yield. The 17.96 yield
increase (a 86.30 percent efficiency improvement) was achieved just by
changing the triage procedure. No aspects of performing the PET/CT
scans were altered. Only recommendations to undergo or not to undergo a
scan were based on PCM-generated probabilities rather than on
conventional guidelines.

3.7 Assessing Cost-Benefit Trade-offs to Select an FDG-PET/CT Recommendation Policy Appropriate for a Particular Medical Institution

Figure 10 has been produced to illustrate in graphical form the equilibrating
analysis just performed for PET/CT scans. Figure 10 is the equivalent of figure
5 produced for the SLNB analysis. Figure 10 relates the resulting yield of
positive scan outcomes (vertical Y-axis) to the number of PET/CT scans that
must be executed in order to generate that yield (horizontal X-axis).

The single point in the northeast region of figure 10 (pointed to as the Actual
CPMC Experience) depicts the consequences of CPMC's actual triage policy. It
resulted in executing 173 PET/CT scans, which generated thirty-six positive
scan outcomes.

CPMC's actual policy was similar to the triage policy adopted by many melanoma
centers during the same historical time period. Patients with primary lesions
in excess of two millimeters thick were regularly recommended to undergo a
PET/CT scan. In addition, some patients with thinner melanomas (no more than
two millimeters) were also recommended to undergo a PET/CT scan based on the
number and severity of any high-risk features with which they presented at
initial diagnosis.

The yield curve in figure 10 shows the consequences of substituting alternative
G1PETPPR cutoff probabilities for the guideline-based triage policy actually
adopted. Each point on the curve identifies the cost and yield consequences of
substituting a separate probability. Alternative G1PETPPR cutoff probabilities
were generated by the PCM prediction algorithm based on four prognostic factors
(patient sex, primary tumor thickness, bleeding of the primary tumor, and
lymphadenopathy).

The result of the equilibrating analysis just performed is represented as the
point where the horizontal line joining thirty-six positive PET/CT scan
outcomes to the single point in the northeast region of figure 10 representing
CPMC's actual experience intersects this yield curve.

Unlike figure 5, however, figure 10 depicts only a single yield curve. A second
curve depicting the consequences of substituting alternative PCPETPPR cutoff
probabilities, instead, seemed unnecessary. The four prognostic factors from
which G1PETPPR probabilities are calculated are either commonly recorded or
easy to obtain by questioning patients.

Substituting a given cutoff probability drawn from the curve means that any patient who is assigned by G1PETPPR that or a higher probability of a positive scan outcome would have been recommended to receive the scan. Any patient assigned a lower probability would have been recommended not to receive the scan. Recommendations are uniformly assumed to have been accepted and executed. Therefore, substituting each cutoff probability implies both a number of scans that would then necessarily have been executed (horizontal X-axis) and either the number of positive scan outcomes that would actually have resulted or the expected number of positive scan outcomes that would likely have resulted (vertical Y-axis).

The curve was produced after first sequencing patients in descending order according to their PCM-generated G1PETPPR probabilities. Thus, the lowest (most southwesterly) point on the curve represents the patient with the highest possible positivity probability. The highest (most northeasterly) point represents the patient with the lowest possible positivity probability.

The curve is actually a sequence of 132 (not necessarily distinct) points. The thirty-six patients who actually underwent PET/CT scans with positive outcomes contributed thirty-six points to it. The ninety-six patients who did not undergo PET/CT scans contributed the remaining ninety-six points. Since tied cutoff probabilities sometimes occurred the 132 points comprising the curve were often but not always distinct.

The ninety-four patients who underwent PET/CT scans with negative outcomes are nowhere represented on the curve. This is because each cutoff probability is being viewed as a candidate substitute criterion for the actual, guideline-based triage policy. No candidate cutoff probability would ever be selected as an appropriate substitute criterion if there existed at least one other cutoff probability on the same curve that produced the same number of positive test results, but from a smaller number of scans required to achieve them. Because executing any scan with a negative outcome always increased the cost of the triage procedure (by one scan) but never the benefit (since no additional positive scan resulted), such outcomes were uniformly ignored. Plotting points to represent these ninety-four patients would only contribute to the clutter, but not to the useful information conveyed by figure 10.

Figure 10 is presented on the next page.

Figure 10

FDG-PET/CT Scan Cost-Benefit Analysis for 269 CPMC Patients
(173 Patients Underwent FDG-PET/CT Scans, while 96 Did Not)

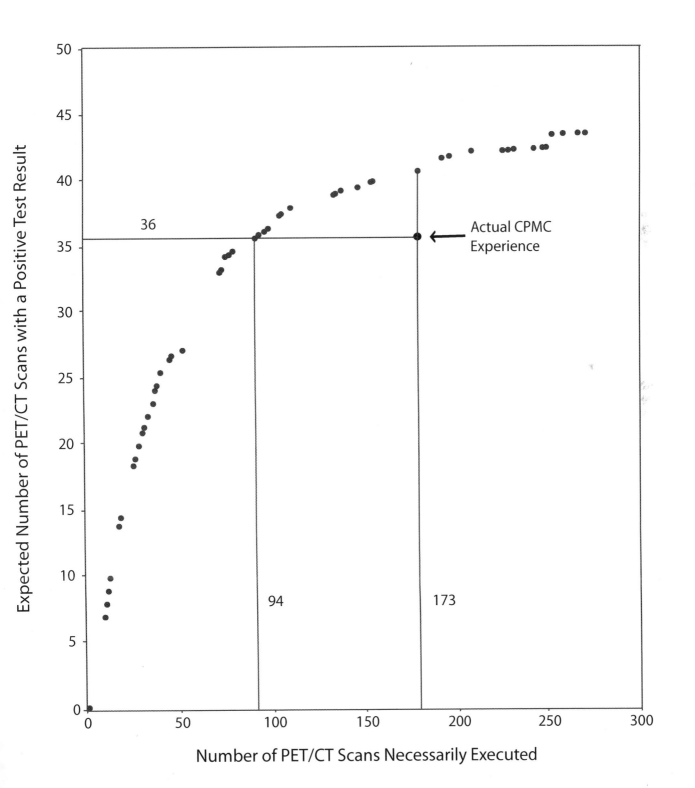

Comparison of figures 5 and 10 shows that all three of the yield curves share the same general shape. Just like both SLNB positivity yield curves shown in figure 5, the positive PET/CT scan yield curve shown in figure 10 rises consistently, but at an ever-decreasing rate as successively lower cutoff probabilities are considered as substitute candidates for the actual triage policy. Choosing each lower cutoff probability simultaneously requires that an ever-increasing number of scans be executed.

Just as figure 4 demonstrated in the case of SLNBs, figure 9 also demonstrated that PET/CT positivity probabilities converge with great fidelity to the actual frequencies of positive test results. Because of this, consistently rising at an ever-decreasing rate is a direct consequence of the manner in which both figure 5 and figure 10 were constructed, in conjunction with the common shape of the underlying probability curves.

Now that we have a methodology to compare the costs with the benefits of executing a PET/CT scan, how can a particular medical institution use G1PETPPR positivity probabilities and the various tables and graphs constructed from them to pick the "best" cutoff probability?

Cost-benefit trade-offs can be made as follows.

1. Pick a G1PETPPR cutoff probability. That means contemplate revising whatever was the institution's historical recommendation policy by substituting use of the just-picked PCM-generated probability.
2. Compare its tabled and graphed benefits and disbenefits relative to the institution's historical recommendation policy.
3. Judge which contemplated revised recommendation policies (i.e., which contemplated cutoff probabilities) deliver, on balance, a net improvement compared to the institution's historical policy.
4. From among the cutoff probabilities that offer a net improvement pick the one offering the maximum net improvement.
5. Optionally, make judicious interpolations to "round off" the cutoff to a more cosmetically pleasing positive FDG-PET/CT outcome probability.

Returning to figure 10, there are several points on the G1PETPPR curve that lie in the northwest quadrant relative to the institution's actual historical experience. All of these northwesterly points promise either less cost without giving up any PET/CT positivity yield or a greater positivity yield without having to execute more PET/CT scans or both. In terms of their triage consequences, therefore, substituting any one of the corresponding cutoff probabilities for the conventional, guideline-based triage procedure actually adopted would appear to have been unequivocally cost-effective.

Coincidentally, all of these northwesterly points are generated by cutoff probabilities in the neighborhood of 10 percent (i.e., between 5.75 percent and 12.08 percent). The coincidence is fortuitous. Unlike the situation with SLNBs, there was no intention to adopt a 10 percent policy or any other policy designed to achieve a specific likelihood of a positive PET/CT scan outcome. What would or should result in terms of any patient's test positivity was never discussed quantitatively.

Nevertheless, it is easy to conclude that the triage procedure could have been improved substantially by adopting a cutoff probability, had such probabilities been historically available. Going forward, abandoning reliance on conventional guidelines in favor of adopting such a cutoff probability would seem eminently wise.

These are exactly the same conclusions we drew from the SLNB analysis.

3.8 Concluding Comments

Regrettably absent from our analysis of PET/CT scans was a split-half reliability test for statistical overfitting by the PCM methodology. Such a test was performed in the SLNB analysis. Its successful results were reported in appendix B. The omission was necessitated here by the small size of the PET/CT sample. Reliable statistical estimates could no longer have been obtained after splitting only 173 patients randomly into two subsamples.

On the other hand, the consequences of omitting a split-half reliability test were mitigated somewhat by the much smaller number of statistical parameters PCM was required to estimate for the PET/CT analysis compared to the SLNB analysis.

The small sample size also precluded stratifying the 173 PET/CT patients into even two separate risk subgroups prior to applying the SPSA algorithm to produce UIRIs. Prior stratification has been shown to make a substantial contribution to improving PCM's predictive accuracy. Fortunately, however, noticeably greater accuracy was still achieved, despite this omission.

Figures 4 and 9 demonstrated the convergence of PCM-generated probabilities to their corresponding observed relative frequencies. Convergence uniformly improves with increasing sample size. Also, the number of separately displayable scale partitions increases with patient sample size, given a constant minimum partition size (e.g., twenty-five patients). Predictive accuracy increases with greater convergence. Predictive accuracy can therefore be improved by increasing both patient and minimum partition sample sizes.

Visual comparison of figures 5 and 10 provides further insight into sample size's pivotal role in the PCM methodology. The shape of the positivity yield curves is regularly-increasing-at-a-decreasing-rate. Since all such curves are really sequences of distinct points (one for each alternative PCM-generated cutoff probability that might be substituted for a conventional, guideline-based triage procedure), there must be an adequate number of such points to give the impression of a smooth curve. A small sample size undermines the apparent smoothness of any diagnostic test's positivity yield curve. This can be seen in the visible jump at the northeast extreme of the PET/CT positivity yield curve in figure 10. Similar jumps occurred throughout figure 5, but they were "smoothed out" (i.e., visually masked) by the increase in sample size from 269 total patients to 1,340 total patients.

The purpose of any equilibrating cutoff probability analysis is to facilitate an institutional audit. An institutional audit is a retrospective procedure to determine whether or not there was substantial room for practical improvement in whatever conventional, guideline-based procedures were actually employed by a medical center in the triage of patients to some diagnostic test. If the audit suggests little room for improvement, traditional procedures need not be altered. On the other hand, if an institutional audit suggests that substantial cost reductions and efficiency improvements are achievable by substituting PCM-generated probabilities for traditional guidelines, it may be worthwhile to complete the cost-benefit analysis and to consider altering the triage procedure accordingly. Conveniently, a complete cost-benefit analysis may be individually tailored to a specific medical center.

PCM is not a small-sample methodology. Our SLNB and PET/CT scan analyses suggest that patient sample sizes must be at least in the hundreds and preferably more than a thousand to support its successful application. Therefore, PCM-based institutional audits would seem to be possible only for at-least-medium-size institutions and for organizations (such as the AJCC) that collect patient records from multiple sources.

Perhaps the most questionable step in the process of applying PCM to the selection of patients for diagnostic test procedures is where a predictive algorithm based on patients who have undergone the procedure is applied to patients who did not undergo it. Successful results of a split-sample reliability test do render this step more credible. A direct test would add still more credibility. Plausible candidates for some diagnostic procedure who would normally be recommended not to undergo it under the conventional, guideline-based triage methodology could be given the test on an experimental basis. Their actual test outcomes could then be used to assess more directly PCM's predictive accuracy in this more questionable context.

Any form of cost-benefit analysis requires that both costs and benefits be measured in some way. Only then can they be compared. In the case of both SLNBs and PET/CT scans the principal medical benefit was presumed to flow from a positive test outcome. A negative test result can be reassuring to both physician and patient, but it does not generally point to any particular therapeutic action.

Therefore, our analyses of both SLNBs and PET/CT scans used the expected number of positive test outcomes as the principal measure of benefit. It was plotted along the vertical axis (Y-axis) of both figure 5 and figure 10. The number of SLNBs or PET/CT scans required to obtain any expected number of positive test outcomes was adopted as the principal measure of cost. It was plotted along the horizontal axis (X-axis) of both figures. The implicit assumption was that any quantification of either costs (e.g., via accounting procedures) or benefits (e.g., by making explicit specific therapeutic consequences of a positive test result) would be ordinally related to these two measures, respectively.

Demonstrating the existence or nonexistence of actionable points on the curves depicted in figures 5 and 10 that lie to the northwest of the point representing what a particular medical center actually achieved in some historical context then became the principal conclusion to be drawn from an institutional audit. Their nonexistence would indicate little or no room for improvement. Their existence would indicate at least some room for improvement.

An equilibrating probability cutoff analysis resolved the existence question. After establishing the existence of such favorable points, the magnitude of their offset in the northwesterly direction served to calibrate both potential cost savings and potential improvements in triage efficiency. Substituting PCM-generated probabilities for conventional, guideline-based triage criteria is the proposed mechanism that renders actionable any northwesterly points on such a curve and, therefore, that renders potentially achievable actual cost savings and efficiency gains.

The cost-benefit concept can be extended to other types of diagnostic test procedures. So can our accompanying analyses be extended. For example, if a negative test outcome possessed some type of medical benefit or disbenefit, test outcome probabilities generated via PCM could be used to compute an expected net benefit from undergoing the test procedure. Diagnostic tests with more than just two possible outcomes (i.e., positive versus negative) could be treated similarly.

4.0 THE DISCRIMINATOR SELECTION AND SEQUENCING ALGORITHM (DSSA)

The early sections of this book have demonstrated how PCM may be applied to predicting the outcomes of existing diagnostic procedures. When a diagnostic test, such as a sentinel lymph node biopsy or a PET/CT scan, is expensive and can produce one or more undesirable side effects it is especially important to select with great care the patients who should and should not undergo it.

PCM's predictions of both these diagnostic test outcomes were shown to be quite accurate. Predictions were based on patient data obtainable prior to actually undergoing each test. Therefore, PCM's predicted test outcome could be compared with its cost in advance. Such a cost-benefit analysis could have both reduced cost and improved triage (patient selection) efficiency in two medical centers.

The remaining sections of this book will present an alternative methodology for generating new diagnostic tests. The alternative methodology is embodied in the Discriminator Selection and Sequencing Algorithm (DSSA).

As an analytical procedure DSSA is similar to regression. Regression analysis produces an explicit regression equation derived from empirical observations gathered for some specific explanatory or predictive purpose.

There are many different versions of regression analysis. They differ in terms of the nature of what is to be explained or predicted, how these things are measured, how explanatory and predictive factors are defined and measured, and the manner of explanation or prediction. Both inputs to and outputs from a regression analysis, however, must always be numerically coded.

Regression analysis produces an algebraic equation. The equation links what is to be explained or predicted (as measured by its dependent output variable) to some mathematical function of its one or more input predictors or explanatory factors (independent variables). The particular mathematical function specifies the particular regression model assumed to connect the explained or predicted outcome with whatever input data are being analyzed.

The regression equation produced may be viewed as a special type of predictive or explanatory algorithm. The numeric value of the dependent variable on the left side of the equation (the explanation or prediction) may be obtained by evaluating the algebraic expression on the right side embodying the mathematical function of the predictors or explanatory factors. The detailed mechanics of expression evaluation are themselves algorithmic in nature.

The concept of an algorithm is used in this book in its less restrictive dictionary sense rather than in its more restrictive mathematical sense. According to the dictionary an algorithm is any well-defined, step-by-step procedure designed to solve some particular problem. In the dictionary sense executing an algorithmic procedure does not necessarily guarantee a "perfect" or "complete" or "optimal" solution. In the more restrictive mathematical sense a procedure must guarantee such a solution to be labeled a genuine algorithm. Various step-by-step procedures included within DSSA generally qualify as algorithmic in the less restrictive dictionary sense but only sometimes in the more restrictive mathematical sense. DSSA is more appropriately characterized, mathematically, as a heuristic rather than as an algorithmic procedure.

The process of generating a regression equation is also algorithmic in nature. It follows a preprogrammed sequence of steps designed to optimize something desirable such as maximizing the likelihood of obtaining an observed correspondence between dependent and independent variables in some training data set. The generating procedure (preprogrammed sequence of steps) is frequently referred to as a regression analysis. The output produced is referred to as its output regression equation or output regression function. Because the likelihood maximization procedure generally guarantees an optimum solution regression analysis also satisfies the more restrictive mathematical definition of a genuine algorithm. When successful, it produces the best possible (maximum likelihood) regression equation.

Similarly, DSSA is an algorithmic generation procedure that produces an explicit diagnostic algorithm tailored to observations of its input factors gathered in some diagnostic context. However, the output of DSSA is not an algebraic equation. Neither is it a mathematical function or an algebraic expression that evaluates to a number. It is an ordered sequence of conditional conclusion-drawing statements. Each statement draws a definite conclusion about the outcome to be diagnosed (the dependent output variable), conditional upon the value of one of its diagnostic indicators (independent variables).

The ordered sequence is organized in the form of a logical flow diagram. The flow diagram represents an explicit diagnostic algorithm that identifies which conclusion (or neither) is to be drawn on the basis of each conclusion-drawing statement. It evaluates the truth of each successive statement in the sequence until either a definite conclusion is eventually reached or it becomes clear that no diagnostic conclusion is possible, given the input data. Thus, DSSA is also an algorithmic generation procedure that produces an explicit diagnostic algorithm (flow diagram) that is analogous to an explicit regression equation.

Unlike regression analysis, however, DSSA does not guarantee an optimum solution. As a heuristic procedure it promises only to generate a pretty good diagnosis most of the time. The good news is that DSSA is also quite capable of generating an excellent diagnosis. This will be demonstrated in section 5.

DSSA can be a useful tool of inference in any context where one wishes to discriminate between two mutually exclusive and collectively exhaustive diagnostic conclusions. Discriminating means choosing one of the two conclusions relevant to that context and rejecting the other.

Examples include choosing:

1. which of two possible conditions or states of the world pertains;
2. which of two interpretive definitions of a situation is more appropriate; and
3. which of two events will occur in the future or whether or not a particular future event will occur.

Being mutually exclusive and collectively exhaustive guarantees that exactly one of the two conclusions must, by construction, apply in a given context. The two possible conclusions are intentionally formulated that way.

DSSA is currently designed to choose one from a set of exactly two possible conclusions. Future versions of the algorithm may be extended to choose one from a set of three or more mutually exclusive and collectively exhaustive possible conclusions, thereby rejecting all but the chosen conclusion.

Conclusion here signifies that the choice is not to be made on the basis of direct and immediate observation. It must be inferred from one or more typically quite imperfect indicators.

In turn, an indicator must encapsulate some kind of empirical evidence. It may be and frequently is derived from direct and immediate observation of some empirical phenomenon, but this is not necessary. An indication may, itself, be inferred indirectly from other indicators. Brownian motion illustrates the point. The irregular oscillatory movement of tiny particles suspended in a fluid is directly observed through a microscope. The irregular oscillatory movement is, itself, taken to be an indication of underlying molecular motion within the fluid.

The important point is that DSSA bases its diagnostic conclusion, however indirectly, on some form of empirical evidence. DSSA is an inductive, evidence-based inference procedure.

Here are some examples.

1. The appropriate condition or state of the world may be unobservable or only partially observable. Thus, whether or not a patient has a specified disease (or has been cured of it) may be diagnosed from the observed pattern of (or absence of) symptoms presented by that patient.
2. How a situation is to be characterized and interpreted may depend on a large number of different factors and how these various factors interact in combination. Thus, interpreting another country's true intentions as bellicose or benign may depend on a myriad of carefully compiled intelligence indicators.
3. Any event that has not yet occurred must be predicted or forecast. Thus, whether or not someone who has just suffered his first heart attack will suffer another one within the next five years may be forecast on the basis of various prognostic indicators included within his family history, his medical record, his diet, and so forth.
4. Whether or not a student applicant will be or should be admitted to a particular university may be indicated by various attributes of the student in conjunction with the historical behavior of that university's admissions committee (e.g., their past decisions concerning whether or not there is a sufficient "match" between a given student applicant and the desired "culture" of the university).
5. Whether or not a loan will be repaid if granted by a commercial bank may be predictable on the basis of especially indicative information contained in the loan application.

The above list is intended to be illustrative only. It is far from exhaustive.

Note, however, a common aspect of all these situations. There is always appreciable uncertainty surrounding the conclusion. In none of the examples does there appear to exist a perfect indicator. A perfect indicator would always point to the correct conclusion with 100 percent accuracy and 100 percent certainty. DSSA would then be unnecessary. Neither DSSA nor any other procedure that incorporates and integrates empirical information from diverse sources could contribute anything of incremental value in the infrequent situation where a perfect indicator is available. Instead, DSSA is designed to deal with the far more frequent situation where we must rely on substantially imperfect indicators to draw the best conclusion we can. It rests on the ability to select and to combine a number of imperfect indicators in such a way as to render diagnostic conclusions more accurate.

4.1 Inputs to DSSA

DSSA receives as inputs various data items that bear upon its choice of one from the two possible diagnostic conclusions. Any kind of data that relates systematically to making this choice may serve as a candidate indicator.

There are two types of candidate indicators that may enter DSSA.

1. Some indicators may initially bear or may be conveniently modeled as bearing a dichotomous, threshold-like relationship to the conclusion being sought. These are called candidate threshold indicators.
2. Other indicators initially bear a different type of relationship to the conclusion being sought. There may be more than two categories or levels of the indicator that relate systematically to the conclusion. The indicator may even possess a full-fledged quantitative relationship to the conclusion throughout the indicator's entire scale (range of numeric indicator values). These are called candidate nonthreshold indicators.

A dichotomous, threshold-like relationship is one where "just enough" of something matters. Beyond that, "more than enough" and "how much more" do not matter. A Geiger counter (scintillator) clicks when it detects at least a minimum threshold of radiation. A neuron fires when it receives at least a minimum threshold of stimulation. There are numerous other examples in both technology and nature.

Although frequently the case, possessing a threshold relationship is not intended to require that more or less of any particular "thing" be measured. Varying intensities of radiation and varying levels of stimulation both denote more or less of something. However, not all dichotomous indicators have this property. Certain dichotomous indicators are unordered. They merely indicate differences. Thus, female mammals are constructed with the biological capacity to bear offspring, while male mammals are not. Males and females are just differently constructed in this sense.

Indicators whose scale values measure nothing more than unordered differences in some sense are called nominal or categorical. Indicators whose scale values measure more or less of something are called ordinal scale indicators.

Possessing a nominal or categorical versus an ordinal scale does not refer to whether an indicator bears a nondirectional versus a directional relationship to some conclusion. It refers instead to the underlying concept measured by the indicator itself. Radiation and stimulation are ordinal concepts. It makes sense to contemplate there being more or less of each. The varying degrees of each can be placed in a natural sequence. In contrast, possessing or not possessing the ability to bear offspring by virtue of being female versus male is a nominal or categorical distinction. It denotes different capacities, but the different capacities do not fall in any natural biological sequence, such as the varying size and complexity of different animal brains.

For an indicator to bear a directional relationship to some conclusion it must first possess an ordinal scale. That is a necessary, though not sufficient precondition. The indicator's successive scale values must fall in a natural order or sequence that reflects the intended meaning of whatever concept the indicator is measuring. It is this natural sequence that subsequently defines the direction of its relationship to whatever conclusion is to be drawn.

Referring to the relationship between indicator and conclusion, any candidate indicator that initially bears or can be conveniently modeled as bearing a threshold relationship to the conclusion qualifies immediately as a threshold indicator. It requires no modification to begin as an admissible indicator, although it may later turn out to be directionally inadmissible or otherwise defective and become inadmissible for those other reasons.

In the commercial loan example it may happen that, based on the experience of the lending bank, the likelihood of repayment depends critically on which of three levels of disposable income the applicant can anticipate during the repayment period:

1. inadequate, suggesting a very low likelihood of repayment;
2. barely adequate, suggesting an intermediate repayment likelihood; or
3. fully adequate, suggesting a much higher likelihood of repayment.

There are more than two possible levels of the applicant's disposable income. Each level appears to exert a different impact on the likelihood of loan repayment. Therefore, disposable income qualifies initially as a nonthreshold indicator of the repayment outcome.

Because the applicant can receive different amounts of income and because these different income levels fall naturally in a definite order or sequence, disposable income is measured on an ordinal scale. The necessary preconditions for being an ordinal indicator of the repayment outcome are thus satisfied.

Because history has suggested that the three levels of disposable income are related in the unidirectional sense shown above to the likelihood of loan repayment, disposable income also satisfies the sufficient conditions. Disposable income would then enter DSSA as a nonthreshold, ordinal indicator.

A great deal of research has shown that the thickness (in millimeters) of their primary lesion is a key indicator with both diagnostic and prognostic significance for melanoma patients. Tumor size is also a prognostically useful ordinal indicator for patients afflicted with other types of cancer, such as breast cancer.

Appendix A presents tumor thickness (Breslow depth) in melanoma as conventionally partitioned by the AJCC into four categories:

1. T1, very thin (no more than 1 millimeter);
2. T2, moderately thin (more than 1, but no more than 2 millimeters);
3. T3, moderately thick (more than 2, but no more than 4 millimeters); and
4. T4, very thick (more than 4 millimeters).

Tumor thickness and tumor size classified into categories such as these have been used extensively in staging both melanoma and breast cancer patients. Because of this, both constitute prime candidates for initial inclusion in DSSA as nonthreshold, ordinal, diagnostic or prognostic indicators.

A most distinctive feature of DSSA is that it relies primarily on the nominal and ordinal properties of its indicators to draw conclusions. DSSA asks not how much more or how much less of something is measured by any indicator. DSSA asks instead whether or not something has been observed or whether more than or less than or exactly some specified amount of something has been observed.

Such a restriction would be crippling in physics and engineering. The important relationships are generally quantitative in these disciplines. Within parts of medicine, economics, and many social sciences, however, little more is known with precision than the ordinal properties of many indicators and just their directional relationships to interesting conclusions. The specific role played by newly discovered genes is an example. It will take some time to fathom the detailed biological mechanisms linking specific genes to specific biological outcomes. In the meantime, analytical procedures such as DSSA can be useful in exploiting the many nominal and ordinal relationships currently identifiable.

4.2   The Three Stages of DSSA: The First Stage

DSSA processes whatever inputs it receives in three sequential stages.

The first stage of DSSA proceeds as follows.

1. Candidate threshold and nonthreshold indicators are collected,
   screened, and, where necessary, modified to produce a subset of N
   admissible threshold indicators.
2. Each indicator so produced either begins in threshold form or is
   immediately converted to threshold form in order to become admissible.
3. A training data set is then obtained. Training data are in the form of
   M historical pairings of the values of the N admissible indicators with
   whichever of the two possible conclusions was appropriate for that
   particular set of N indicator values.
4. The training data set may be represented as a data table with M rows
   and N+1 columns. The first N columns contain values of the N admissible
   indicators in some arbitrary sequence. The N+1st column records which
   of the two discriminating conclusions was known historically to have
   been appropriate in each case (i.e., paired with the particular N
   indicator values falling in each of the M rows of the data table).

The first stage then selects a subset (possibly all) of the N admissible
threshold indicators, decomposes them in a special way to be described later,
and sequences the decomposed indicators so as to achieve the most favorable
quantity and quality of historically accurate discriminations over the M
pairings in the training set.

Perhaps more than anything else it is the distinctive manner in which:

1. its nonthreshold indicators are modified to corresponding threshold
   form;
2. the modified nonthreshold indicators are then combined with initial
   threshold indicators;
3. the N resulting admissible threshold indicators are decomposed and
   sequenced to make conditional dichotomous discriminations; and
4. all dichotomous discriminations are based solely on nominal and ordinal
   relationships linking decomposed indicators to diagnostic conclusions

that differentiates DSSA from other inductive inference procedures trying to
accomplish a similar objective.

The output of DSSA's first stage is a discriminating algorithm produced by the
preceding steps. This may be applied to one or more separate test data sets
containing (similarly coded) data on (at least a subset of) these same N
admissible threshold indicators. The discriminating algorithm is constructed by
sequencing in an optimal manner conditional statements referring to the values
of the decomposed N admissible threshold indicators.

It is possible to execute the first stage of DSSA separately on more than one
set of training data. This would be appropriate if different data sets were
heterogeneous in terms of impact relationships. Heterogeneity of impact would
occur if either the directions of or the constant, accelerating, or
decelerating shapes of relationships linking each indicator to the diagnostic
conclusion being sought were to differ among separate sets of training data.

Separate training data sets generate different discriminating algorithms.
Collectively, the different algorithms so generated could be viewed as a

single, conditional algorithm separately tailorable to heterogeneous (i.e., to differentially impacting) strata of a single, merged target population. Each separate training data set would then be viewed as a separate stratum of the single, merged population. The ability to accomplish this is another distinctive design feature of DSSA. It, too, will be demonstrated in section 5.

The second stage applies the (possibly conditional) discriminating algorithm produced in the first stage to one or more test data sets. Its ability to draw conclusions (e.g., to make dichotomous diagnoses, prognoses, predictions, characterizations, etc.) appropriate to the test data is assessed.

The assessment question asks how effectively the discriminating algorithm produced from and optimized on the basis of the training data operates on separate data drawn from one or more (possibly unrelated) test sets. How accurate are the conclusions it draws?

A training data set and one or more test data sets may be generated by randomly partitioning a single historical data set into two or more subsets. One subset is designated the training subset. These training data are used to produce a discriminating algorithm. Data from the other subset or subsets are used to test or validate independently the discriminating algorithm.

Random partitioning is often employed by DSSA, but it is not required. DSSA may also obtain separate test data from sources unrelated to the training data set. Whenever possible, DSSA adopts the latter procedure, if only as a supplement to random partitioning.

The third stage of DSSA is not always executed. In some circumstances it is both possible to detect and desirable to characterize (at least in terms of shape) connections between various indicators and the conclusion being sought. If and when appropriate, this is accomplished by means of PCM's SPSA procedure. SPSA converts into DSSA-usable form whatever relationships beyond nominal and ordinal link the two possible conclusions to the same set of N indicators.

4.2.1 Obtaining N Admissible Threshold Indicators

The first stage of DSSA makes its choice of one from the two possible conclusions on the basis of N admissible threshold indicators, each of which must be unidirectionally related to the choice being made.

A candidate indicator is admissible to the first stage of DSSA and, therefore, may be incorporated in decomposed form within the DSSA discriminating algorithm produced if:

1. its relationship to the conclusion being sought is, may be conveniently modeled as, or may be modified so as to become dichotomous and threshold-like, and
2. either it possesses a measurement scale that consists of exactly two mutually exclusive and collectively exhaustive, unordered scale values capable of providing no more than a same-versus-different indication in the sense or meaning of the indicator itself (i.e., it is a nominal or categorical indicator),
3. or it possesses a measurement scale that consists of at least two mutually exclusive and collectively exhaustive values that fall in a natural order or sequence in the sense or meaning of the indicator itself (i.e., it is an ordinal scale indicator that specifies an ordered sequence of degrees or amounts of "something" and, therefore,

mediates an ordinal characterization of that "something"), where
4. either one of the two unordered scale values or scale values at one end
   of the ordered sequence are systematically associated with one of the
   two discriminating conclusions, while
5. either the other unordered scale value or scale values at the opposite
   end of the ordered sequence are systematically associated with the
   opposite conclusion, and where
6. this association is unidirectional (i.e., does not change direction) as
   one passes through successive scale values of the indicator if its
   scale possesses an ordered sequence of more than two values.

Some candidate nonthreshold indicators may be systematically related to the
pair of discriminating conclusions, but not initially in a unidirectional
manner. This can sometimes be corrected by partitioning the measurement scale
of the original indicator into subscales, each of which is unidirectionally
related to the pair of discriminating conclusions. After partitioning, DSSA may
accept each partitioned subscale as if it belonged to a separate and
unidirectional candidate indicator, even though not all partitioned subscales
now point in the same direction.

Other candidate indicators may begin in nonthreshold form but prove to be
conveniently modifiable in a different manner. If its overall measurement scale
can be partitioned into an ordered sequence of three or more subscales (i.e.,
distinct subsequences of contiguous scale values), a set of dichotomous dummy
indicators may be substituted for the original nonthreshold indicator.

If the nonthreshold indicator possesses K (at least three) ordered subscales
and if there are no missing observations on that indicator, K-1 dichotomous
dummy indicators are created as follows.

1. The first dummy indicator is assigned a value of 1 if the value of the
   nonthreshold indicator falls in the second-lowest partitioned subscale;
   0, if it falls in a different subscale.
2. The second dummy indicator is assigned a value of 1 if the value of the
   nonthreshold indicator falls in the third-lowest subscale; 0, if it
   falls in a different subscale.
3. Additional dummy indicators may be defined in a similar manner to form
   a total of K-1.
4. An entity whose original indicator value falls in the lowest subscale
   is assigned 0 on all K-1 dummies, while an entity whose original
   indicator value falls in any but the lowest subscale is assigned 1 on
   exactly one of the K-1 dummies.
5. Assuming clear distinguishability and proper ordering of the impact of
   the K-1 subscales on the conclusion to be drawn, DSSA may then
   incorporate each of these K-1 dummies as a separate threshold indicator
   in the set of N admissible indicators. The K-1 dummies (or a subset
   thereof) are substituted for the original nonthreshold indicator.

Alternatively, if the nonthreshold indicator possesses K (at least three)
ordered subscales and some missing observations, K dichotomous dummy indicators
are created as follows.

1. The first dummy indicator is assigned a value of 1 if the value of the
   nonthreshold indicator falls in the lowest partitioned subscale; 0,
   otherwise (0 is also assigned to all missing observations).
2. The second dummy indicator is assigned a value of 1 if the value of the
   nonthreshold indicator falls in the second-lowest subscale; 0,
   otherwise (0 is also assigned to all missing observations).
3. Additional dummy indicators are defined in a similar manner to form a

total of K.
4. Any entity whose original indicator value is undefined (missing observation) is assigned 0 on all K dummies, while every entity whose original indicator value possesses a defined value is assigned 1 on exactly one of the K dummies.
5. Assuming clear distinguishability and proper ordering of the impact of the K subscales on the conclusion to be drawn, DSSA may then incorporate each of these K dummies as a separate threshold indicator in the set of N admissible indicators. The K dummies (or a subset thereof) are again substituted for the original nonthreshold indicator.

In both of the above modification procedures there remain the twin questions of distinguishability and proper ordering of the impact of the partitioned subscales on the conclusion to be drawn. Both questions can be answered by logistic regression analysis. The two possible conclusions that might be drawn are numerically coded as 0 and 1, respectively. These become logistic regression's dependent variable. Each of the K-1 or K dummy variables just constructed becomes a separate independent variable.

The regression analysis estimates values for each of the K-1 or K regression coefficients. The signed algebraic magnitudes of the regression coefficients indicate the ordering of the impacts of the K-1 or K subscales. The analysis also assigns just-achievable statistical significance levels (i.e., p values) to each dummy variable's estimated regression coefficient.

The estimated regression coefficients and the p value assigned to each coefficient are not interpreted here in the traditional (Neyman-Pearson) statistical hypothesis testing context. They are regarded as strictly descriptive statistics. A monotonic algebraic sequence of successive regression coefficients is interpreted as confirming a unidirectional impact of the indicator (i.e., its sequence of partitioned subscales) on the conclusion being sought. Numerically small p values are interpreted as suggesting substantially distinguishable impacts associated with belonging to successive subscales. Through trial and error, these descriptive statistics can suggest an improved way to partition the scale of the indicator. Applying the SPSA algorithm to the indicator's raw measurement scale is a convenient way to initiate the trial-and-error process.

Whether or not a candidate indicator is modified in one of the above ways or in any other manner prior to entering as an input to DSSA, an optimal cut point within its set of observed values is always identified. This is done by DSSA automatically and separately for each indicator. Optimal means that, if the indicator were converted via its cut point to a dichotomous diagnostic test for drawing the appropriate discriminating conclusion, the weighted average of the sensitivity and specificity of that diagnostic test would be maximized. An indicator's discriminating cut point, its sensitivity, and its specificity are described below.

A candidate indicator that enters DSSA already in threshold form possesses only one logically possible cut point. That unique cut point constitutes the indicator's discriminating cut point and its optimal cut point. Such would be the case for each of the K-1 or K dummy variables created for logistic regression analysis. Each dummy variable possesses two observable values.

When a candidate indicator enters DSSA in nonthreshold form, it is dichotomized by means of its optimal cut point. The procedure to accomplish this is illustrated in the following purely hypothetical example.

Suppose that a diagnostic test for pregnancy has been developed. A positive test result is supposed to indicate that the woman taking the test is pregnant. A negative test result is supposed to indicate nonpregnancy. The two diagnostic conclusions are actual pregnancy versus actual nonpregnancy. The two test results are positive for pregnancy versus negative for pregnancy.

Suppose, further, that test results are based on the concentration in the blood of a certain hormone known to be associated with pregnancy. The concentration of this hormone is a candidate nonthreshold ordinal indicator. Relatively high concentrations indicate pregnancy, while relatively low concentrations indicate nonpregnancy. The task is to identify a discriminating cut point within some set of observed concentrations that distinguishes operationally a positive from a negative test result. Any but the lowest-valued observed concentration can serve as the discriminating cut point.

Relative to any given cut point the sensitivity of the pregnancy test is defined as the proportion of actually pregnant test takers who obtain a (correct) positive (at or above the cut point) test result. The specificity of the pregnancy test is defined as the proportion of actually nonpregnant test takers who obtain a (correct) negative (below the cut point) test result. The other two possible (incorrect) test outcomes are referred to as false positives and false negatives, respectively.

Notice that neither the sensitivity nor the specificity of the pregnancy test depends in any way on the relative number of test takers who are actually pregnant versus actually nonpregnant. Sensitivity is defined as the proportion of pregnant test takers who get a correct (positive) test result. Specificity is defined as the proportion of nonpregnant test takers who get a correct (negative) test result.

These observations are important for two reasons.

1. The ability of the test to indicate correctly actual pregnancy versus nonpregnancy, when defined conditionally in terms of sensitivity and specificity, can be assessed by means of observations on test takers whose relative composition of pregnant versus nonpregnant women is arbitrary—chosen as a matter of convenience. The assessment data set need not be compositionally representative in this sense of any target population of interest (e.g., the population of women who might eventually use the pregnancy test on a continuing basis).

   Consequently, if DSSA adopts as its goal optimizing something defined in terms of sensitivity and specificity, its training (assessment) data set need not be compositionally representative in the same sense of any (typically more interesting) test data sets. Only its sensitivity and specificity need be representative. These are both proportions, thus allowing significant flexibility in the choice of a training data set. Conveniently accessible data may be used for this purpose.

2. The training data are compositionally representative of the test data in the special case where a single historical data set is randomly partitioned into training and test subsets. This eliminates undue concern for representativeness.

The first stage of DSSA adopts a maximum weighted average of various sensitivity and specificity measures (as opposed to a simple, unweighted mean) as its optimizing criterion. Assigning unequal weights permits DSSA to adjust the optimizing procedure selectively in the direction of achieving either higher sensitivity or higher specificity.

The relative merits of sensitivity and specificity are generally quite context-dependent. Assessing whether it is more important for an indicator to be sensitive or specific relative to drawing a particular conclusion requires comparing the consequences of a false positive and a false negative indication in some particular context.

A married woman who has been attempting for a long time to become pregnant is likely to be primarily averse to false positive test outcomes. Obtaining a false positive result (only to learn later that the test was incorrect) could be emotionally devastating. From a practical standpoint, obtaining a false positive test result and then terminating, prematurely, whatever measures were being taken to enhance the likelihood of pregnancy would be counterproductive.

In contrast, the consequences of a false negative test result could be discouraging and might induce the expenditure of wasted time, energy, and other resources; but she might well judge these to be the lesser of the two evils.

A recent rape victim is likely to be primarily averse to false negative test outcomes. Falsely concluding that the rape had not resulted in pregnancy (only to learn later that the test was incorrect) would also be emotionally devastating. Even worse, foregoing whatever corrective measures might have been appropriate in the false belief of nonpregnancy could be especially serious.

In contrast, the consequences of a false positive test result would also be discouraging and might also induce the expenditure of wasted time, energy, and other resources; but these might also be judged the lesser of the two evils.

Once the design and the operating characteristics of a pregnancy test have been determined, it is no longer possible to improve its accuracy. Superior methods of measuring hormone concentration and substitution of a different hormone with superior discrimination ability are no longer realistic options. However, the discriminating cut point distinguishing a positive from a negative test result can still be raised or lowered, depending on the context in which the test will be used. It is possible to tailor the test to different contexts by selectively adjusting its cut point.

Lowering the test's discriminating cut point will increase the number of positive results it generates. This increases its sensitivity (true positive results), but it also produces more false positive results.

Raising the test's discriminating cut point will increase the number of negative results it generates. This increases its specificity (true negative results), but it also produces more false negative results.

Trading off more false positive results against more false negative results and, concurrently, increased sensitivity against increased specificity is a judgmental exercise. The likely consequences of the different types of errors may be compared by means of a careful cost-benefit analysis. Then separate versions of the test with different discriminating cut points (producing different sensitivities, specificities, false positives, and false negatives) can be designed for use by hopeful mothers as opposed to anxious rape victims.

Once the design and operation of a test are determined, improving either its sensitivity or its specificity by adjusting its discriminating cut point generally occurs at the expense of the other. For any given test these two proportions are defined in such a way that increasing either one can never increase (and generally decreases) the other. The exact rates at which such trade-offs occur depend on the particular way the test is designed and carried out.

Adjusting the weights assigned by DSSA to sensitivity and specificity when calculating various weighted averages to be maximized is analogous to altering the discriminating cut point of a pregnancy test. It is analogous in the sense that it provides a mechanism to make desirable trade-offs. DSSA's conclusions can be nudged toward improvements in the direction of either sensitivity (avoiding false negatives) or specificity (avoiding false positives).

An entirely different goal can also be achieved by adjusting DSSA's sensitivity and specificity weights. Its accuracy (i.e., number of correct discriminating conclusions) can generally be maximized by choosing weights according to the relative composition of a training data set. For example, setting the sensitivity weight equal to the proportion of actually pregnant women in the data set used to assess the pregnancy test's accuracy and then adjusting its discriminating cut point so as to maximize the test's weighted average sensitivity and specificity would generally maximize the number of correct discriminations it makes in that particular data set.

Across separate applications of the DSSA algorithm the weighted average sensitivity and specificity may be numerically reduced according to (i.e., multiplied by one minus) the proportion of entities the discriminating algorithm fails to classify. Failure to draw a conclusion can occur when no indicators possess a potent impact on the conclusion to be drawn. Failure to draw a conclusion can also occur in the face of an overwhelming quantity of missing indicator data. By using the numerically reduced weighted average as an overall optimizing criterion DSSA can make implicit trade-offs between quantity and quality of discrimination.

The weights assigned to sensitivity and specificity, respectively, are two numbers greater than zero and less than one that add exactly to one. If sensitivity were regarded as twice as important as specificity to achieve in some particular context, the sensitivity weight would be two-thirds. The specificity weight would be one-third.

If no weights are explicitly specified, DSSA assumes equal weights of one-half each, and the simple, unweighted mean of various sensitivity and specificity measures is maximized. This is DSSA's default execution procedure.

The same weights, whether explicitly assigned or assumed by default, apply uniformly to selecting an optimal cut point for each of the N admissible indicators and to optimizing the remainder of the first stage procedure. It is through the judicious choice of weights that DSSA can influence the selection of optimal cut points and can balance thereby trade-offs among sensitivity, specificity, false positives, and false negatives.

There are other ways beside maximizing a weighted average to optimize DSSA's first stage procedure. Examples of alternative optimizing criteria include:

1. choosing cut points that maximize the specificity of an indicator or set of indicators, subject to achieving at least a minimum sensitivity; and
2. choosing cut points that maximize the sensitivity of an indicator or set of indicators, subject to achieving at least a minimum specificity.

DSSA could be modified to achieve these and other optimizing goals. At present, however, DSSA relies on sensitivity and specificity weights.

Prior to identifying an optimal cut point for each candidate indicator, its directional relationship with the pair of discriminating conclusions over the M pairings within the training data set is verified. A Mann-Whitney statistical test (also called a Wilcoxon two-sample test) is performed. Any indicator whose direction of relationship with the pair of discriminating conclusions is opposite to what previous research has established as appropriate is culled. Any candidate indicator whose optimal cut point cannot be properly identified is also culled.

4.2.2 Minimum Requirements Imposed by DSSA upon Its Training Data Table

A training data set contains historical data. As previously stated, it may be represented as a data table with M rows and N+1 columns.

The first N columns contain observed values of the N admissible threshold indicators (after culling). The N+1st column records which of the two discriminating conclusions was known historically to have been applicable to each set of N indicator values.

Each of the M rows of the table records a distinct historical pairing of the N values of the N admissible indicators (one value for each indicator) with the corresponding conclusion in the N+1st column.

The M rows correspond, respectively, to M distinct entities. An entity is the "thing" about which one of the two possible conclusions must be drawn. That same entity is also the "thing" relative to which each of the N admissible indicators provides an indication. Returning to the five illustrative examples previously offered:

1. entities are distinct patients about whom a diagnostic conclusion must be drawn concerning whether or not each one has (or has been cured of) a specified disease, and the N symptoms (or lack of symptoms) provide N items of information with diagnostic significance relative to each patient;
2. entities are distinct countries in specified historical contexts to which either of two interpretive characterizations is applicable, and the N pieces of intelligence information describe N aspects of what each country was about in that historical context;
3. entities are distinct patients who have just suffered their first heart attack about whom a prognostic conclusion must be drawn concerning whether or not each one will suffer another attack within the next five years, and the N indicators provide N items of information with prognostic significance relative to each patient;
4. entities are distinct student applicants about whom a conclusion must be drawn concerning whether or not each one will or should be admitted to a particular university, and the N indicators include responses to questions in the student's application for admission and descriptions of the admission committee's historical admission decisions; and
5. entities are distinct loans about which a conclusion must be drawn concerning whether or not each one is likely to be repaid if granted by the commercial bank, and the N indicators are N responses to questions in each loan application.

Based on the admissibility requirements and the need to establish optimal cut points for each admissible indicator DSSA requires its training data table to possess the following characteristics.

1. There must be at least one admissible threshold indicator. Otherwise, DSSA cannot even get started. This implies that N must be at least one.
2. All M data items in the N+1st column of the training data table must be

fully defined. No missing or undefined values are permitted. Otherwise, there would be no historically known conclusion for the entity in the undefined row of the table to pair with values of that entity's N admissible indicators.

3. There must be at least one instance of each of the two possible conclusions recorded in the N+1st column of the data table. Otherwise, there would be no historical discriminations to exploit in the training process. This implies that M must be at least two.

4. Looking down each of the first N columns in the data table, there must be at least two distinct values of each indicator. Otherwise, no optimal cut point can be established for that indicator. This also implies that M must be at least two.

5. Looking across each of the M rows, missing or undefined values are permitted within some but not all of the first N columns. Otherwise, if all N values were undefined, there would be no indicator values to pair with the conclusion in the N+1st column known historically to have been applicable to that entity.

6. Finally, after establishing initial optimal cut points and after satisfying all of the preceding requirements, a comparison of each of the first N columns in the data table with the N+1st column must produce at least one pairing of an above-the-cut-point indicator value with one of the two conclusions and at least one pairing of a below-the-cut-point indicator value with the other conclusion. Otherwise, that indicator possesses no discriminatory power relative to the conclusion to be drawn.

At this point, DSSA checks the training data set to ensure that all of the minimum requirements are satisfied. Additional rows (entities) and columns (admissible indicators) may need to be culled. DSSA continues only after all minimum requirements are satisfied. Otherwise, it terminates unsuccessfully.

4.2.3   Casting the N Indicators and the Two Conclusions in Canonical Form

In many contexts, one of the two discriminating conclusions naturally commands greater interest and attention than the other. Concluding that one has become pregnant would normally be the interesting conclusion. More dramatically, concluding that an asteroid will collide with the earth during the next year is far greater cause for interest and concern than concluding that no such collision will occur.

DSSA requires that the state or event or situation referenced by one of its two conclusions be labeled FOCAL. The other one must be labeled ALTERNATIVE. The FOCAL state, event, or situation is the one that seems to command greater interest and on which greater attention is appropriately focused. The ALTERNATIVE state, event, or situation is simply its logical complement. If it is not obvious how to assign these labels, the assignment may be arbitrary, but DSSA requires that a definite assignment be made.

When originally obtained or created, indicators need not be numerically coded. A candidate indicator may possess a measurement scale whose component values are not numbers. Thus, the final rank of a retiring military officer may be Lieutenant, Major, or General. That indicator may provide a reasonable basis for concluding whether the officer's length of military service is likely to have been relatively long or relatively short.

Even though DSSA exploits only the nominal (categorically distinguishing) and ordinal (rank-orderable) properties inherent in the raw measurement values of its indicators, all indicators are subject to recoding prior to determining their optimal cut points. This is done for computational convenience.

1. If a candidate indicator is not already coded numerically, numbers are substituted for its nonnumeric scale values such that algebraically higher numbers correspond to relatively higher degrees, levels, or amounts of the "something" being measured (e.g., hormone concentration, military rank, etc.), while algebraically lower numbers correspond to relatively lower degrees, levels, or amounts.

2. Positive integers (and possibly zero) are frequently useful as recoding values. They are assigned sequentially so as to preserve the ordering of the original scale values and, therefore, the ordinal "sense" of the indicator.

3. Recoding in terms of nonnegative integers, though convenient, is not essential. Any properly sequenced (i.e., order-preserving) numeric assignment will suffice, including the use of fractions, decimals, and negative numbers.

4. The resulting numeric scale of each recoded indicator (its original scale, if numeric and no recoding is necessary) is then compared with the FOCAL vs. ALTERNATIVE assignment. By convention (but only by convention) DSSA requires that algebraically higher indicator scale values be associated with the FOCAL state, event, or situation and that lower values be associated with the ALTERNATIVE. If this does not occur naturally all scale values can be subtracted from the maximum numerically assigned value to make it occur. Uniform subtraction serves to reverse the direction of the ordinal scale.

5. The opposite convention could just as easily have been adopted with no loss in procedural effectiveness.

6. In the special case where the candidate indicator possesses a measurement scale that consists of exactly two unordered scale values capable of providing no more than a same-versus-different indication, a pair of numbers (e.g., 0 and 1) is assigned as the indicator's recoded scale in a manner consistent with the above convention.

Each of the (possibly recoded) admissible threshold indicators remaining in the training data table may now be associated with the FOCAL and ALTERNATIVE states, events, or situations in a standard manner. The standard manner is by means of a conceptual two-by-two cross-table (frequency cross-tabulation) in canonical form.

1. The first row of the canonical table holds algebraically lower values of the indicator (all scale values strictly below its optimal cut point).

2. The second row of the canonical table holds algebraically higher values of the indicator (all scale values at or above its optimal cut point).

3. The ALTERNATIVE state, event, or situation heads the first column of the canonical table.

4. Specificity is defined as the proportion of entities in the first column (for which the ALTERNATIVE conclusion is actually appropriate) that are also in the first row (i.e., in the northwest cell of the two-by-two cross-table) because they are assigned indicator values algebraically lower than the cut point.

5. The FOCAL state, event, or situation heads the second column of the canonical table.

6. Sensitivity is defined as the proportion of entities in the second column (for which the FOCAL conclusion is actually appropriate) that are also in the second row (i.e., in the southeast cell of the two-by-two cross-table) because they are assigned indicator values at least as high, algebraically, as the cut point.

7. In a typical diagnostic context, the first row of the canonical table would be identified as a test result NEGATIVE with respect to the FOCAL state, event, or situation; while the second row would be identified as a test result POSITIVE with respect to the FOCAL state, event, or situation.

As with the convention of associating higher scale values with FOCAL and lower scale values with ALTERNATIVE states, events, or situations, the numeric scale of each indicator could just as easily have been partitioned by its optimal cut point into values strictly greater than versus values equal to or less than the cut point. The procedural effectiveness of DSSA is not affected by this arbitrary choice, either.

Data from the training data table are then cross-tabulated to produce actual two-by-two canonical tables—one for each of the N admissible indicators. Whichever cut point maximizes the weighted average sensitivity and specificity is identified as the optimal cut point for every indicator.

By virtue of having executed all of the previously described steps the historical frequencies appearing in each canonical cross-table will concentrate along its major diagonal (i.e., within its top-left or northwest cell and its bottom-right or southeast cell). This concentration of historical frequencies along the major diagonal provides visual confirmation of the conventionally defined, unidirectional impact of each indicator on the ALTERNATIVE versus FOCAL state, event, or situation. Relatively lower historical frequencies will occupy each table's off-diagonal (i.e., its top-right or northeast [false negative] and its bottom-left or southwest [false positive]) cells.

The product of the two major-diagonal (true or correct) frequencies in each canonical table must equal or exceed (usually exceed) the product of its two off-diagonal (false or incorrect) frequencies. This means that if a canonical table of cross-tabulated frequencies were regarded as a two-by-two matrix, it would always possess a nonnegative determinant (difference between these two products). The magnitude of its determinant serves as a measure of the strength of impact of each indicator on the conclusion to be drawn.

4.2.4 Decomposing the N Admissible Threshold Indicators into 2xN Discriminators

The data table has been converted to the proper format. Each of its N remaining columns now contains numerically coded values of a fully admissible ordinal threshold indicator in canonical form. Consequently, each indicator may now be related to the FOCAL versus ALTERNATIVE conclusion according to a conditional statement of the following standard form.

If the numeric value of the indicator falls below that indicator's optimal cut point, choose the ALTERNATIVE conclusion. Otherwise, if the numeric value falls at or above its optimal cut point, choose the FOCAL conclusion.

When applied to the M entities in the training data table each such conditional statement:

1. either draws the ALTERNATIVE conclusion about that entity; or
2. draws the FOCAL conclusion about that entity; or
3. draws no conclusion about that entity.

Exactly one of the two conclusions applies to every entity that possesses a defined value of the indicator in question. No conclusion will be drawn concerning entities whose values of the indicator are undefined (e.g., missing data).

DSSA then decomposes each conditional statement in standard form into a matched pair of related conditional statements, also in standard form. These are called discriminators.

If the numeric value of the indicator falls below that indicator's optimal cut point, choose the ALTERNATIVE conclusion.

If the numeric value of the indicator falls at or above its optimal cut point, choose the FOCAL conclusion.

N admissible indicators always produce N matched pairs of discriminators for a total of 2xN discriminators.

When applied to the M entities in the training data table the first discriminator in each matched pair:

1. either draws the ALTERNATIVE conclusion about that entity; or
2. draws no conclusion about that entity.

The ALTERNATIVE conclusion will be drawn for every entity that possesses a defined value of the indicator that falls below the indicator's optimal cut point. No conclusion will be drawn for entities whose values of the indicator are either undefined or are defined but fall at or above the indicator's optimal cut point.

When applied to the same M entities in the training data table the second discriminator in each matched pair:

1. either draws the FOCAL conclusion about that entity; or
2. draws no conclusion about that entity.

The FOCAL conclusion is drawn for every entity that possesses a defined value of the indicator that falls at or above the indicator's optimal cut point. No conclusion will be drawn for entities whose values of the indicator are either undefined or are defined but fall below the indicator's optimal cut point.

A discriminating algorithm is then defined by DSSA as the application of any sequence of discriminators contained within a nonempty subset of the complete set of the above 2xN discriminators to some collection of relevant entities.

1. If all 2xN discriminators are included in the sequence there are (2xN)! [2xN factorial] logically possible sequences and, therefore, (2xN)! logically possible discriminating algorithms that may be constructed from the N admissible threshold indicators.
2. Applying such a sequence of 2xN discriminators to a collection of M relevant entities (e.g., to the M entities in the training data table) means:

a. picking one of the M entities;
b. proceeding through the sequence of 2xN discriminators until the first one is encountered that draws a definite conclusion about that entity;
c. classifying that entity accordingly (i.e., drawing that conclusion about that entity); and

      d. repeating this process for the next entity until all M entities
        have been classified.

   3. Because of the manner in which the 2xN discriminators were constructed
      a definite conclusion will be drawn about all M entities in the
      training set. No entities will remain unclassified when all 2xN
      discriminators are included in the sequence.
   4. There is no guarantee, however, that any of the conclusions will be
      correct.
   5. The number of correct conclusions and, therefore, correct
      classifications will vary with the sequence in which discriminators are
      applied.
   6. DSSA's task is to identify the "best" way to sequence the 2xN
      discriminators so as to draw the most "appropriate" conclusions.

If fewer than all 2xN discriminators are included in the sequence (say P of
them) there are P! [P factorial] logically possible sequences and, therefore,
P! logically possible discriminating algorithms. Now DSSA's task is twofold.

   1. First pick the "best" subset of P discriminators.
   2. Then determine the "best" way to sequence them.

When fewer than all 2xN discriminators are included in the sequence it is no
longer guaranteed that a definite conclusion will be drawn about all entities
in the training set. DSSA must also be "trained" how to trade off drawing an
incorrect conclusion about an entity against drawing no conclusion at all. That
trade-off is part of the intended meaning of "best."

4.2.5 Selecting and Sequencing Discriminators from the Training Data Table

The overall purpose of DSSA's first stage is to produce the "best" possible
discriminating algorithm relative to the M entities in the training data table.

Discriminating means drawing either the FOCAL or the ALTERNATIVE conclusion in
the "best" possible way concerning as many entities as possible.

"Best" is defined in terms of the weighted average of the overall sensitivity
and specificity of the resulting diagnosis. The same weights used to determine
optimal cut points are reused for this purpose.

Equal weights will tend to maximize the simple (unweighted) mean of sensitivity
and specificity. Alternatively, unequal weights may be chosen either:

   1. to nudge the diagnosis in the direction of relatively more sensitivity;
      or
   2. to nudge the diagnosis in the direction of relatively more specificity;
      or
   3. to draw the greatest number of correct diagnostic conclusions, without
      regard to either sensitivity or specificity.

Selecting the subset of the 2xN discriminators to include in the final
discriminating algorithm proceeds somewhat in the manner of stepwise
regression, but with several important differences.

   1. At the outset, none of the N admissible indicators and, therefore, none
      of the 2xN discriminators is regarded as included in the final
      algorithm.

2. The selection procedure is iterative. At each successive iteration an additional discriminator is selected to enter into the algorithm. The next discriminator selected is the one judged "best" from among the remaining, as-yet-unselected discriminators.
3. The "best" discriminator is the one that does the "best" job of drawing correct conclusions about whichever entities have not yet been classified (correctly or incorrectly) by discriminators already entered into the algorithm during previous iterations.
4. When a discriminator is selected, the indicator from which it was decomposed is simultaneously regarded as having been selected to enter the algorithm (at least partially).
5. Once entered, neither a discriminator nor its associated indicator can later be removed from the final algorithm (this is different from stepwise regression).
6. Whenever one discriminator in a pair enters the algorithm, its matching discriminator must either enter the algorithm during a later iteration defined in terms of the same optimal cut point, or it may never enter the algorithm.
7. Iterations continue until:

   a. either all 2xN discriminators (and, therefore, all N indicators) have been fully entered into the algorithm;
   b. or it is determined that DSSA cannot make additional diagnostic improvements by entering additional discriminators;
   c. or conclusions have already been drawn about all M entities in the training data set;
   d. whichever occurs first, at which point the procedure terminates successfully.

8. At successful termination, the discriminators entered constitute the subset selected for the final discriminating algorithm being produced. The sequence in which they were entered determines the sequence in which they will subsequently be applied to successive entities.

DSSA can terminate successfully but prematurely. This occurs when a next discriminator is permitted to enter the final algorithm only when it improves the overall weighted average sensitivity and specificity. Premature termination means before selecting all 2xN discriminators and, possibly, before conclusions have been drawn concerning all M entities.

When zero or negative improvements are permitted the "least bad" next discriminator is uniformly selected at each iteration. Then DSSA will not terminate until all 2xN discriminators have been entered (in some definite sequence) and a definite (although not necessarily correct) conclusion has been drawn concerning all M entities in the training set.

DSSA contains a logical "control knob" that either allows premature termination or forces the algorithm production process to proceed to completion. Unless explicitly precluded DSSA allows premature termination as its default option.

4.2.6   Interpreting and Applying the Final Discriminating Algorithm

DSSA then applies the discriminating algorithm just produced to the training data. The number and percentage of correct discriminations made is calculated. The number and percentage of entities, if any, for which no conclusion could be drawn is also calculated. Overall sensitivity and specificity proportions are calculated for the subset of M entities in the training table concerning which the discriminating algorithm drew a definite conclusion. A ROC/AUC analysis is performed on this same subset of M entities, and its AUC value is estimated.

4.3   The Second Stage of DSSA

DSSA's next task is to apply the discriminating algorithm just produced to one or more test data sets. Comparable weighted average sensitivities and specificities and AUC scores are calculated for each test set. So are the number and percentage of correct discriminations. The number and percentage of entities for which no conclusion can be drawn are also noted for each set.

The weighted average sensitivity and specificity and AUC score calculated for test data sets and the percentage of correct discriminations tend to be lower than for the training set. This is because the first stage of DSSA attempts to optimize only with respect to the training data. It cannot do so with respect to any test data. It has no access to test data.

An important question is by how much DSSA has capitalized on spurious (i.e., nonsystematic and nonreproducible) relationships within the training data. This would be characterized as overfitting the final discriminating algorithm to the training data. It is the same problem discussed in section 2.6 and illustrated via the split-sample reliability analysis presented in appendix B.

Evidence of overfitting would include a large drop in the weighted average sensitivity and specificity from training to test data sets, a large drop in estimated AUC score, a large drop in the percentage of correct discriminations, or some combination of all three. Tolerably small drops and (occasional) increases are good news. A substantial increase in the percentage of entities for which no conclusion can be drawn could also indicate overfitting.

A reasonable way to confirm or disconfirm suspected overfitting would be to execute an explicit split-sample reliability analysis, as was done for PCM.

Comparison with alternative inference procedures is also appropriate. For example, the same N admissible threshold indicators might be analyzed via a classification tree or a carefully constructed neural net. Weighted average sensitivity and specificity, estimated AUC, and the number and percentage of correct discriminations can then be compared.

Some novel features of DSSA have already been mentioned.

1. DSSA can produce a discriminating algorithm especially tailored to almost any training data set and associated test sets.

   a. Tailoring is accomplished by partitioning training data obtained from a heterogeneous population into separate, relatively homogeneous subsamples drawn, respectively, from separate, relatively homogeneous strata of their heterogeneous parent population;
   b. by then generating separate discriminating algorithms from each training subsample; and
   c. by then combining the separate algorithms into a single, composite algorithm that may be applied to the original training data set and to all associated test data sets.

2. The discriminating algorithm produced can be intentionally weighted in the direction of achieving either greater sensitivity or greater

specificity, but necessarily at the expense of the other. It can also be weighted to maximize the number of correct conclusions drawn from the training data set.

3. An implicit trade-off can be made between quantity and quality of discriminatory efficacy by reducing the weighted average sensitivity and specificity to account for the percentage of entities for which no diagnosis can be made.

4. Substantial quantities of missing indicator data are handled by DSSA in a simple and straightforward manner. Whenever an entity possesses no value of some indicator, the discriminating algorithm simply proceeds to the next discriminator in the ordered sequence that possesses a defined value applicable to that particular entity. When an entity possesses no values on any indicators, DSSA can draw no diagnostic conclusion about it either in the training or in any test data set.

Another feature of DSSA is its ability to combine collections of indicators into an index via some arithmetic expression or other mathematical function while still retaining each component indicator in its original form as a separate input. For example, the presumed interaction between two quantitative indicators may be modeled by multiplying their separate numeric values and appending the computed product to the same indicator list.

How well such a strategy succeeds can be judged by how early in the sequence of discriminators constituting the final discriminating algorithm either of the two discriminators generated as a matched pair from the computed product appears, how many entities are so classified, its impact on the weighted average sensitivity and specificity, and its contribution to the number and percentage of correct discriminations. If the pair of discriminators associated with the calculated product ends up classifying no entities, while discriminators associated, separately, with the two original indicators that were multiplied together do end up classifying (correctly) at least some entities, the presumed interaction may not exist—at least not in the presumed multiplicative form.

The ability to adopt such a strategy is not novel. Many forms of regression analysis can append this type of interaction term to their list of independent variables. What is novel is DSSA's ability to include linear combinations of indicators in a single collection of diagnostic inputs. For example, the (weighted) sum of or difference between two indicators may be included along with the same two indicators entered separately. No form of regression is able to accept linear combinations of input variables. Section 5 will document a diagnostic application of DSSA that illustrates dramatically its capacity to analyze linearly interdependent indicators.

Still another novel feature is DSSA's ability both to compare its performance with and to incorporate, selectively, the best features of alternative inference procedures that operate on the same N admissible threshold indicators. The operating characteristics of such an alternative procedure (e.g., a classification tree) may be encapsulated in a special function that assigns the conclusions drawn by that procedure (FOCAL versus ATLERNATIVE classification) to each of the M entities in the training data table. The special function may then be treated by DSSA as just another diagnostic indicator in dichotomous form. The discriminating algorithm produced by DSSA with this special function included in its collection of indicators will then utilize the two discriminators produced from it to classify as many entities in the training set as are appropriate. How many entities these discriminators classify, which ones, how correctly, and how early in the discriminating algorithm sequence either or both of the two discriminators fall provide rich comparative detail.

4.4 The Optional Third Stage of DSSA

As stated previously, portions of a PCM analysis can be performed on the same training data diagnosed by DSSA. Applying SPSA to partition more finely the measurement scale of selected indicators can sometimes improve DSSA's diagnostic accuracy. Indicators believed to exert a genuine quantitative impact on the FOCAL and ALTERNATIVE conclusions (in addition to the nominal and ordinal impacts identified by DSSA) would be appropriate candidates on which to execute this optional third-stage procedure. Section 5.10 will demonstrate how useful such additional fine-tuning can sometimes be.

5.0 USING DSSA TO DIAGNOSE MELANOMA MALIGNANCY WITH FIVE GENETIC BIOMARKERS

The human genome contains approximately twenty-five thousand (or more) distinct genes. Most genes are involved in neither the initial development nor the subsequent progress of melanoma. In 2004 we tried to isolate a subset of these genes that are so involved. We used a statistical technique called Significance Analysis of Microarrays (SAM) to generate candidates.

Human tissue obtained from benign nevi (moles) was compared with tissue obtained from malignant melanomas. The purpose was to identify genes that could be used in their differential diagnosis. Our SAM analysis produced several hundred promising candidates, along with a directional indication of each gene's biological role in melanoma progression. Any gene that appeared either systematically overexpressed or systematically underexpressed in malignant melanomas compared to benign nevi constituted a promising candidate.

From the several hundred promising candidates we selected five specific genes to serve as biomarkers in diagnosing malignant melanomas. Selections were based on two criteria. Each gene must have demonstrated a statistically significant expression difference between the two types of tissue in the SAM analysis, and commercially available antibodies had to exist in the marketplace in 2006 to calibrate via immunohistochemistry the degree of protein expression associated with each gene's overexpression or underexpression.

The five specific genes we selected were the first five in the group of nine molecular factors listed as nontraditional prognostic factors in section 2.4 of this book. All five genes were systematically overexpressed in malignant melanomas compared to benign nevi. The five genes were:

1. WNT2;
2. ARPC2;
3. SPP1 (also referred to as osteopontin or OPN);
4. RGS1; and
5. FN1.

Melanoma diagnosis is typically based on a pathological evaluation of biopsied tissue. Biopsied tissue can be obtained either from a primary tumor or from subsequent metastases.

There is reasonable consensus among pathologists concerning many histopathological features signaling malignancy in melanocytic neoplasms. However, the diagnosis of melanoma remains problematic with respect to several special cases. These include dysplastic nevi and Spitz nevi. Both can appear atypical under the microscope, but are otherwise benign. With respect to these two problem cases there is far less diagnostic concordance among separate pathologists. Not everybody weights atypical observational criteria identically in drawing final diagnostic conclusions.

The importance to patients of early and accurate diagnosis of melanoma cannot be overemphasized. Melanoma is a life-threatening malignancy. It has a very poor prognosis in its later stages of development. It accounts for 80 percent of deaths due to skin cancer. Skin cancer is one of the more common forms of cancer in humans. Melanoma patients fare much better when accurately diagnosed and properly treated early in the disease's progression.

No genes or other molecular biomarkers were routinely used in 2006 for diagnostic purposes in melanoma. Neither were any molecular biomarkers used to deal with the two problem cases. Our central task was to fill both gaps.

Following is a step-by-step description of our attempt to exploit the differentiating capacity of our five selected genes in producing a multimarker assay to distinguish malignant melanomas from benign nevi. Progress was achieved in a sequence of four distinct stages. They unfolded much like four successive acts in an ongoing play. Hence, our analysis will be described as if it progressed in this four-act sequence.

5.1 Act I: Confirmation of the SAM Analysis Using Conventional Methodology

Tissue obtained from their primary malignant lesions was available for patients diagnosed with melanoma by the University of California at San Francisco (UCSF) prior to April 2007. Tissue was also available from benign nevi collected from other UCSF patients prior to April 2007. Immunohistochemical analysis of these two tissue sets designed to compare the systematic overexpression or underexpression of our five selected genes would serve either to confirm or to disconfirm the directional indications obtained from the SAM analysis.

With the aid of commercially obtained antibodies lesions from both tissue sets were stained for the presence of proteins associated, respectively, with each of the five genes. One of the authors (Dr. Richard W. Sagebiel) read all stained lesions under a microscope. Staining intensities of each lesion were recorded separately for each of the five genes on a four-point numeric scale as either: absent (0); light (1); moderate (2); or intense (3).

The pathologist (Dr. Sagebiel) was not always able to evaluate staining intensity. Sometimes a score could not be assigned to a lesion for one or more of the five genes. The inability to assign a definite intensity score for a given gene to any lesion was treated as a missing observation. This produced a noticeable quantity of missing data.

Any lesion in either tissue set that possessed a definite intensity score on at least one of the five genes was deemed eligible for inclusion in the initial training data set. Training data were thus obtained from:

1. 421 malignant melanomas (primary tumors of patients diagnosed with melanoma); and
2. 98 benign nevi (nonmalignant moles belonging to other patients);
3. constituting a total of 519 separate lesions; of which
4. 213 (41.04 percent) possessed complete data on all five genes; while
5. 306 (58.96 percent) possessed a missing observation on at least one gene.

The two problem cases were intentionally excluded from the initial training data. Tissue was also collected from sixty patients with benign dysplastic nevi and from twenty-one patients with benign Spitz nevi. None of their eighty-one lesions was included. These difficult-to-diagnose lesions were excluded because neither of the two problem cases was included in the original SAM analysis.

Each of the five genes was then evaluated individually for its ability to discriminate between a benign nevus and a malignant melanoma. Discriminations were based on the four-point numeric staining intensity scores assigned by the pathologist. The ability to make correct diagnostic discriminations was uniformly assessed both by a univariate logistic regression analysis and by an accompanying receiver-operating-characteristic (ROC) analysis. Results of all five univariate analyses, including cross-tabulations of input data, details on missing observations, logistic regression statistics, and accompanying area-under-the-curve (AUC) scores, are displayed on the next few pages.

Univariate Analyses of WNT2

VALUE OF ATTRIBUTE WNT2	VALUE OF ATTRIBUTE FINALDX		
	BENIGN NEVUS	MALIGNANT MELANOMA	TOTAL
0	18	14	32
1	20	91	111
2	1	157	158
3	0	75	75
*	59	84	143
TOTAL	98	421	519

Note: There were 59/98 = 60.20 percent missing WNT2 intensity scores among benign nevi and 84/421 = 19.95 percent missing WNT2 scores among malignant melanomas, resulting in complete data for 376/519 = 72.45 percent of the lesions in the training data set.

RESULTS OF LOGISTIC REGRESSION ANALYSIS (LINEAR MODEL)

The dependent variable is a binary-coded numeric variable whose values are either 0 or 1. It is embodied in the first expression (parameter) of the LOGREG command, which is 0 IF FINALDX="BENIGN NEVUS" ELSE 1 IF FINALDX="MALIGNANT MELANOMA".

The independent variable WNT2 is just the attribute WNT2, optimally partitioned into four subscales (0 IF WNT2=0 ELSE 1 IF WNT2=1 ELSE 2 IF WNT2=2 ELSE 3 IF WNT2=3: the entire raw intensity scale is utilized).

Likelihood ratio chi-square statistic: 86.634, 2-tail p value: .0000 (based on 1 degree of freedom and 376 complete observations).

INDEPENDENT VARIABLE	REGRESSION COEFFICIENT	STANDARD DEVIATION	CHI-SQUARE (DF = 1)	2-TAIL P VALUE	ODDS RATIO MULTIPLIER
intercept	-.5085	.3290	2.3898	.1221	.6014
WNT2	2.2776	.3187	51.0580	.0000	9.7532

GOODNESS OF STATISTICAL FIT OF LOGISTIC REGRESSION MODEL

Pearson chi-square fit statistic (based on 2 degrees of freedom): 2.823, p value: .2438.

Deviance chi-square fit statistic (based on 2 degrees of freedom): 3.234, p value: .1985.

RESULT OF RECEIVER-OPERATING-CHARACTERISTIC (ROC) ANALYSIS

The area under the complete ROC curve is estimated to be AUC = 0.8859.

Univariate Analyses of ARPC2

VALUE OF ATTRIBUTE ARPC2	VALUE OF ATTRIBUTE FINALDX		
	BENIGN NEVUS	MALIGNANT MELANOMA	TOTAL
0	4	3	7
1	34	95	129
2	45	143	188
3	4	78	82
*	11	102	113
TOTAL	98	421	519

Note: There were 11/98 = 11.22 percent missing ARPC2 intensity scores among benign nevi and 102/421 = 24.23 percent missing ARPC2 scores among malignant melanomas, resulting in complete data for 406/519 = 78.23 percent of the lesions in the training data set.

RESULTS OF LOGISTIC REGRESSION ANALYSIS (LINEAR MODEL)

The dependent variable is a binary-coded numeric variable whose values are either 0 or 1. It is embodied in the first expression (parameter) of the LOGREG command, which is 0 IF FINALDX="BENIGN NEVUS" ELSE 1 IF FINALDX="MALIGNANT MELANOMA".

The independent variable ARPC2 is just the attribute ARPC2, optimally partitioned into three subscales (0 IF ARPC2=0 ELSE 1 IF ARPC2=1 OR ARPC2=2 ELSE 2 IF ARPC2=3).

Likelihood ratio chi-square statistic: 24.154, 2-tail p value: .0000 (based on 1 degree of freedom and 406 complete observations).

INDEPENDENT VARIABLE	REGRESSION COEFFICIENT	STANDARD DEVIATION	CHI-SQUARE (DF = 1)	2-TAIL P VALUE	ODDS RATIO MULTIPLIER
intercept	−.6005	.4513	1.7709	.1833	.5485
ARPC2	1.7210	.4166	17.0660	.0000	5.5899

GOODNESS OF STATISTICAL FIT OF LOGISTIC REGRESSION MODEL

Pearson chi-square fit statistic (based on 1 degree of freedom): .251, p value: .6164.

Deviance chi-square fit statistic (based on 1 degree of freedom): .249, p value: .6179.

RESULT OF RECEIVER-OPERATING-CHARACTERISTIC (ROC) ANALYSIS

The area under the complete ROC curve is estimated to be AUC = 0.6122.

Univariate Analyses of OPN

VALUE OF ATTRIBUTE OPN	VALUE OF ATTRIBUTE FINALDX		
	BENIGN NEVUS	MALIGNANT MELANOMA	TOTAL
0	9	32	41
1	43	101	144
2	24	119	143
3	7	63	70
*	15	106	121
TOTAL	98	421	519

Note: There were 15/98 = 15.31 percent missing OPN intensity scores among benign nevi and 106/421 = 25.18 percent missing OPN scores among malignant melanomas, resulting in complete data for 398/519 = 76.69 percent of the lesions in the training data set. OPN stands for osteopontin, which is an alternative designator of the SPP1 gene.

RESULTS OF LOGISTIC REGRESSION ANALYSIS (LINEAR MODEL)

The dependent variable is a binary-coded numeric variable whose values are either 0 or 1. It is embodied in the first expression (parameter) of the LOGREG command, which is 0 IF FINALDX="BENIGN NEVUS" ELSE 1 IF FINALDX="MALIGNANT MELANOMA".

The independent variable OPN is just the attribute OPN, optimally partitioned into three subscales (0 IF OPN=0 OR OPN=1 ELSE 1 IF OPN=2 ELSE 2 IF OPN=3).

Likelihood ratio chi-square statistic: 12.880, 2-tail p value: .0003 (based on 1 degree of freedom and 398 complete observations).

INDEPENDENT VARIABLE	REGRESSION COEFFICIENT	STANDARD DEVIATION	CHI-SQUARE (DF = 1)	2-TAIL P VALUE	ODDS RATIO MULTIPLIER
intercept	.9437	.1579	35.6955	.0000	2.5694
OPN	.6404	.1882	11.5818	.0007	1.8973

GOODNESS OF STATISTICAL FIT OF LOGISTIC REGRESSION MODEL

Pearson chi-square fit statistic (based on 1 degree of freedom): .011, p value: .9156.

Deviance chi-square fit statistic (based on 1 degree of freedom): .011, p value: .9157.

RESULT OF RECEIVER-OPERATING-CHARACTERISTIC (ROC) ANALYSIS

The area under the complete ROC curve is estimated to be AUC = 0.6151.

Univariate Analyses of RGS1

VALUE OF ATTRIBUTE RGS1	VALUE OF ATTRIBUTE FINALDX		
	BENIGN NEVUS	MALIGNANT MELANOMA	TOTAL
0	1	18	19
1	18	69	87
2	37	108	145
3	7	76	83
*	35	150	185
TOTAL	98	421	519

Note: There were 35/98 = 35.71 percent missing RGS1 intensity scores among benign nevi and 150/421 = 35.63 percent missing RGS1 scores among malignant melanomas, resulting in complete data for 334/519 = 64.35 percent of the lesions in the training data set.

RESULTS OF LOGISTIC REGRESSION ANALYSIS (LINEAR MODEL)

The dependent variable is a binary-coded numeric variable whose values are either 0 or 1. It is embodied in the first expression (parameter) of the LOGREG command, which is 0 IF FINALDX="BENIGN NEVUS" ELSE 1 IF FINALDX="MALIGNANT MELANOMA".

The independent variable RGS1 is just the attribute RGS1, optimally partitioned into two subscales (0 IF RGS1=0 OR RGS1=1 OR RGS1=2 ELSE 1 IF RGS1=3).

Likelihood ratio chi-square statistic: 8.977, 2-tail p value: .0027 (based on 1 degree of freedom and 334 complete observations).

INDEPENDENT VARIABLE	REGRESSION COEFFICIENT	STANDARD DEVIATION	CHI-SQUARE (DF = 1)	2-TAIL P VALUE	ODDS RATIO MULTIPLIER
intercept	1.2476	.1516	67.7225	.0000	3.4821
RGS1	1.1372	.4231	7.2244	.0072	3.1179

GOODNESS OF STATISTICAL FIT OF LOGISTIC REGRESSION MODEL

Analysis impossible, since there were too few distinct values of the independent variable (partitioned subscales of the RGS1 attribute).

RESULT OF RECEIVER-OPERATING-CHARACTERISTIC (ROC) ANALYSIS

The area under the complete ROC curve is estimated to be AUC = 0.5847.

Univariate Analyses of FN1

VALUE OF ATTRIBUTE FN1	VALUE OF ATTRIBUTE FINALDX		
	BENIGN NEVUS	MALIGNANT MELANOMA	TOTAL
0	29	75	104
1	33	144	177
2	18	63	81
3	0	9	9
*	18	130	148
TOTAL	98	421	519

Note: There were 18/98 = 18.37 percent missing FN1 intensity scores among benign nevi and 130/421 = 30.88 percent missing FN1 scores among malignant melanomas, resulting in complete data for 371/519 = 71.48 percent of the lesions in the training data set.

RESULTS OF LOGISTIC REGRESSION ANALYSIS (LINEAR MODEL)

The dependent variable is a binary-coded numeric variable whose values are either 0 or 1. It is embodied in the first expression (parameter) of the LOGREG command, which is 0 IF FINALDX="BENIGN NEVUS" ELSE 1 IF FINALDX="MALIGNANT MELANOMA".

The independent variable FN1 is just the attribute FN1, optimally partitioned into three subscales (0 IF FN1=0 ELSE 1 IF FN1=1 OR FN1=2 ELSE 2 IF FN1=3).

Likelihood ratio chi-square statistic: 4.746, 2-tail p value: .0294 (based on 1 degree of freedom and 371 complete observations).

INDEPENDENT VARIABLE	REGRESSION COEFFICIENT	STANDARD DEVIATION	CHI-SQUARE (DF = 1)	2-TAIL P VALUE	ODDS RATIO MULTIPLIER
intercept	.8998	.2121	17.9999	.0000	2.4591
FN1	.5540	.2534	4.7789	.0288	1.7402

GOODNESS OF STATISTICAL FIT OF LOGISTIC REGRESSION MODEL

Pearson chi-square fit statistic (based on 1 degree of freedom): 1.376, p value: .2407.

Deviance chi-square fit statistic (based on 1 degree of freedom): 2.435, p value: .1187.

RESULT OF RECEIVER-OPERATING-CHARACTERISTIC (ROC) ANALYSIS

The area under the complete ROC curve is estimated to be AUC = 0.5622.

Multivariate Analysis of All Five Genes

The five genes were then combined to produce a multimarker diagnostic assay. A multivariate logistic regression analysis was executed with the same dependent variable used in each univariate analysis and with the five optimally partitioned staining intensity scores as independent variables. Complete data existed for 213/519 = 41.04 percent of the lesions.

RESULTS OF LOGISTIC REGRESSION ANALYSIS (LINEAR MODEL)

The dependent variable is a binary-coded numeric variable whose values are either 0 or 1. It is embodied in the first expression (parameter) of the LOGREG command, which is 0 IF FINALDX="BENIGN NEVUS" ELSE 1 IF FINALDX="MALIGNANT MELANOMA".

The independent variable WNT2 is the optimally partitioned attribute WNT2.
The independent variable ARPC2 is the optimally partitioned attribute ARPC2.
The independent variable OPN is the optimally partitioned attribute OPN.
The independent variable RGS1 is the optimally partitioned attribute RGS1.
The independent variable FN1 is the optimally partitioned attribute FN1.

Likelihood ratio chi-square statistic: 70.569, 2-tail p value: .0000 (based on 5 degrees of freedom and 213 complete observations).

INDEPENDENT VARIABLE	REGRESSION COEFFICIENT	STANDARD DEVIATION	CHI-SQUARE (DF = 1)	2-TAIL P VALUE	ODDS RATIO MULTIPLIER
intercept	-2.1665	1.0306	4.4196	.0355	.1146
WNT2	2.5462	.4938	26.5896	.0000	12.7582
ARPC2	.4675	.8543	.2995	.5842	1.5960
OPN	.1314	.3808	.1190	.7301	1.1404
RGS1	1.1746	.7672	2.3439	.1258	3.2367
FN1	.1753	.5393	.1057	.7451	1.1916

GOODNESS OF STATISTICAL FIT OF LOGISTIC REGRESSION MODEL

Pearson chi-square fit statistic (based on 55 degrees of freedom): 31.565, p value: .9953.

Deviance chi-square fit statistic (based on 55 degrees of freedom): 29.327, p value: .9982.

RESULT OF RECEIVER-OPERATING-CHARACTERISTIC (ROC) ANALYSIS

The area under the complete ROC curve is estimated to be AUC = 0.9067.

The probability of being a malignant melanoma (as opposed to a benign nevus) was computed from the above multivariate output statistics for each of the 213 lesions with no missing observations. Probabilities were computed according to the procedure described in sections 2.3 and 2.4 of this book. These probabilities ranged from 0.1546 to 0.9996, with a mean of 0.8545.

An optimum separation probability was also identified. It was optimum in the sense that, when all lesions with equal or higher probability were diagnosed as malignant while all lesions with lower probability were diagnosed as benign, the simple average (i.e., unweighted mean) of the resulting sensitivity and specificity of diagnostic discrimination was maximized.

The optimum separation probability was 0.8288. The resulting sensitivity was 138/182 = 75.82 percent, the resulting specificity was 29/31 = 93.55 percent, and adopting the optimizing probability as a separation criterion produced (138+29)/213 = 78.40 percent correct diagnoses.

Regrettably, only 213/519 = 41.04 percent of the training lesions possessed complete data. The remaining 306/519 = 58.96 percent could not be diagnosed using the conventional methodology just illustrated. Its effective success rate was thereby reduced to (138+29)/519 = 32.18 percent.

The directional indications of the SAM analysis were fully confirmed. All five univariate logistic regression analyses assigned positive regression coefficients to the five genes. The multivariate logistic regression analysis combining all five genes into an extraordinarily close-fitting multimarker diagnostic assay also assigned positive regression coefficients to each of the five genes. A relatively greater expression of each gene was thereby confirmed as pointing to a malignant melanoma rather than to a benign nevus.

The foregoing analyses were exploratory. The proper way to measure and calibrate gene expression as an indicator of anything related to melanoma had not yet been established. That is why the training data were used to partition optimally each gene's four-point staining intensity scale so as to reflect as closely as possible that gene's univariate relationship to malignancy.

Because of this the usual hypothesis-testing interpretation of chi-square statistics and accompanying p values were rendered inappropriate both in the five univariate and in the multivariate logistic regression analyses. One cannot legitimately partition measurement scales to improve their relationship to malignancy and then use the same partitioned scale values either to test whether or not such a relationship really exists or to judge the goodness of its statistical fit with an assumed linear regression model. With the aid of such optimizing scale partitioning, however, one can conclude that apparent relationships in the predicted direction were uniformly detected and that the multivariate linear regression model fit the data extraordinarily closely.

Only when a diagnostic algorithm is derived from these training data and subsequently tested against independently gathered validation data can formal hypothesis tests be performed in the traditional manner. Exactly that will be accomplished and reported, following some additional analyses.

5.2 Act II: Exploiting a Serendipitous Discovery

The pathologist noticed an intriguing pattern while scoring the staining intensity of WNT2 (the first gene processed). This pattern was detected after observing approximately the first fifty lesions under the microscope. It appeared that protein staining was systematically more intense in the junctional zone of a benign nevus compared with a noticeable loss of intensity at its base. In contrast, staining intensity was observed to be more uniform between the junctional zone and the base of each malignant melanoma.

To see if the same pattern persisted lesions were then rescored for staining intensity both at the top (junctional zone) and at the bottom (base) of each melanocytic neoplasm whose top-to-bottom orientation was clearly discernible. The training data set was thereby doubled in size. It now included both top and bottom intensity scores assigned, separately, to each of the 519 lesions for each of the five genes. (Note: Act I analyses and results were derived primarily from the bottom intensity scores of all five genes.)

Univariate Top-to-Bottom Difference Analyses of WNT2

Top and bottom intensity scores were cross-tabulated, as shown below.

VALUE OF ATTRIBUTE WNT2BOT	VALUE OF ATTRIBUTE WNT2TOP				
	0	1	2	3	TOTAL
0	6	8	10	0	24
1	0	28	18	2	48
2	0	0	53	1	54
3	0	0	0	18	18
TOTAL	6	36	81	21	144

Note: There were 287/519 = 55.30 percent missing WNT2TOP intensity scores and 143/519 = 27.55 percent missing WNT2BOT intensity scores, resulting in complete data for 144/519 = 27.75 percent of the training lesions.

Top-to-bottom difference scores could then be calculated for these 144 lesions and cross-tabulated with the final (assumed correct) diagnosis of each lesion.

VALUE OF ATTRIBUTE WTBDIFF	VALUE OF ATTRIBUTE FINALDX		
	BENIGN NEVUS	MALIGNANT MELANOMA	TOTAL
-2	12	0	12
-1	27	0	27
0	0	105	105
TOTAL	39	105	144

Note: Each top score is subtracted from its corresponding bottom score to obtain a top-to-bottom difference. Negative WTBDIFF scores (top staining intensity greater than bottom staining intensity) are associated with benign nevi, while zero or positive WTBDIFF scores (more uniform top and bottom intensity) are associated with malignant melanomas.

	BENIGN NEVUS	MALIGNANT MELANOMA	TOTAL
WTBDIFF LESS THAN 0	39	0	39
WTBDIFF AT LEAST 0	0	105	105
TOTAL	39	105	144

Note: The diagnostic cross-table shown above uses WTBDIFF scores with a cutoff value of 0 to discriminate between benign nevi and malignant melanomas. When their value of WTBDIFF is less than 0 lesions are diagnosed as benign. When their value of WTBDIFF is at least 0 lesions are diagnosed as malignant. This results in a diagnostic sensitivity of 105/105 = 100.00 percent and a diagnostic specificity of 39/39 = 100.00 percent (i.e., a 100 percent perfect diagnostic discrimination).

A Fisher exact test of the diagnostic cross-table produced a significant result in the direction hypothesized by the pathologist, with a two-tailed p value less than 0.00005. A ROC analysis of the same WTBDIFF data produced an area under the complete ROC curve estimated to be AUC = 1.0000 (equivalently indicating a 100 percent perfect diagnostic discrimination).

Univariate Top-to-Bottom Difference Analyses of ARPC2

Top and bottom intensity scores were cross-tabulated, as shown below.

VALUE OF ATTRIBUTE ARPC2BOT	VALUE OF ATTRIBUTE ARPC2TOP			
	1	2	3	TOTAL
0	2	3	0	5
1	30	24	4	58
2	0	70	11	81
3	0	0	25	25
TOTAL	32	97	40	169

Note: There were 297/519 = 57.23 percent missing ARPC2TOP intensity scores and 113/519 = 21.77 percent missing ARPC2BOT intensity scores, resulting in complete data for 169/519 = 32.56 percent of the training lesions.

Top-to-bottom difference scores could then be calculated for these 169 lesions and cross-tabulated with the final (assumed correct) diagnosis of each lesion.

VALUE OF ATTRIBUTE ATBDIFF	VALUE OF ATTRIBUTE FINALDX		
	BENIGN NEVUS	MALIGNANT MELANOMA	TOTAL
-2	6	1	7
-1	34	3	37
0	27	98	125
TOTAL	67	102	169

Note: Each top score is subtracted from its corresponding bottom score to obtain a top-to-bottom difference. Negative ATBDIFF scores (top staining intensity greater than bottom staining intensity) are associated with benign nevi, while zero or positive ATBDIFF scores (more uniform top and bottom intensity) are associated with malignant melanomas.

	BENIGN NEVUS	MALIGNANT MELANOMA	TOTAL
ATBDIFF LESS THAN 0	40	4	44
ATBDIFF AT LEAST 0	27	98	125
TOTAL	67	102	169

Note: The diagnostic cross-table shown above uses ATBDIFF scores with a cutoff value of 0 to discriminate between benign nevi and malignant melanomas. When their value of ATBDIFF is less than 0 lesions are diagnosed as benign. When their value of ATBDIFF is at least 0 lesions are diagnosed as malignant. This results in a diagnostic sensitivity of 98/102 = 96.08 percent and a diagnostic specificity of 40/67 = 59.70 percent.

A Fisher exact test of the diagnostic cross-table produced a significant result in the direction hypothesized by the pathologist, with a two-tailed p value less than 0.00005. A ROC analysis of the same ATBDIFF data produced an area under the complete ROC curve estimated to be AUC = 0.7777.

Univariate Top-to-Bottom Difference Analyses of OPN

Top and bottom intensity scores were cross-tabulated, as shown below.

VALUE OF ATTRIBUTE OPNBOT	VALUE OF ATTRIBUTE OPNTOP				
	0	1	2	3	TOTAL
0	11	3	4	0	18
1	0	40	18	5	63
2	0	1	51	11	63
3	0	0	0	25	25
TOTAL	11	44	73	41	169

Note: There were 313/519 = 60.31 percent missing OPNTOP intensity scores and 121/519 = 23.31 percent missing OPNBOT intensity scores, resulting in complete data for 169/519 = 32.56 percent of the training lesions.

Top-to-bottom difference scores could then be calculated for these 169 lesions and cross-tabulated with the final (assumed correct) diagnosis of each lesion.

VALUE OF ATTRIBUTE OTBDIFF	VALUE OF ATTRIBUTE FINALDX		
	BENIGN NEVUS	MALIGNANT MELANOMA	TOTAL
-2	9	0	9
-1	31	1	32
0	24	103	127
1	1	0	1
TOTAL	65	104	169

Note: Each top score is subtracted from its corresponding bottom score to obtain a top-to-bottom difference. Negative OTBDIFF scores (top staining intensity greater than bottom staining intensity) are associated with benign nevi, while zero or positive OTBDIFF scores (more uniform top and bottom intensity) are associated with malignant melanomas.

	BENIGN NEVUS	MALIGNANT MELANOMA	TOTAL
OTBDIFF LESS THAN 0	40	1	41
OTBDIFF AT LEAST 0	25	103	128
TOTAL	65	104	169

Note: The diagnostic cross-table shown above uses OTBDIFF scores with a cutoff value of 0 to discriminate between benign nevi and malignant melanomas. When their value of OTBDIFF is less than 0 lesions are diagnosed as benign. When their value of OTBDIFF is at least 0 lesions are diagnosed as malignant. This results in a diagnostic sensitivity of 103/104 = 99.04 percent and a diagnostic specificity of 40/65 = 61.54 percent.

A Fisher exact test of the diagnostic cross-table produced a significant result in the direction hypothesized by the pathologist, with a two-tailed p value less than 0.00005. A ROC analysis of the same OTBDIFF data produced an area under the complete ROC curve estimated to be AUC = 0.7959.

Univariate Top-to-Bottom Difference Analyses of RGS1

Top and bottom intensity scores were cross-tabulated, as shown below.

VALUE OF ATTRIBUTE RGS1BOT	\	\	\	\	\
	0	1	2	3	TOTAL
0	8	0	0	0	8
1	0	28	9	1	38
2	0	1	55	6	62
3	0	0	0	33	33
TOTAL	8	29	64	40	141

Note: There were 341/519 = 65.70 percent missing RGS1TOP intensity scores and 185/519 = 35.65 percent missing RGS1BOT intensity scores, resulting in complete data for 141/519 = 27.17 percent of the training lesions.

Top-to-bottom difference scores could then be calculated for these 141 lesions and cross-tabulated with the final (assumed correct) diagnosis of each lesion.

VALUE OF ATTRIBUTE RTBDIFF	VALUE OF ATTRIBUTE FINALDX		
	BENIGN NEVUS	MALIGNANT MELANOMA	TOTAL
-2	1	0	1
-1	14	1	15
0	29	95	124
1	1	0	1
TOTAL	45	96	141

Note: Each top score is subtracted from its corresponding bottom score to obtain a top-to-bottom difference. Negative RTBDIFF scores (top staining intensity greater than bottom staining intensity) are associated with benign nevi, while zero or positive RTBDIFF scores (more uniform top and bottom intensity) are associated with malignant melanomas.

	BENIGN NEVUS	MALIGNANT MELANOMA	TOTAL
RTBDIFF LESS THAN 0	15	1	16
RTBDIFF AT LEAST 0	30	95	125
TOTAL	45	96	141

Note: The diagnostic cross-table shown above uses RTBDIFF scores with a cutoff value of 0 to discriminate between benign nevi and malignant melanomas. When their value of RTBDIFF is less than 0 lesions are diagnosed as benign. When their value of RTBDIFF is at least 0 lesions are diagnosed as malignant. This results in a diagnostic sensitivity of 95/96 = 98.96 percent and a diagnostic specificity of 15/45 = 33.33 percent.

A Fisher exact test of the diagnostic cross-table produced a significant result in the direction hypothesized by the pathologist, with a two-tailed p value equal to 0.0014. A ROC analysis of the same RTBDIFF data produced an area under the complete ROC curve estimated to be AUC = 0.6506.

Univariate Top-to-Bottom Difference Analyses of FN1

Top and bottom intensity scores were cross-tabulated, as shown below.

VALUE OF ATTRIBUTE FN1BOT	VALUE OF ATTRIBUTE FN1TOP				
	0	1	2	3	TOTAL
0	26	10	0	0	36
1	3	57	1	0	61
2	0	2	30	0	32
3	0	0	0	2	2
TOTAL	29	69	31	2	131

Note: There were 330/519 = 63.58 percent missing FN1TOP intensity scores and 148/519 = 28.52 percent missing FN1BOT intensity scores, resulting in complete data for 131/519 = 25.24 percent of the training lesions.

Top-to-bottom difference scores could then be calculated for these 131 lesions and cross-tabulated with the final (assumed correct) diagnosis of each lesion.

VALUE OF ATTRIBUTE FTBDIFF	VALUE OF ATTRIBUTE FINALDX		
	BENIGN NEVUS	MALIGNANT MELANOMA	TOTAL
-1	10	1	11
0	29	86	115
1	4	1	5
TOTAL	43	88	131

Note: Each top score is subtracted from its corresponding bottom score to obtain a top-to-bottom difference. Negative FTBDIFF scores (top staining intensity greater than bottom staining intensity) are associated with benign nevi, while zero or positive FTBDIFF scores (more uniform top and bottom intensity) are associated with malignant melanomas.

	BENIGN NEVUS	MALIGNANT MELANOMA	TOTAL
FTBDIFF LESS THAN 0	10	1	11
FTBDIFF AT LEAST 0	33	87	120
TOTAL	43	88	131

Note: The diagnostic cross-table shown above uses FTBDIFF scores with a cutoff value of 0 to discriminate between benign nevi and malignant melanomas. When their value of FTBDIFF is less than 0 lesions are diagnosed as benign. When their value of FTBDIFF is at least 0 lesions are diagnosed as malignant. This results in a diagnostic sensitivity of 87/88 = 98.86 percent and a diagnostic specificity of 10/43 = 23.26 percent.

A Fisher exact test of the diagnostic cross-table produced a significant result in the direction hypothesized by the pathologist, with a two-tailed p value equal to 0.0101. A ROC analysis of the same FTBDIFF data produced an area under the complete ROC curve estimated to be AUC = 0.5690.

The next task was to combine the five top-to-bottom difference scores into a multimarker diagnostic assay analogous to the multimarker assay obtained by combining separate (primarily bottom) intensity scores for all five genes.

Review of the univariate top-to-bottom difference analyses of WNT2 shows a 100 percent perfect diagnostic discrimination. The two distributions of difference scores for benign nevi and malignant melanomas, respectively, were perfectly separated. Among the 144 lesions where top-to-bottom differences were clearly discernible each of the thirty-nine nevi lost expression intensity from its junctional zone to its base. Each of the 105 melanomas displayed uniform expression intensity between its junctional zone and its base. This triggered a strictly computational failure. Logistic regression's maximum likelihood procedure for estimating multivariate regression coefficients and their associated chi-square and p values failed to produce precise numeric results in the face of WNT2's perfect top-to-bottom difference discrimination.

Such perfect discrimination presents no problem for DSSA. In addition, DSSA is specifically designed to handle the very large amount of partially missing data among top-to-bottom difference scores. Logistic regression typically excludes any lesion possessing less than complete data on all five differences.

At least one of the five top-to-bottom difference scores could be calculated for 235 of the 519 training lesions. DSSA analyses of top-to-bottom differences drawn from these 235 lesions are shown below and on the next page.

The diagnostic algorithm produced by DSSA was:

"DIAGNOSED MALIGNANT: WTBDIFF>=0" IF WTBDIFF>=0 ELSE
"DIAGNOSED BENIGN: WTBDIFF<0" IF WTBDIFF<0 ELSE
"DIAGNOSED BENIGN: OTBDIFF<0" IF OTBDIFF<0 ELSE
"DIAGNOSED BENIGN: RTBDIFF<0" IF RTBDIFF<0 ELSE
"DIAGNOSED BENIGN: FTBDIFF<0" IF FTBDIFF<0 ELSE
"DIAGNOSED BENIGN: ATBDIFF<0" IF ATBDIFF<0 ELSE
"DIAGNOSED MALIGNANT: RTBDIFF>=0" IF RTBDIFF>=0 ELSE
"DIAGNOSED MALIGNANT: FTBDIFF>=0" IF FTBDIFF>=0 ELSE
"DIAGNOSED MALIGNANT: OTBDIFF>=0" IF OTBDIFF>=0 ELSE
"DIAGNOSED MALIGNANT: SINCE ATBDIFF>=0" IF ATBDIFF>=0 ELSE
"NO DIAGNOSTIC CONCLUSION"

Results of applying this diagnostic algorithm to the 519 training lesions were:

| | CORRECT DIAGNOSIS OF LESION | | |
DSSA-GENERATED DIAGNOSTIC CONCLUSION	BENIGN	MALIGNANT	TOTAL
DIAGNOSED MALIGNANT: WTBDIFF>=0	0	105	105
DIAGNOSED BENIGN: WTBDIFF<0	39	0	39
DIAGNOSED BENIGN: OTBDIFF<0	17	0	17
DIAGNOSED BENIGN: RTBDIFF<0	4	0	4
DIAGNOSED BENIGN: FTBDIFF<0	2	0	2
DIAGNOSED BENIGN: ATBDIFF<0	5	2	7
DIAGNOSED MALIGNANT: RTBDIFF>=0	5	14	19
DIAGNOSED MALIGNANT: FTBDIFF>=0	6	20	26
DIAGNOSED MALIGNANT: OTBDIFF>=0	2	7	9
DIAGNOSED MALIGNANT: ATBDIFF>=0	3	4	7
NO DIAGNOSTIC CONCLUSION	15	269	284
TOTAL	98	421	519

A summarized version of the same diagnostic algorithm was:

```
"POSITIVE TEST: INDICATES MALIGNANT" IF WTBDIFF>=0 ELSE
"NEGATIVE TEST: INDICATES BENIGN" IF WTBDIFF<0 ELSE
"NEGATIVE TEST: INDICATES BENIGN" IF OTBDIFF<0 ELSE
"NEGATIVE TEST: INDICATES BENIGN" IF RTBDIFF<0 ELSE
"NEGATIVE TEST: INDICATES BENIGN" IF FTBDIFF<0 ELSE
"NEGATIVE TEST: INDICATES BENIGN" IF ATBDIFF<0 ELSE
"POSITIVE TEST: INDICATES MALIGNANT" IF RTBDIFF>=0 ELSE
"POSITIVE TEST: INDICATES MALIGNANT" IF FTBDIFF>=0 ELSE
"POSITIVE TEST: INDICATES MALIGNANT" IF OTBDIFF>=0 ELSE
"POSITIVE TEST: INDICATES MALIGNANT" IF ATBDIFF>=0 ELSE
"NO DIAGNOSTIC CONCLUSION"
```

Results of applying the summarized algorithm to the same 519 lesions were:

	CORRECT DIAGNOSIS OF LESION		
DSSA-GENERATED DIAGNOSTIC CONCLUSION	BENIGN	MALIGNANT	TOTAL
NEGATIVE TEST: INDICATES BENIGN	67	2	69
POSITIVE TEST: INDICATES MALIGNANT	16	150	166
NO DIAGNOSTIC CONCLUSION	15	269	284
TOTAL	98	421	519

Accuracy measures for the 235 lesions about which DSSA was able to draw a definite diagnostic conclusion were then computed. Notice that definite, but proportionately unhelpful conclusions were drawn for the seven lesions at the very end of the algorithm (when ATBDIFF>=0). DSSA was instructed to draw a definite (even if incorrect) conclusion concerning all 519 lesions.

For these 235 lesions DSSA's analysis of top-to-bottom difference scores achieved a sensitivity of $150/(150+2) = 98.68$ percent. This compared to a sensitivity of 75.82 percent achieved by the five-marker assay of the 213 lesions possessing complete data analyzed by multivariate logistic regression in Act I. The DSSA analysis also achieved a specificity of $67/(67+16) = 80.72$ percent, compared to a 93.55 percent specificity in ACT I; $(150+67)/235 = 92.34$ percent correct diagnoses, compared to 78.40 percent correct diagnoses achieved in Act I; and an AUC of 0.8970, compared to an AUC of 0.9067 achieved in Act I.

Top-to-bottom difference scores analyzed by DSSA in Act II produced a decidedly higher percentage of correct diagnoses (92.34 versus 78.40 percent) for a slightly larger number of training lesions (235 versus 213) when compared to the five-marker assay obtained from multivariate logistic regression in Act I. Much more interesting, however, was the very different sensitivity and specificity produced by these two different sets of scores. Analysis of top-to-bottom intensity differences achieved much superior sensitivity in Act II. Analysis of primarily bottom expression intensity achieved noticeably superior specificity in Act I. This strongly suggested combining the results of both sets of scores to exploit each one's separate type of diagnostic potency.

Review of the univariate top-to-bottom difference analyses of all five genes also showed a definite, though less-than-perfect positive correlation between top scores and bottom scores associated with each gene. Act III will therefore attempt to combine and integrate the apparently useful information contained, separately, in top expression intensity, bottom expression intensity, and top-to-bottom intensity difference scores into a single diagnostic algorithm.

5.3 Act III: Combining and Integrating Top Intensity Scores, Bottom Intensity
         Scores, and Top-to-Bottom Intensity Difference Scores into a
         Single Diagnostic Algorithm

It was not possible to include top intensity scores, bottom intensity scores,
and top-to-bottom intensity difference scores as independent variables in a
single multivariate regression analysis. These three sets of scores are defined
in such a way as to be linearly interdependent. No form of regression analysis
can accept as inputs linearly interdependent diagnostic indicators. This is a
strictly logical problem. Act III required a different methodology for this
reason, as well as due to the perfect separation of WTBDIFF scores.

DSSA was specifically designed to accept as possible inputs linearly
interdependent diagnostic indicators. Therefore, DSSA was applied to all three
sets of scores describing the 519 training lesions in order to distinguish
between the ninety-eight benign nevi and the 421 malignant melanomas.

The following conventions were adopted in applying DSSA to the training data.

1. DSSA first checked for the proper diagnostic directionality of all its
   input indicators. We know from previous analyses that all five bottom
   intensity scores and all five top-to-bottom intensity difference scores
   pointed in the proper direction (i.e., in the direction previously
   observed during the SAM analysis and in the direction hypothesized by
   the pathologist, respectively). DSSA verified proper directionality for
   each of these ten indicators.
2. Initial directionality checks of the five top intensity scores revealed
   that only WNT2TOP and FN1TOP pointed in the same (SAM-observed)
   direction as their corresponding bottom scores. ARPC2TOP, OPNTOP, and
   RGS1TOP scores pointed in the opposite direction. Univariate logistic
   regression analyses strongly suggested that the opposite directionality
   of these top scores was systematic—not due to random noise in the
   data. ARPC2TOP's two-tailed p value was 0.0004. OPNTOP's two-tailed p
   value was less than 0.00005. RGS1TOP's two-tailed p value was 0.0178.
3. Since the maximum score assigned by the pathologist to each indicator
   was 3 (signifying intense expression), each indicator's top intensity
   score was subtracted from 3 to reverse its directional orientation.
   That produced fifteen directionally compatible indicators from which
   DSSA could then construct fifteen matched pairs of discriminators
   (thirty discriminators in all).
4. DSSA was again required to make a definite diagnosis of all 519
   training lesions, even when adding relatively impotent discriminators
   to the end of the diagnostic algorithm reduced overall accuracy. Doing
   so guaranteed an algorithm applicable to all conceivable lesions.
5. After several trial-and-error runs, DSSA's weight on sensitivity was
   raised from a balanced value of 0.50 to 0.55 to nudge the diagnosis in
   the direction of slightly more sensitive than specific discriminations.

Results of this DSSA analysis are presented on the next three pages.

The diagnostic algorithm produced by DSSA was:

```
"DIAGNOSED BENIGN: WTBDIFF<0" IF WTBDIFF<0 ELSE
"DIAGNOSED MALIGNANT: WTBDIFF>=0" IF WTBDIFF>=0 ELSE
"DIAGNOSED MALIGNANT: WNT2BOT>=2" IF WNT2BOT>=2 ELSE
"DIAGNOSED BENIGN: OTBDIFF<0" IF OTBDIFF<0 ELSE
"DIAGNOSED BENIGN: RTBDIFF<0" IF RTBDIFF<0 ELSE
"DIAGNOSED MALIGNANT: 3-RGS1TOP>=2" IF 3-RGS1TOP>=2 ELSE
"DIAGNOSED BENIGN: FTBDIFF<0" IF FTBDIFF<0 ELSE
"DIAGNOSED BENIGN: ATBDIFF<0" IF ATBDIFF<0 ELSE
"DIAGNOSED BENIGN: 3-OPNTOP<1" IF 3-OPNTOP<1 ELSE
"DIAGNOSED MALIGNANT: RGS1BOT>=3" IF RGS1BOT>=3 ELSE
"DIAGNOSED MALIGNANT: 3-ARPC2TOP>=2" IF 3-ARPC2TOP>=2 ELSE
"DIAGNOSED BENIGN: FN1TOP<1" IF FN1TOP<1 ELSE
"DIAGNOSED BENIGN: WNT2TOP<2" IF WNT2TOP<2 ELSE
"DIAGNOSED MALIGNANT: RTBDIFF>=0" IF RTBDIFF>=0 ELSE
"DIAGNOSED MALIGNANT: FN1TOP>=1" IF FN1TOP>=1 ELSE
"DIAGNOSED MALIGNANT: FTBDIFF>=0" IF FTBDIFF>=0 ELSE
"DIAGNOSED BENIGN: 3-ARPC2TOP<2" IF 3-ARPC2TOP<2 ELSE
"DIAGNOSED MALIGNANT: ATBDIFF>=0" IF ATBDIFF>=0 ELSE
"DIAGNOSED MALIGNANT: 3-OPNTOP>=1" IF 3-OPNTOP>=1 ELSE
"DIAGNOSED MALIGNANT: OTBDIFF>=0" IF OTBDIFF>=0 ELSE
"DIAGNOSED MALIGNANT: FN1BOT>=1" IF FN1BOT>=1 ELSE
"DIAGNOSED BENIGN: ARPC2BOT<1" IF ARPC2BOT<1 ELSE
"DIAGNOSED MALIGNANT: OPNBOT>=2" IF OPNBOT>=2 ELSE
"DIAGNOSED MALIGNANT: WNT2TOP>=2" IF WNT2TOP>=2 ELSE
"DIAGNOSED MALIGNANT: ARPC2BOT>=1" IF ARPC2BOT>=1 ELSE
"DIAGNOSED BENIGN: RGS1BOT<3" IF RGS1BOT<3 ELSE
"DIAGNOSED BENIGN: FN1BOT<1" IF FN1BOT<1 ELSE
"DIAGNOSED BENIGN: 3-RGS1TOP<2" IF 3-RGS1TOP<2 ELSE
"DIAGNOSED BENIGN: WNT2BOT<2" IF WNT2BOT<2 ELSE
"DIAGNOSED BENIGN: OPNBOT<2" IF OPNBOT<2 ELSE
"NO DIAGNOSTIC CONCLUSION"
```

Results of applying this diagnostic algorithm to all 519 training lesions were:

DSSA-GENERATED DIAGNOSTIC CONCLUSION	CORRECT DIAGNOSIS OF LESION		
	BENIGN	MALIGNANT	TOTAL
DIAGNOSED BENIGN: WTBDIFF<0	39	0	39
DIAGNOSED MALIGNANT: WTBDIFF>=0	0	105	105
DIAGNOSED MALIGNANT: WNT2BOT>=2	0	161	161
DIAGNOSED BENIGN: OTBDIFF<0	17	0	17
DIAGNOSED BENIGN: RTBDIFF<0	4	0	4
DIAGNOSED MALIGNANT: 3-RGS1TOP>=2	0	13	13
DIAGNOSED BENIGN: FTBDIFF<0	2	0	2
DIAGNOSED BENIGN: ATBDIFF<0	5	1	6
DIAGNOSED BENIGN: 3-OPNTOP<1	3	2	5
DIAGNOSED MALIGNANT: RGS1BOT>=3	1	24	25
DIAGNOSED MALIGNANT: 3-ARPC2TOP>=2	1	17	18
DIAGNOSED BENIGN: FN1TOP<1	3	6	9
DIAGNOSED BENIGN: WNT2TOP<2	13	7	20
DIAGNOSED MALIGNANT: RTBDIFF>=0	0	2	2
DIAGNOSED MALIGNANT: FN1TOP>=1	1	16	17
DIAGNOSED BENIGN: 3-ARPC2TOP<2	2	6	8
DIAGNOSED MALIGNANT: 3-OPNTOP>=1	1	5	6
DIAGNOSED MALIGNANT: FN1BOT>=1	1	29	30
DIAGNOSED MALIGNANT: OPNBOT>=2	1	9	10

```
DIAGNOSED MALIGNANT: WNT2TOP>=2              0          2          2
DIAGNOSED MALIGNANT: ARPC2BOT>=1             3         12         15
DIAGNOSED BENIGN: RGS1BOT<3                  1          1          2
DIAGNOSED BENIGN: 3-RGS1TOP<2                0          1          1
DIAGNOSED BENIGN: WNT2BOT<2                  0          1          1
DIAGNOSED BENIGN: OPNBOT<2                   0          1          1

TOTAL                                       98        421        519
```

A summarized version of the same diagnostic algorithm was:

```
"NEGATIVE TEST: INDICATES BENIGN" IF WTBDIFF<0 ELSE
"POSITIVE TEST: INDICATES MALIGNANT" IF WTBDIFF>=0 ELSE
"POSITIVE TEST: INDICATES MALIGNANT" IF WNT2BOT>=2 ELSE
"NEGATIVE TEST: INDICATES BENIGN" IF OTBDIFF<0 ELSE
"NEGATIVE TEST: INDICATES BENIGN" IF RTBDIFF<0 ELSE
"POSITIVE TEST: INDICATES MALIGNANT" IF 3-RGS1TOP>=2 ELSE
"NEGATIVE TEST: INDICATES BENIGN" IF FTBDIFF<0 ELSE
"NEGATIVE TEST: INDICATES BENIGN" IF ATBDIFF<0 ELSE
"NEGATIVE TEST: INDICATES BENIGN" IF 3-OPNTOP<1 ELSE
"POSITIVE TEST: INDICATES MALIGNANT" IF RGS1BOT>=3 ELSE
"POSITIVE TEST: INDICATES MALIGNANT" IF 3-ARPC2TOP>=2 ELSE
"NEGATIVE TEST: INDICATES BENIGN" IF FN1TOP<1 ELSE
"NEGATIVE TEST: INDICATES BENIGN" IF WNT2TOP<2 ELSE
"POSITIVE TEST: INDICATES MALIGNANT" IF RTBDIFF>=0 ELSE
"POSITIVE TEST: INDICATES MALIGNANT" IF FN1TOP>=1 ELSE
"POSITIVE TEST: INDICATES MALIGNANT" IF FTBDIFF>=0 ELSE
"NEGATIVE TEST: INDICATES BENIGN" IF 3-ARPC2TOP<2 ELSE
"POSITIVE TEST: INDICATES MALIGNANT" IF ATBDIFF>=0 ELSE
"POSITIVE TEST: INDICATES MALIGNANT" IF 3-OPNTOP>=1 ELSE
"POSITIVE TEST: INDICATES MALIGNANT" IF OTBDIFF>=0 ELSE
"POSITIVE TEST: INDICATES MALIGNANT" IF FN1BOT>=1 ELSE
"NEGATIVE TEST: INDICATES BENIGN" IF ARPC2BOT<1 ELSE
"POSITIVE TEST: INDICATES MALIGNANT" IF OPNBOT>=2 ELSE
"POSITIVE TEST: INDICATES MALIGNANT" IF WNT2TOP>=2 ELSE
"POSITIVE TEST: INDICATES MALIGNANT" IF ARPC2BOT>=1 ELSE
"NEGATIVE TEST: INDICATES BENIGN" IF RGS1BOT<3 ELSE
"NEGATIVE TEST: INDICATES BENIGN" IF FN1BOT<1 ELSE
"NEGATIVE TEST: INDICATES BENIGN" IF 3-RGS1TOP<2 ELSE
"NEGATIVE TEST: INDICATES BENIGN" IF WNT2BOT<2 ELSE
"NEGATIVE TEST: INDICATES BENIGN" IF OPNBOT<2 ELSE
"NO DIAGNOSTIC CONCLUSION"
```

Results of applying the summarized algorithm to the same 519 lesions were:

DSSA-GENERATED DIAGNOSTIC CONCLUSION	CORRECT DIAGNOSIS OF LESION		
	BENIGN	MALIGNANT	TOTAL
NEGATIVE TEST: INDICATES BENIGN	89	26	115
POSITIVE TEST: INDICATES MALIGNANT	9	395	404
TOTAL	98	421	519

DSSA produced a definite diagnostic conclusion for all 519 training lesions.

1. It achieved a sensitivity of 395/421 = 93.82 percent. This compared to a sensitivity of 75.82 percent achieved by the five-marker assay based on (bottom) expression intensities of only the 213 lesions possessing

complete data analyzed by multivariate logistic regression in Act I and to a sensitivity of 98.68 percent achieved by DSSA analyzing top-to-bottom differences of only the 235 lesions possessing complete data in Act II.

2. It achieved a specificity of 89/98 = 90.82 percent. This compared to a specificity of 93.55 percent in ACT I and to a specificity of 80.72 percent in Act II.

3. It made (89+395)/519 = 93.26 percent correct diagnoses of 519 lesions. This compared to 78.40 percent correct diagnoses of 213 lesions achieved in Act I and to 92.34 percent correct diagnoses of 235 lesions achieved in Act II.

4. It achieved an AUC of 0.9232. This compared to an AUC of 0.9067 in Act I and to an AUC of 0.8970 in Act II. When derived from applying the DSSA diagnostic algorithms produced in Acts II and III, estimated AUC values were based on each lesion's diagnosis as either benign or malignant. This defined a single diagnostic cut point in the ROC/AUC analysis. The AUC value was then the area of the polygon whose northwest corner point was defined by that single cut point.

On balance, DSSA's Act III analysis of all fifteen directionally compatible indicators applied to all 519 training lesions achieved more accurate diagnoses of more lesions than the Act I analysis of only 213 expression intensities and the Act II analysis of only 235 top-to-bottom intensity differences. Combining and integrating all three sets of indicators via DSSA proved to be quite successful.

5.4 By How Much Did Removing Problem Cases Improve DSSA's Diagnostic Accuracy?

As mentioned previously, dysplastic and Spitz nevi regularly cause problems for pathologists in distinguishing accurately between benign nevi and malignant melanomas. Therefore, neither type of lesion was included among the 519 training lesions just diagnosed by DSSA. Excluding both was presumed to eliminate diagnostic difficulties specifically attributable to the two problem cases. This was an additional reason to exclude them. The initial reason was that no lesions of either variety were included in the SAM analysis.

Underlying our presumption was the same reasoning underlying the fundamental design of PCM. PCM's initial step is always to partition some population of interest into relatively homogeneous strata. The principle of stratification is based on whatever factor or index best predicts whatever has been selected as the focal end point. When the interesting population is heterogeneous in this predictive sense the increased within-stratum homogeneity produced by stratification generally improves predictive accuracy.

DSSA is similarly designed. Removing problem cases such as dysplastic and Spitz nevi should have the same effect of homogenizing the diagnosis and improving, thereby, its accuracy.

The benign nevi originally obtained from patient tissue were collected from 179 separate patients. Of these, sixty provided tissue containing lesions of a dysplastic nature. Twenty-one provided tissue containing Spitz nevi. These eighty-one were removed. Only the remaining ninety-eight nondysplastic and non-Spitz lesions were included in the 519-lesion training data just analyzed.

Now we shall see by how much excluding the sixty dysplastic nevi and the twenty-one Spitz nevi improved DSSA's diagnostic accuracy. We shall combine the sixty dysplastic nevi, the twenty-one Spitz nevi, and the other ninety-eight benign nevi into a total set of 179 benign nevi; compare them with the same 421 malignant melanomas; and reanalyze via DSSA the total of 600 lesions.

All 600 lesions will again require a definite diagnosis, and the same slightly higher weight of 0.55 will be placed on achieving a more sensitive than specific diagnosis to enable comparability of results.

To enable the combined reanalysis both top and bottom readings were also made under the microscope of each dysplastic nevus' and each Spitz nevus' level of expression intensity for each of our five genes. These readings were made by the same pathologist (Dr. Richard W. Sagebiel). The corresponding eighty-one top-to-bottom difference scores were also calculated separately for each gene.

Results of the reanalysis are shown below and on the next two pages.

The diagnostic algorithm produced by DSSA was:

```
"DIAGNOSED BENIGN: WTBDIFF<0" IF WTBDIFF<0 ELSE
"DIAGNOSED BENIGN: OTBDIFF<0" IF OTBDIFF<0 ELSE
"DIAGNOSED MALIGNANT: WNT2BOT>=3" IF WNT2BOT>=3 ELSE
"DIAGNOSED BENIGN: FTBDIFF<0" IF FTBDIFF<0 ELSE
"DIAGNOSED BENIGN: RTBDIFF<0" IF RTBDIFF<0 ELSE
"DIAGNOSED MALIGNANT: 3-RGS1TOP>=2" IF 3-RGS1TOP>=2 ELSE
"DIAGNOSED BENIGN: ATBDIFF<0" IF ATBDIFF<0 ELSE
"DIAGNOSED MALIGNANT: RGS1BOT>=3" IF RGS1BOT>=3 ELSE
"DIAGNOSED BENIGN: WNT2TOP<1" IF WNT2TOP<1 ELSE
"DIAGNOSED BENIGN: 3-OPNTOP<1" IF 3-OPNTOP<1 ELSE
"DIAGNOSED MALIGNANT: 3-ARPC2TOP>=2" IF 3-ARPC2TOP>=2 ELSE
"DIAGNOSED BENIGN: FN1TOP<1" IF FN1TOP<1 ELSE
"DIAGNOSED MALIGNANT: FN1BOT>=2" IF FN1BOT>=2 ELSE
"DIAGNOSED MALIGNANT: OPNBOT>=2" IF OPNBOT>=2 ELSE
"DIAGNOSED MALIGNANT: FN1TOP>=1" IF FN1TOP>=1 ELSE
"DIAGNOSED MALIGNANT: ARPC2BOT>=3" IF ARPC2BOT>=3 ELSE
"DIAGNOSED MALIGNANT: RTBDIFF>=0" IF RTBDIFF>=0 ELSE
"DIAGNOSED MALIGNANT: FTBDIFF>=0" IF FTBDIFF>=0 ELSE
"DIAGNOSED MALIGNANT: WTBDIFF>=0" IF WTBDIFF>=0 ELSE
"DIAGNOSED BENIGN: 3-ARPC2TOP<2" IF 3-ARPC2TOP<2 ELSE
"DIAGNOSED MALIGNANT: ATBDIFF>=0" IF ATBDIFF>=0 ELSE
"DIAGNOSED MALIGNANT: 3-OPNTOP>=1" IF 3-OPNTOP>=1 ELSE
"DIAGNOSED MALIGNANT: OTBDIFF>=0" IF OTBDIFF>=0 ELSE
"DIAGNOSED BENIGN: 3-RGS1TOP<2" IF 3-RGS1TOP<2 ELSE
"DIAGNOSED MALIGNANT: WNT2TOP>=1" IF WNT2TOP>=1 ELSE
"DIAGNOSED BENIGN: RGS1BOT<3" IF RGS1BOT<3 ELSE
"DIAGNOSED BENIGN: FN1BOT<2" IF FN1BOT<2 ELSE
"DIAGNOSED BENIGN: ARPC2BOT<3" IF ARPC2BOT<3 ELSE
"DIAGNOSED BENIGN: OPNBOT<2" IF OPNBOT<2 ELSE
"DIAGNOSED BENIGN: WNT2BOT<3" IF WNT2BOT<3 ELSE
"NO DIAGNOSTIC CONCLUSION"
```

Results of applying this diagnostic algorithm to all 600 lesions were:

DSSA-GENERATED DIAGNOSTIC CONCLUSION	CORRECT DIAGNOSIS OF LESION		
	BENIGN	MALIGNANT	TOTAL
DIAGNOSED BENIGN: WTBDIFF<0	57	0	57
DIAGNOSED BENIGN: OTBDIFF<0	27	1	28
DIAGNOSED MALIGNANT: WNT2BOT>=3	0	75	75
DIAGNOSED BENIGN: FTBDIFF<0	8	1	9

```
DIAGNOSED BENIGN: RTBDIFF<0                    6        1        7
DIAGNOSED MALIGNANT: 3-RGS1TOP>=2              1       36       37
DIAGNOSED BENIGN: ATBDIFF<0                    5        2        7
DIAGNOSED MALIGNANT: RGS1BOT>=3                2       60       62
DIAGNOSED BENIGN: WNT2TOP<1                    4        1        5
DIAGNOSED BENIGN: 3-OPNTOP<1                   7        8       15
DIAGNOSED MALIGNANT: 3-ARPC2TOP>=2             4       28       32
DIAGNOSED BENIGN: FN1TOP<1                    22        9       31
DIAGNOSED MALIGNANT: FN1BOT>=2                 3       32       35
DIAGNOSED MALIGNANT: OPNBOT>=2                 9       60       69
DIAGNOSED MALIGNANT: FN1TOP>=1                 9       27       36
DIAGNOSED MALIGNANT: ARPC2BOT>=3               0       12       12
DIAGNOSED MALIGNANT: RTBDIFF>=0                0        1        1
DIAGNOSED MALIGNANT: WTBDIFF>=0                1        7        8
DIAGNOSED BENIGN: 3-ARPC2TOP<2                 5        4        9
DIAGNOSED MALIGNANT: 3-OPNTOP>=1               1        7        8
DIAGNOSED BENIGN: 3-RGS1TOP<2                  0        3        3
DIAGNOSED MALIGNANT: WNT2TOP>=1                3        4        7
DIAGNOSED BENIGN: RGS1BOT<3                    2       22       24
DIAGNOSED BENIGN: FN1BOT<2                     1        7        8
DIAGNOSED BENIGN: ARPC2BOT<3                   2        3        5
DIAGNOSED BENIGN: OPNBOT<2                     0        4        4
DIAGNOSED BENIGN: WNT2BOT<3                    0        6        6

TOTAL                                        179      421      600
```

A summarized version of the same diagnostic algorithm was:

```
"NEGATIVE TEST: INDICATES BENIGN" IF WTBDIFF<0 ELSE
"NEGATIVE TEST: INDICATES BENIGN" IF OTBDIFF<0 ELSE
"POSITIVE TEST: INDICATES MALIGNANT" IF WNT2BOT>=3 ELSE
"NEGATIVE TEST: INDICATES BENIGN" IF FTBDIFF<0 ELSE
"NEGATIVE TEST: INDICATES BENIGN" IF RTBDIFF<0 ELSE
"POSITIVE TEST: INDICATES MALIGNANT" IF 3-RGS1TOP>=2 ELSE
"NEGATIVE TEST: INDICATES BENIGN" IF ATBDIFF<0 ELSE
"POSITIVE TEST: INDICATES MALIGNANT" IF RGS1BOT>=3 ELSE
"NEGATIVE TEST: INDICATES BENIGN" IF WNT2TOP<1 ELSE
"NEGATIVE TEST: INDICATES BENIGN" IF 3-OPNTOP<1 ELSE
"POSITIVE TEST: INDICATES MALIGNANT" IF 3-ARPC2TOP>=2 ELSE
"NEGATIVE TEST: INDICATES BENIGN" IF FN1TOP<1 ELSE
"POSITIVE TEST: INDICATES MALIGNANT" IF FN1BOT>=2 ELSE
"POSITIVE TEST: INDICATES MALIGNANT" IF OPNBOT>=2 ELSE
"POSITIVE TEST: INDICATES MALIGNANT" IF FN1TOP>=1 ELSE
"POSITIVE TEST: INDICATES MALIGNANT" IF ARPC2BOT>=3 ELSE
"POSITIVE TEST: INDICATES MALIGNANT" IF RTBDIFF>=0 ELSE
"POSITIVE TEST: INDICATES MALIGNANT" IF FTBDIFF>=0 ELSE
"POSITIVE TEST: INDICATES MALIGNANT" IF WTBDIFF>=0 ELSE
"NEGATIVE TEST: INDICATES BENIGN" IF 3-ARPC2TOP<2 ELSE
"POSITIVE TEST: INDICATES MALIGNANT" IF ATBDIFF>=0 ELSE
"POSITIVE TEST: INDICATES MALIGNANT" IF 3-OPNTOP>=1 ELSE
"POSITIVE TEST: INDICATES MALIGNANT" IF OTBDIFF>=0 ELSE
"NEGATIVE TEST: INDICATES BENIGN" IF 3-RGS1TOP<2 ELSE
"POSITIVE TEST: INDICATES MALIGNANT" IF WNT2TOP>=1 ELSE
"NEGATIVE TEST: INDICATES BENIGN" IF RGS1BOT<3 ELSE
"NEGATIVE TEST: INDICATES BENIGN" IF FN1BOT<2 ELSE
"NEGATIVE TEST: INDICATES BENIGN" IF ARPC2BOT<3 ELSE
"NEGATIVE TEST: INDICATES BENIGN" IF OPNBOT<2 ELSE
"NEGATIVE TEST: INDICATES BENIGN" IF WNT2BOT<3 ELSE
"NO DIAGNOSTIC CONCLUSION"
```

Results of applying the summarized algorithm to the same 600 lesions were:

DSSA-GENERATED DIAGNOSTIC CONCLUSION	CORRECT DIAGNOSIS OF LESION		
	BENIGN	MALIGNANT	TOTAL
NEGATIVE TEST: INDICATES BENIGN	146	72	218
POSITIVE TEST: INDICATES MALIGNANT	33	349	382
TOTAL	179	421	600

The reanalysis showed a substantial deterioration in diagnostic accuracy.

1. It achieved a sensitivity of 349/421 = 82.90 percent. This compared to a sensitivity of 93.82 percent achieved by DSSA's analysis of the 519 training lesions. Removing the eighty-one problem cases (i.e., the sixty dysplastic nevi and the twenty-one Spitz nevi) improved the diagnostic sensitivity by 93.82 - 82.90 = 10.92 percentage points.
2. It achieved a specificity of 146/179 = 81.56 percent. This compared to a specificity of 90.82 percent achieved by DSSA's analysis of the 519 training lesions. Removing the problem cases also improved the specificity of the diagnosis by 90.82 - 81.56 = 9.26 percentage points.
3. It made (146+349)/600 = 82.50 percent correct diagnoses of 600 lesions. This compared to 93.26 percent correct diagnoses of 519 training lesions. Removing the problem cases improved the percentage of correct diagnoses by 93.26 - 82.50 = 10.76 percentage points.
4. It achieved an AUC of 0.8223. This compared to an AUC of 0.9232 achieved by DSSA's analysis of the 519 training lesions. Removing the problem cases improved the AUC by 0.9232 - 0.8223 = 0.1009.

By every measure excluding the sixty dysplastic nevi and the twenty-one Spitz nevi from the original 179 benign nevi in order to eliminate known problem cases improved DSSA's diagnostic accuracy. Homogenizing the 519-lesion training data in this manner was definitely beneficial.

Homogeneity means that the various diagnostic indicators entering DSSA bear a similar relationship to all types of benign lesions; a similar relationship to all types of malignant melanomas; but a distinguishable relationship to the set of all benign versus the set of all malignant lesions. All benign lesions can then be treated as if they were "the same." All malignant lesions can be treated as if they, too, were "the same."

Heterogeneity means that at least some indicators bear distinguishable relationships to selected subsets of lesions within a total set. For example, heterogeneity would suggest that a single diagnostic algorithm may not be appropriate for all benign nevi; or that a single diagnostic algorithm may not be appropriate for all malignant melanomas; or, possibly, both. There may exist distinct, though internally homogeneous subsets within either or both sets of lesions that need to be diagnosed separately, thereby generating separate diagnostic algorithms.

Dysplastic nevi and Spitz nevi may be heterogeneous in this sense both compared to each other and to other benign nevi. That could explain, at least in part, why they constitute problem cases. If so, DSSA might be able to improve its accuracy of discrimination by diagnosing the two difficult-to-diagnose nevi separately from each other and separately from the easier-to-diagnose other benign nevi and malignant melanomas. We decided to explore this possibility.

The pathologist was asked to articulate how he made his differential diagnoses. Except in the two problem cases, he relied on a standard collection of twenty-two distinguishing features of each lesion visible under the microscope. In the case of lesions initially displaying either a dysplastic-like or a Spitzoid appearance, however, he adopted a different approach. His different approach was based on different observable criteria. This was encouraging.

In order to mimic the pathologist's different approach, DSSA's next task will be to produce two preliminary diagnostic algorithms tailored just to detect dysplastic and just to detect Spitz nevi, respectively. These two preliminary algorithms will then be merged with the homogenized DSSA algorithm already obtained from the 519 training lesions. The result will be a single, composite algorithm applicable to all 600 training lesions.

To the extent that dysplastic and Spitz nevi are problem cases because of heterogeneity the composite algorithm should improve diagnostic accuracy still further. That would be consistent with and tend to support our homogeneity versus heterogeneity interpretation of the problem.

Section 4.3 outlined the second stage of DSSA. During its second stage the discriminating algorithm generated by DSSA can be intentionally weighted in the direction of achieving either greater sensitivity or greater specificity. Weighting in either direction, however, is necessarily at the expense of the other. The algorithm can also be weighted to maximize the number of correct conclusions drawn from any training data set. We can exploit these capabilities to mimic the pathologist's tailored approach to dysplastic and Spitz nevi.

Each new lesion can first be inspected for any dysplastic or Spitzoid features. A tentative initial diagnosis would result, depicting the lesion as either:

1. dysplastic-like (lesion possesses at least some dysplastic features); or
2. Spitzoid (lesion possesses at least some Spitzoid features); or
3. neither (lesion possesses neither dysplastic nor Spitzoid features).
4. [Clarifying comment: In the pathologist's experience lesions did not possess both dysplastic-like and Spitzoid features simultaneously.]

The idea is then to invoke a DSSA-generated diagnostic algorithm specifically designed either to confirm or to disconfirm the pathologist's tentative initial diagnosis. It would be invoked if, but only if the tentative diagnosis identified either dysplastic-like or Spitzoid features. Otherwise, a lesion displaying neither type of feature would be referred straightaway to the homogenized DSSA algorithm already obtained from the 519 training lesions.

When either confirmatory algorithm is invoked, a confirmed tentative diagnosis becomes the final diagnosis. A nonconfirmed tentatively diagnosed lesion would then be referred to the same homogenized DSSA algorithm already obtained from the 519 training lesions.

5.5 A DSSA-Generated Confirmatory Algorithm Designed Just for Dysplastic Nevi

Fifteen univariate logistic regression analyses of top, bottom, and top-to-bottom difference scores assigned to all five genetic markers for all 600 lesions were executed. The common outcome predicted by each of the fifteen indicators was encapsulated in a 0/1 dummy variable (DYSDUMMY) identifying whether or not each of the 600 lesions was finally diagnosed as a dysplastic nevus. Of the 600 lesions sixty were so diagnosed, while 540 were not.

The purpose of these fifteen analyses was twofold:

1. to determine which indicators provided a statistically significant discrimination between those lesions finally diagnosed as dysplastic and all remaining lesions otherwise diagnosed; and
2. to determine from the sign of its statistically significant regression coefficient in which direction each such indicator pointed; where
3. an indicator had to point in either direction with a two-tailed p value at most 0.10 in order to qualify as statistically significant.

Seven of the fifteen indicators qualified as significant identifiers of dysplastic nevi. They are listed below, along with their directions of indication and accompanying two-tailed p values.

A dysplastic nevus was separately indicated by:

1. a higher as opposed to lower WTBDIFF score (p = 0.0262);
2. a higher as opposed to lower ARPC2TOP score (p < 0.00005);
3. a higher as opposed to lower ARPC2BOT score (p < 0.00005);
4. a higher as opposed to lower ATBDIFF score (p = 0.0030);
5. a higher as opposed to lower OTBDIFF score (p = 0.0131);
6. a lower as opposed to higher FN1TOP score (p < 0.00005); and
7. a lower as opposed to higher FN1BOT score (p < 0.00005).

The DSSA procedure was then applied to these seven significant indicators scored by the pathologist on all 600 lesions. They constituted DSSA's independent variable data inputs. DSSA's dependent variable was the dichotomous final diagnostic variable DYSDX denoting either dysplastic or not dysplastic.

DSSA's weight on sensitivity was varied by trial and error to just achieve 100 percent confirmation of the sixty lesions finally diagnosed as dysplastic, but with a minimum concomitant loss in specificity. There is no guarantee that any weight, no matter how extreme, will suffice to produce complete confirmation. Fortunately, complete confirmation did turn out to be easily achievable in this instance.

The confirmatory algorithm generated by DSSA is displayed below.

```
"DYSPLASTIC DISCONFIRMED: FN1BOT>=2" IF FN1BOT>=2 ELSE
"DYSPLASTIC DISCONFIRMED: 1-WTBDIFF>=2.5" IF 1-WTBDIFF>=2.5 ELSE
"DYSPLASTIC DISCONFIRMED: 1-OTBDIFF>=2.5" IF 1-OTBDIFF>=2.5 ELSE
"DYSPLASTIC CONFIRMED: 1-ATBDIFF<2" IF 1-ATBDIFF<2 ELSE
"DYSPLASTIC DISCONFIRMED: 3-ARPC2TOP>=2" IF 3-ARPC2TOP>=2 ELSE
"DYSPLASTIC DISCONFIRMED: FN1TOP>=3" IF FN1TOP>=3 ELSE
"DYSPLASTIC CONFIRMED: 1-WTBDIFF<2.5" IF 1-WTBDIFF<2.5 ELSE
"DYSPLASTIC CONFIRMED: 1-OTBDIFF<2.5" IF 1-OTBDIFF<2.5 ELSE
"DYSPLASTIC CONFIRMED: 3-ARPC2TOP<2" IF 3-ARPC2TOP<2 ELSE
"DYSPLASTIC DISCONFIRMED: 3-ARPC2BOT>=2" IF 3-ARPC2BOT>=2 ELSE
"DYSPLASTIC DISCONFIRMED: 1-ATBDIFF>=2" IF 1-ATBDIFF>=2 ELSE
"DYSPLASTIC CONFIRMED: FN1TOP<3" IF FN1TOP<3 ELSE
"DYSPLASTIC CONFIRMED: FN1BOT<2" IF FN1BOT<2 ELSE
"DYSPLASTIC CONFIRMED: 3-ARPC2BOT<2" IF 3-ARPC2BOT<2 ELSE
"NO DIAGNOSTIC CONCLUSION"
```

Notice that the algorithm contains all fourteen discriminators. This is because DSSA was instructed to diagnose all 600 lesions (even if incorrectly), and no discriminator's diagnostic impact was permitted to remain undisclosed.

Since the purpose of this algorithm is only to confirm or not to confirm as actually dysplastic a lesion initially identified by the pathologist as possessing one or more dysplastic-like features the seven disconfirmatory discriminators were purged. That left the following reduced algorithm.

```
"DYSPLASTIC CONFIRMED: 1-ATBDIFF<2" IF 1-ATBDIFF<2 ELSE
"DYSPLASTIC CONFIRMED: 1-WTBDIFF<2.5" IF 1-WTBDIFF<2.5 ELSE
"DYSPLASTIC CONFIRMED: 1-OTBDIFF<2.5" IF 1-OTBDIFF<2.5 ELSE
"DYSPLASTIC CONFIRMED: 3-ARPC2TOP<2" IF 3-ARPC2TOP<2 ELSE
"DYSPLASTIC CONFIRMED: FN1TOP<3" IF FN1TOP<3 ELSE
"DYSPLASTIC CONFIRMED: FN1BOT<2" IF FN1BOT<2 ELSE
"DYSPLASTIC CONFIRMED: 3-ARPC2BOT<2" IF 3-ARPC2BOT<2 ELSE
"NO DIAGNOSTIC CONCLUSION"
```

Applying the reduced confirmatory algorithm to the 600 lesions produced the following results.

VALUE OF DESIGNATED EXPRESSION	ABSOLUTE FREQUENCIES (COUNTS)	RELATIVE FREQUENCIES (PROPORTIONS)	CUMULATIVE RELATIVE FREQUENCIES
DYSPLASTIC CONFIRMED: 1-ATBDIFF<2	55	.0917	.0917
DYSPLASTIC CONFIRMED: 1-WTBDIFF<2.5	1	.0017	.0933
DYSPLASTIC CONFIRMED: 1-OTBDIFF<2.5	1	.0017	.0950
DYSPLASTIC CONFIRMED: 3-ARPC2TOP<2	2	.0033	.0983
DYSPLASTIC CONFIRMED: FN1TOP<3	1	.0017	.1000
NO DIAGNOSTIC CONCLUSION	540	.9000	1.0000
TOTAL	600	1.0000	

Notes:

1. Complete confirmation turned out to be achievable with five of our fifteen indicators (ATBDIFF, WTBDIFF, OTBDIFF, ARPC2TOP, and FN1TOP) involving four of our five genes (ARPC2, WNT2, SPP1 also called OPN, and FN1). All sixty dysplastic lesions were successfully confirmed by selecting a just-extreme-enough sensitivity weight, but with the least possible concomitant reduction in specificity.
2. The reason for purging the seven disconfirming discriminators from the fourteen-discriminator confirmatory algorithm originally generated by DSSA can now be fully appreciated. When any one of the 600 lesions to which the reduced algorithm is later applied is not confirmed as being dysplastic, no diagnostic conclusion will be drawn. The algorithm will continue to process the next discriminator in the sequence. That next discriminator may be part of the confirmatory algorithm for dysplastic nevi; part of the confirmatory algorithm for Spitz nevi; or part of the homogenized DSSA algorithm previously obtained from the 519 training lesions. Equally importantly, the same benefit will be realized if and when this confirmatory algorithm is later applied to a distinct sample of validation lesions. Prepartitioning every input indicator to DSSA into a corresponding matched pair of discriminators enabled DSSA to emulate quite precisely the pathologist's diagnostic routine.
3. The first four staining intensity scores in the algorithm were subtracted from either their highest possible or highest occurring numeric score to satisfy DSSA's requirement that all input indicators be coded in the directionally appropriate manner. This permitted their uniform transformation to canonical form, as described in section 4.2.3.
4. Two of the critical cutoff scores (right-hand sides of the

algebraic inequalities) in the algorithm were not integers. The
pathologist occasionally indicated his sense that a staining
intensity fell right at the borderline between two adjacent levels
by assigning a halfway-between score. Thus, a score of 2.5 would
signify being borderline between the moderate (2) and intense (3)
levels of staining intensity.

5. Remarkably, the two discriminating statements based on ARPC2 scores
   accounted for fifty-seven of the sixty successful confirmations.
   WNT2 accounted for only one additional confirmation of a dysplastic
   nevus. This stands in sharp contrast to the relative potency of
   these two genes in discriminating between benign nevi and malignant
   melanomas in the homogenized DSSA algorithm previously obtained from
   the 519 training lesions. The same gene can play separate roles of
   dramatically different potency in different diagnostic settings.

6. Recalling that ATBDIFF is defined as ARPC2TOP subtracted from
   ARPC2BOT, and after performing some algebra, the top-ranked
   discriminator statement 1-ATBDIFF<2 is shown to be equivalent to the
   statement ARPC2BOT>=ARPC2TOP. This is just the reverse of the
   typical top-to-bottom staining intensity differential of benign
   nevi compared to malignant melanomas uniformly replicated with
   respect to all five of our genes.

7. The other ARPC2-related discriminator statement 3-ARPC2BOT<2 is
   equivalent to the statement ARPC2BOT>1. The direction of impact of
   ARPC2BOT in confirming a dysplastic nevus is also just the reverse
   of its usual direction when indicating a benign nevus as opposed to
   a malignant melanoma. Not all benign lesions can be treated as if
   they were "the same" with respect to a given gene in all diagnostic
   settings. The underlying biology may not be "the same" at all.

8. ARPC2 appears to play an important, though highly specialized role
   in the context of dysplastic nevi. This deserves further scrutiny.

5.6 A DSSA-Generated Confirmatory Algorithm Designed Just for Spitz Nevi

Fifteen univariate logistic regression analyses of top, bottom, and
top-to-bottom difference scores assigned to all five genetic markers for all
600 lesions were executed. The common outcome predicted by each of the fifteen
indicators was encapsulated in a 0/1 dummy variable (SPIDUMMY) identifying
whether or not each of the 600 lesions was finally diagnosed as a Spitz nevus.
Of the 600 lesions twenty-one were so diagnosed, while 579 were not.

The purpose of these fifteen analyses was twofold:

1. to determine which indicators provided a statistically significant
   discrimination between those lesions finally diagnosed as Spitz nevi
   and all remaining lesions otherwise diagnosed; and
2. to determine from the sign of its statistically significant regression
   coefficient in which direction each such indicator pointed; where
3. an indicator had to point in either direction with a two-tailed p value
   at most 0.10 in order to qualify as statistically significant.

Nine of the fifteen indicators qualified as significant identifiers of Spitz
nevi. They are listed on the next page, along with their directions of
indication and accompanying two-tailed p values.

A Spitz nevus was separately indicated by:

    1. a higher as opposed to lower WNT2TOP score ($p = 0.0367$);
    2. a lower as opposed to higher WNT2BOT score ($p = 0.0005$);
    3. a lower as opposed to higher WTBDIFF score ($p = 0.0001$);
    4. a lower as opposed to higher OPNBOT score ($p < 0.00005$);
    5. a lower as opposed to higher OTBDIFF score ($p < 0.00005$);
    6. a lower as opposed to higher RGS1BOT score ($p = 0.0659$);
    7. a lower as opposed to higher RTBDIFF score ($p = 0.0004$);
    8. a lower as opposed to higher FN1BOT score ($p = 0.0009$); and
    9. a lower as opposed to higher FTBDIFF score ($p = 0.0001$).

The DSSA procedure was then applied to these nine significant indicators scored by the pathologist on all 600 lesions. They constituted DSSA's independent variable data inputs. DSSA's dependent variable was the dichotomous final diagnostic variable SPIDX denoting either Spitz or not Spitz.

DSSA's weight on sensitivity was varied by trial and error to just achieve 100 percent confirmation of the twenty-one lesions finally diagnosed as Spitz nevi, but with a minimum concomitant loss in specificity. There is no guarantee that any weight, no matter how extreme, will suffice to produce complete confirmation. Fortunately, complete confirmation did turn out to be easily achievable in this instance.

The confirmatory algorithm generated by DSSA is displayed below.

```
"SPITZ CONFIRMED: FTBDIFF<0" IF FTBDIFF<0 ELSE
"SPITZ DISCONFIRMED: OPNBOT>=1.5" IF OPNBOT>=1.5 ELSE
"SPITZ CONFIRMED: RTBDIFF<0" IF RTBDIFF<0 ELSE
"SPITZ CONFIRMED: WTBDIFF<-.5" IF WTBDIFF<-.5 ELSE
"SPITZ DISCONFIRMED: OTBDIFF>=-1" IF OTBDIFF>=-1 ELSE
"SPITZ DISCONFIRMED: 3-WNT2TOP>=2" IF 3-WNT2TOP>=2 ELSE
"SPITZ CONFIRMED: OTBDIFF<-1" IF OTBDIFF<-1 ELSE
"SPITZ DISCONFIRMED: FN1BOT>=1" IF FN1BOT>=1 ELSE
"SPITZ DISCONFIRMED: RGS1BOT>=2" IF RGS1BOT>=2 ELSE
"SPITZ DISCONFIRMED: RTBDIFF>=0" IF RTBDIFF>=0 ELSE
"SPITZ CONFIRMED: 3-WNT2TOP<2" IF 3-WNT2TOP<2 ELSE
"SPITZ DISCONFIRMED: WNT2BOT>=1" IF WNT2BOT>=1 ELSE
"SPITZ DISCONFIRMED: FTBDIFF>=0" IF FTBDIFF>=0 ELSE
"SPITZ DISCONFIRMED: WTBDIFF>=-.5" IF WTBDIFF>=-.5 ELSE
"SPITZ CONFIRMED: WNT2BOT<1" IF WNT2BOT<1 ELSE
"SPITZ CONFIRMED: RGS1BOT<2" IF RGS1BOT<2 ELSE
"SPITZ CONFIRMED: FN1BOT<1" IF FN1BOT<1 ELSE
"SPITZ CONFIRMED: OPNBOT<1.5" IF OPNBOT<1.5 ELSE
"NO DIAGNOSTIC CONCLUSION"
```

Notice that the algorithm contains all eighteen discriminators. This is because DSSA was instructed to diagnose all 600 lesions (even if incorrectly), and no discriminator's diagnostic impact was permitted to remain undisclosed.

Since the purpose of this algorithm is only to confirm or not to confirm as actually a Spitz nevus a lesion initially identified by the pathologist as possessing one or more Spitzoid features the nine disconfirmatory discriminators were purged. That left the following reduced algorithm.

```
"SPITZ CONFIRMED: FTBDIFF<0" IF FTBDIFF<0 ELSE
"SPITZ CONFIRMED: RTBDIFF<0" IF RTBDIFF<0 ELSE
"SPITZ CONFIRMED: WTBDIFF<-.5" IF WTBDIFF<-.5 ELSE
"SPITZ CONFIRMED: OTBDIFF<-1" IF OTBDIFF<-1 ELSE
```

```
"SPITZ CONFIRMED: 3-WNT2TOP<2" IF 3-WNT2TOP<2 ELSE
"SPITZ CONFIRMED: WNT2BOT<1" IF WNT2BOT<1 ELSE
"SPITZ CONFIRMED: RGS1BOT<2" IF RGS1BOT<2 ELSE
"SPITZ CONFIRMED: FN1BOT<1" IF FN1BOT<1 ELSE
"SPITZ CONFIRMED: OPNBOT<1.5" IF OPNBOT<1.5 ELSE
"NO DIAGNOSTIC CONCLUSION"
```

Applying the reduced confirmatory algorithm to the 600 lesions produced the following results.

VALUE OF DESIGNATED EXPRESSION	ABSOLUTE FREQUENCIES (COUNTS)	RELATIVE FREQUENCIES (PROPORTIONS)	CUMULATIVE RELATIVE FREQUENCIES
SPITZ CONFIRMED: FTBDIFF<0	9	.0150	.0150
SPITZ CONFIRMED: RTBDIFF<0	3	.0050	.0200
SPITZ CONFIRMED: WTBDIFF<-.5	6	.0100	.0300
SPITZ CONFIRMED: OTBDIFF<-1	1	.0017	.0317
SPITZ CONFIRMED: 3-WNT2TOP<2	2	.0033	.0350
NO DIAGNOSTIC CONCLUSION	579	.9650	1.0000
TOTAL	600	1.0000	

Notes:

1. Complete confirmation turned out to be achievable with five of our eighteen indicators (FTBDIFF, RTBDIFF, WTBDIFF, OTBDIFF, and WNT2TOP) involving four of our five genes (FN1, RGS1, WNT2, and SPP1 also called OPN). All twenty-one Spitz nevi were successfully confirmed by selecting a just-extreme-enough sensitivity weight, but with the least possible concomitant reduction in specificity.

2. The last staining intensity score in the algorithm (WNT2TOP) was subtracted from its highest possible numeric score to satisfy DSSA's requirement that all input indicators be coded in the directionally appropriate manner. This permitted its transformation to canonical form, as described in section 4.2.3.

3. One of the critical cutoff scores (right-hand sides of the algebraic inequalities) in the algorithm was not an integer. The pathologist occasionally indicated his sense that a staining intensity fell right at the borderline between two adjacent levels by assigning a halfway-between score. Thus, a score of 0.5 would signify being borderline between the absent (0) and slight (1) levels of staining intensity.

4. The WNT2-related discriminator statement 3-WNT2TOP<2 is equivalent to the statement WNT2TOP>1. The direction of impact of WNT2TOP in confirming a Spitz nevus is just the reverse of its usual direction when indicating a benign nevus as opposed to a malignant melanoma. The other four discriminator statements point in the expected direction.

5. FN1 and WNT2 appear to play important roles in the context of identifying Spitz nevi. Together, they account for seventeen of the twenty-one successful confirmations. Notice the contrast with identifying dysplastic nevi. There, ARPC2 was the most potent identifier, accounting for fifty-seven of the sixty successful confirmations.

6. Top-to-bottom differences appear to play a very important identifying role. Collectively, they account for nineteen of the twenty-one successful confirmations.

5.7   ACT III: DSSA's Final Composite Diagnostic Training Algorithm

The pathologist inspected all 600 of the lesions used to train DSSA to produce a composite diagnostic algorithm. He was able to classify all but one of them anatomically. His classification was taken to be his tentative initial diagnosis (TDX).

If his classification was dysplastic or if it made reference to any dysplastic-like features observed, his initial diagnosis was tentatively called dysplastic (TDX=DY). If his classification was Spitz or if it made reference to any Spitzoid features observed, his initial diagnosis was tentatively called Spitz (TDX=SP). In all other cases there was no initial diagnosis (TDX remained undefined).

The two confirmatory algorithms just produced were then merged with the homogenized algorithm already obtained from the 519 training lesions to create the following final composite diagnostic training algorithm.

```
"DYSPLASTIC CONFIRMED: 1-ATBDIFF<2" IF TDX=DY AND 1-ATBDIFF<2 ELSE
"DYSPLASTIC CONFIRMED: 1-WTBDIFF<2.5" IF TDX=DY AND 1-WTBDIFF<2.5 ELSE
"DYSPLASTIC CONFIRMED: 1-OTBDIFF<2.5" IF TDX=DY AND 1-OTBDIFF<2.5 ELSE
"DYSPLASTIC CONFIRMED: 3-ARPC2TOP<2" IF TDX=DY AND 3-ARPC2TOP<2 ELSE
"DYSPLASTIC CONFIRMED: FN1TOP<3" IF TDX=DY AND FN1TOP<3 ELSE
"DYSPLASTIC CONFIRMED: FN1BOT<2" IF TDX=DY AND FN1BOT<2 ELSE
"DYSPLASTIC CONFIRMED: 3-ARPC2BOT<2" IF TDX=DY AND 3-ARPC2BOT<2 ELSE
"SPITZ CONFIRMED: FTBDIFF<0" IF TDX=SP AND FTBDIFF<0 ELSE
"SPITZ CONFIRMED: RTBDIFF<0" IF TDX=SP AND RTBDIFF<0 ELSE
"SPITZ CONFIRMED: WTBDIFF<-.5" IF TDX=SP AND WTBDIFF<-.5 ELSE
"SPITZ CONFIRMED: OTBDIFF<-1" IF TDX=SP AND OTBDIFF<-1 ELSE
"SPITZ CONFIRMED: 3-WNT2TOP<2" IF TDX=SP AND 3-WNT2TOP<2 ELSE
"SPITZ CONFIRMED: WNT2BOT<1" IF TDX=SP AND WNT2BOT<1 ELSE
"SPITZ CONFIRMED: RGS1BOT<2" IF TDX=SP AND RGS1BOT<2 ELSE
"SPITZ CONFIRMED: FN1BOT<1" IF TDX=SP AND FN1BOT<1 ELSE
"SPITZ CONFIRMED: OPNBOT<1.5" IF TDX=SP AND OPNBOT<1.5 ELSE
"DIAGNOSED BENIGN: WTBDIFF<0" IF WTBDIFF<0 ELSE
"DIAGNOSED MALIGNANT: WTBDIFF>=0" IF WTBDIFF>=0 ELSE
"DIAGNOSED MALIGNANT: WNT2BOT>=2" IF WNT2BOT>=2 ELSE
"DIAGNOSED BENIGN: OTBDIFF<0" IF OTBDIFF<0 ELSE
"DIAGNOSED BENIGN: RTBDIFF<0" IF RTBDIFF<0 ELSE
"DIAGNOSED MALIGNANT: 3-RGS1TOP>=2" IF 3-RGS1TOP>=2 ELSE
"DIAGNOSED BENIGN: FTBDIFF<0" IF FTBDIFF<0 ELSE
"DIAGNOSED BENIGN: ATBDIFF<0" IF ATBDIFF<0 ELSE
"DIAGNOSED BENIGN: 3-OPNTOP<1" IF 3-OPNTOP<1 ELSE
"DIAGNOSED MALIGNANT: RGS1BOT>=3" IF RGS1BOT>=3 ELSE
"DIAGNOSED MALIGNANT: 3-ARPC2TOP>=2" IF 3-ARPC2TOP>=2 ELSE
"DIAGNOSED BENIGN: FN1TOP<1" IF FN1TOP<1 ELSE
"DIAGNOSED BENIGN: WNT2TOP<2" IF WNT2TOP<2 ELSE
"DIAGNOSED MALIGNANT: RTBDIFF>=0" IF RTBDIFF>=0 ELSE
"DIAGNOSED MALIGNANT: FN1TOP>=1" IF FN1TOP>=1 ELSE
"DIAGNOSED MALIGNANT: FTBDIFF>=0" IF FTBDIFF>=0 ELSE
"DIAGNOSED BENIGN: 3-ARPC2TOP<2" IF 3-ARPC2TOP<2 ELSE
"DIAGNOSED MALIGNANT: ATBDIFF>=0" IF ATBDIFF>=0 ELSE
"DIAGNOSED MALIGNANT: 3-OPNTOP>=1" IF 3-OPNTOP>=1 ELSE
"DIAGNOSED MALIGNANT: OTBDIFF>=0" IF OTBDIFF>=0 ELSE
"DIAGNOSED MALIGNANT: FN1BOT>=1" IF FN1BOT>=1 ELSE
"DIAGNOSED BENIGN: ARPC2BOT<1" IF ARPC2BOT<1 ELSE
"DIAGNOSED MALIGNANT: OPNBOT>=2" IF OPNBOT>=2 ELSE
"DIAGNOSED MALIGNANT: WNT2TOP>=2" IF WNT2TOP>=2 ELSE
```

```
"DIAGNOSED MALIGNANT: ARPC2BOT>=1" IF ARPC2BOT>=1 ELSE
"DIAGNOSED BENIGN: RGS1BOT<3" IF RGS1BOT<3 ELSE
"DIAGNOSED BENIGN: FN1BOT<1" IF FN1BOT<1 ELSE
"DIAGNOSED BENIGN: 3-RGS1TOP<2" IF 3-RGS1TOP<2 ELSE
"DIAGNOSED BENIGN: WNT2BOT<2" IF WNT2BOT<2 ELSE
"DIAGNOSED BENIGN: OPNBOT<2" IF OPNBOT<2 ELSE
"NO DIAGNOSTIC CONCLUSION"
```

The final composite algorithm was applied to all 600 training lesions. That produced the following results.

DSSA-GENERATED DIAGNOSTIC CONCLUSION	CORRECT DIAGNOSIS OF LESION		
	BENIGN	MALIGNANT	TOTAL
DYSPLASTIC CONFIRMED: 1-ATBDIFF<2	55	0	55
DYSPLASTIC CONFIRMED: 1-WTBDIFF<2.5	1	0	1
DYSPLASTIC CONFIRMED: 1-OTBDIFF<2.5	1	0	1
DYSPLASTIC CONFIRMED: 3-ARPC2TOP<2	2	0	2
DYSPLASTIC CONFIRMED: FN1TOP<3	1	0	1
SPITZ CONFIRMED: FTBDIFF<0	9	0	9
SPITZ CONFIRMED: RTBDIFF<0	3	0	3
SPITZ CONFIRMED: WTBDIFF<-.5	6	0	6
SPITZ CONFIRMED: OTBDIFF<-1	1	0	1
SPITZ CONFIRMED: 3-WNT2TOP<2	2	0	2
DIAGNOSED BENIGN: WTBDIFF<0	39	0	39
DIAGNOSED MALIGNANT: WTBDIFF>=0	0	105	105
DIAGNOSED MALIGNANT: WNT2BOT>=2	0	161	161
DIAGNOSED BENIGN: OTBDIFF<0	17	0	17
DIAGNOSED BENIGN: RTBDIFF<0	4	0	4
DIAGNOSED MALIGNANT: 3-RGS1TOP>=2	0	13	13
DIAGNOSED BENIGN: FTBDIFF<0	2	0	2
DIAGNOSED BENIGN: ATBDIFF<0	5	1	6
DIAGNOSED BENIGN: 3-OPNTOP<1	3	2	5
DIAGNOSED MALIGNANT: RGS1BOT>=3	1	24	25
DIAGNOSED MALIGNANT: 3-ARPC2TOP>=2	1	17	18
DIAGNOSED BENIGN: FN1TOP<1	3	6	9
DIAGNOSED BENIGN: WNT2TOP<2	13	7	20
DIAGNOSED MALIGNANT: RTBDIFF>=0	0	2	2
DIAGNOSED MALIGNANT: FN1TOP>=1	1	16	17
DIAGNOSED BENIGN: 3-ARPC2TOP<2	2	6	8
DIAGNOSED MALIGNANT: 3-OPNTOP>=1	1	5	6
DIAGNOSED MALIGNANT: FN1BOT>=1	1	29	30
DIAGNOSED MALIGNANT: OPNBOT>=2	1	9	10
DIAGNOSED MALIGNANT: WNT2TOP>=2	0	2	2
DIAGNOSED MALIGNANT: ARPC2BOT>=1	3	12	15
DIAGNOSED BENIGN: RGS1BOT<3	1	1	2
DIAGNOSED BENIGN: 3-RGS1TOP<2	0	1	1
DIAGNOSED BENIGN: WNT2BOT<2	0	1	1
DIAGNOSED BENIGN: OPNBOT<2	0	1	1
TOTAL	179	421	600

A summarized version of the same final composite diagnostic algorithm was:

```
"NEGATIVE TEST: INDICATES BENIGN" IF TDX=DY AND 1-ATBDIFF<2 ELSE
"NEGATIVE TEST: INDICATES BENIGN" IF TDX=DY AND 1-WTBDIFF<2.5 ELSE
"NEGATIVE TEST: INDICATES BENIGN" IF TDX=DY AND 1-OTBDIFF<2.5 ELSE
"NEGATIVE TEST: INDICATES BENIGN" IF TDX=DY AND 3-ARPC2TOP<2 ELSE
"NEGATIVE TEST: INDICATES BENIGN" IF TDX=DY AND FN1TOP<3 ELSE
```

```
"NEGATIVE TEST: INDICATES BENIGN" IF TDX=DY AND FN1BOT<2 ELSE
"NEGATIVE TEST: INDICATES BENIGN" IF TDX=DY AND 3-ARPC2BOT<2 ELSE
"NEGATIVE TEST: INDICATES BENIGN" IF TDX=SP AND FTBDIFF<0 ELSE
"NEGATIVE TEST: INDICATES BENIGN" IF TDX=SP AND RTBDIFF<0 ELSE
"NEGATIVE TEST: INDICATES BENIGN" IF TDX=SP AND WTBDIFF<-.5 ELSE
"NEGATIVE TEST: INDICATES BENIGN" IF TDX=SP AND OTBDIFF<-1 ELSE
"NEGATIVE TEST: INDICATES BENIGN" IF TDX=SP AND 3-WNT2TOP<2 ELSE
"NEGATIVE TEST: INDICATES BENIGN" IF TDX=SP AND WNT2BOT<1 ELSE
"NEGATIVE TEST: INDICATES BENIGN" IF TDX=SP AND RGS1BOT<2 ELSE
"NEGATIVE TEST: INDICATES BENIGN" IF TDX=SP AND FN1BOT<1 ELSE
"NEGATIVE TEST: INDICATES BENIGN" IF TDX=SP AND OPNBOT<1.5 ELSE
"NEGATIVE TEST: INDICATES BENIGN" IF WTBDIFF<0 ELSE
"POSITIVE TEST: INDICATES MALIGNANT" IF WTBDIFF>=0 ELSE
"POSITIVE TEST: INDICATES MALIGNANT" IF WNT2BOT>=2 ELSE
"NEGATIVE TEST: INDICATES BENIGN" IF OTBDIFF<0 ELSE
"NEGATIVE TEST: INDICATES BENIGN" IF RTBDIFF<0 ELSE
"POSITIVE TEST: INDICATES MALIGNANT" IF 3-RGS1TOP>=2 ELSE
"NEGATIVE TEST: INDICATES BENIGN" IF FTBDIFF<0 ELSE
"NEGATIVE TEST: INDICATES BENIGN" IF ATBDIFF<0 ELSE
"NEGATIVE TEST: INDICATES BENIGN" IF 3-OPNTOP<1 ELSE
"POSITIVE TEST: INDICATES MALIGNANT" IF RGS1BOT>=3 ELSE
"POSITIVE TEST: INDICATES MALIGNANT" IF 3-ARPC2TOP>=2 ELSE
"NEGATIVE TEST: INDICATES BENIGN" IF FN1TOP<1 ELSE
"NEGATIVE TEST: INDICATES BENIGN" IF WNT2TOP<2 ELSE
"POSITIVE TEST: INDICATES MALIGNANT" IF RTBDIFF>=0 ELSE
"POSITIVE TEST: INDICATES MALIGNANT" IF FN1TOP>=1 ELSE
"POSITIVE TEST: INDICATES MALIGNANT" IF FTBDIFF>=0 ELSE
"NEGATIVE TEST: INDICATES BENIGN" IF 3-ARPC2TOP<2 ELSE
"POSITIVE TEST: INDICATES MALIGNANT" IF ATBDIFF>=0 ELSE
"POSITIVE TEST: INDICATES MALIGNANT" IF 3-OPNTOP>=1 ELSE
"POSITIVE TEST: INDICATES MALIGNANT" IF OTBDIFF>=0 ELSE
"POSITIVE TEST: INDICATES MALIGNANT" IF FN1BOT>=1 ELSE
"NEGATIVE TEST: INDICATES BENIGN" IF ARPC2BOT<1 ELSE
"POSITIVE TEST: INDICATES MALIGNANT" IF OPNBOT>=2 ELSE
"POSITIVE TEST: INDICATES MALIGNANT" IF WNT2TOP>=2 ELSE
"POSITIVE TEST: INDICATES MALIGNANT" IF ARPC2BOT>=1 ELSE
"NEGATIVE TEST: INDICATES BENIGN" IF RGS1BOT<3 ELSE
"NEGATIVE TEST: INDICATES BENIGN" IF FN1BOT<1 ELSE
"NEGATIVE TEST: INDICATES BENIGN" IF 3-RGS1TOP<2 ELSE
"NEGATIVE TEST: INDICATES BENIGN" IF WNT2BOT<2 ELSE
"NEGATIVE TEST: INDICATES BENIGN" IF OPNBOT<2 ELSE
"NO DIAGNOSTIC CONCLUSION"
```

Applying the summarized composite algorithm to the same 600 lesions produced:

DSSA-GENERATED DIAGNOSTIC CONCLUSION	CORRECT DIAGNOSIS OF LESION		
	BENIGN	MALIGNANT	TOTAL
NEGATIVE TEST: INDICATES BENIGN	170	26	196
POSITIVE TEST: INDICATES MALIGNANT	9	395	404
TOTAL	179	421	600

DSSA produced a definite diagnostic conclusion for all 600 training lesions.

1. It achieved a sensitivity of 395/421 = 93.82 percent. This was unchanged from the 519-lesion analysis performed without adding the sixty dysplastic and the twenty-one Spitz nevi, since all eighty-one lesions added for confirmation were benign.
2. It achieved a specificity of 170/179 = 94.97 percent. This compared to a specificity of 89/98 = 90.82 percent without adding the eighty-one difficult-to-diagnose nevi, all of which were accurately confirmed as either dysplastic or Spitz, respectively.
3. It made (170+395)/600 = 94.17 percent correct diagnoses. This was an improvement over the (89+395)/519 = 93.26 percent correct diagnoses achieved by the 519-lesion analysis performed without the eighty-one nevi added for confirmation.
4. It achieved an AUC of 0.9440 compared to an AUC of 0.9232 achieved by the 519-lesion analysis.

By every measure diagnosing the eighty-one problem cases separately and adding the two algorithms designed to confirm their separate diagnoses achieved either the same level of accuracy or more accurate diagnoses. First partitioning the 600 lesions into more homogeneous strata, producing separate diagnostic algorithms via DSSA for each separate stratum, and then merging the results into a final, composite diagnostic algorithm proved to be quite helpful.

Our homogeneous versus heterogeneous explanation of why dysplastic and Spitz nevi are problem cases now appears quite plausible. We do not pretend to have explained the underlying biology. Nevertheless, the noticeably different roles played by our five genes in diagnosing dysplastic versus Spitz nevi may provide useful clues in eventually understanding their biological differences.

5.8 ACT III Validation: Thirty-Eight Malignant Melanomas Arising from a Benign Nevus

Validation of a DSSA-generated diagnostic algorithm means applying it to a completely distinct collection of lesions. We obtained two separate data sets for purposes of validation. None of the lesions nor any of the patients involved in either validation set were included in the 600-lesion training data. Consequently, any accuracy in diagnostic discriminations achieved by applying the composite algorithm to either validation sample cannot be attributed to statistical overfitting.

Thirty-eight instances of a primary melanoma arising from a benign nevus were obtained from patient records. This first validation sample contained thirty-eight matched pairs of lesions. The pathologist was able to evaluate seventy-five of the seventy-six total lesions. He identified four of the nevi in the thirty-seven usable matched pairs as dysplastic, but none as a Spitz nevus.

The reason for selecting melanomas arising from a nevus was to exploit the variance-reducing statistical properties of a matched-pair analysis. Many factors that might confound the differential diagnosis were thereby controlled via matching. Potentially confounding factors include patient sex, anatomical location of the primary lesion, histological subtype, and genetic influences.

Results of applying the composite algorithm to the seventy-five lesions in the thirty-seven matched pairs are shown on the next page.

DSSA-GENERATED DIAGNOSTIC CONCLUSION	CORRECT DIAGNOSIS OF LESION		
	BENIGN	MALIGNANT	TOTAL
DYSPLASTIC CONFIRMED: 1-ATBDIFF<2	3	0	3
DYSPLASTIC CONFIRMED: 1-OTBDIFF<2.5	1	0	1
DIAGNOSED BENIGN: WTBDIFF<0	26	0	26
DIAGNOSED MALIGNANT: WTBDIFF>=0	0	35	35
DIAGNOSED MALIGNANT: WNT2BOT>=2	2	0	2
DIAGNOSED BENIGN: OTBDIFF<0	2	0	2
DIAGNOSED BENIGN: RTBDIFF<0	2	0	2
DIAGNOSED BENIGN: FTBDIFF<0	0	1	1
DIAGNOSED BENIGN: FN1TOP<1	0	1	1
DIAGNOSED BENIGN: ARPC2BOT<1	1	0	1
DIAGNOSED BENIGN: WNT2BOT<2	1	0	1
TOTAL	38	37	75

Results of applying the summarized version of the composite algorithm to the same seventy-five lesions in the thirty-seven matched pairs are shown below.

DSSA-GENERATED DIAGNOSTIC CONCLUSION	CORRECT DIAGNOSIS OF LESION		
	BENIGN	MALIGNANT	TOTAL
NEGATIVE TEST: INDICATES BENIGN	36	2	38
POSITIVE TEST: INDICATES MALIGNANT	2	35	37
TOTAL	38	37	75

Accuracy statistics comparable to our previous analyses can be obtained by regarding diagnoses of the seventy-five lesions separately.

1. DSSA produced a definite diagnostic conclusion for all seventy-five evaluable validation lesions.
2. It successfully confirmed all four of the dysplastic nevi.
3. It achieved a sensitivity of 35/37 = 94.59 percent.
4. It achieved a specificity of 36/38 = 94.74 percent.
5. It made (35+36)/75 = 94.67 percent correct diagnoses.
6. It achieved an AUC of 0.9467.

Applying the composite algorithm to any matched pair of lesions can result in:

1. a completely accurate diagnosis where the melanoma portion of tissue is diagnosed malignant, while the nevus portion is diagnosed benign;
2. a partially accurate diagnosis where only one portion of the tissue is correctly diagnosed but the other portion is misdiagnosed; or
3. a completely inaccurate diagnosis where both portions of tissue are misdiagnosed.

Since only four of the seventy-five lesions were misdiagnosed, at least thirty-three of the thirty-seven matched pairs must have been diagnosed with complete accuracy. A sign test based on the rather optimistic random hypothesis that complete accuracy is fifty percent likely on each matched pair assigned a p value less than 0.0001 to the observed or any more accurate diagnostic result. A hypothesized less-than-50-percent likelihood would have been far more reasonable. If used, it would have generated an even more convincing (i.e., more significant) p value.

A diagnostic algorithm originally fitted to lesions obtained from a sample of 600 patients and later applied to separate lesions obtained from thirty-eight distinct patients would normally result in some accuracy deterioration. That is not what happened. Except for a small reduction in specificity from 94.97 percent to 94.74 percent, all other accuracy statistics improved relative to the training data. Perhaps the pairing of benign and malignant tissue matched for each patient accounted, in part, for this unusual result. In any case the first validation was very successful.

5.9   ACT III Validation: Twenty-Four Initially Misdiagnosed Lesions Reassessed

A second validation sample was obtained. It was designed to pose an especially difficult challenge to DSSA. Medical records at UCSF were searched for melanoma patients who had originally been misdiagnosed but whose diagnoses were later corrected on the basis of subsequent observations. Such cases were few and far between. A concerted effort was required to find them.

Eventually, we identified six patients whose lesions were initially misdiagnosed as melanomas and were later reclassified as benign nevi by a consensus dermatopathology review. We also identified eighteen patients whose lesions were initially misdiagnosed as benign or ambiguous that later recurred locally or metastasized. Together, these represented twenty-four initially misdiagnosed and subsequently corrected cases. The challenge for DSSA was to apply the composite algorithm to the twenty-four originally misdiagnosed lesions to see how many could have been correctly diagnosed at the outset.

Below are listed the initial misdiagnoses (FIRSTDX) and the corrected final diagnoses (FINALDX) of these twenty-four lesions.

VALUE OF ATTRIBUTE FIRSTDX	VALUE OF ATTRIBUTE FINALDX
BENIGN NEVUS (SPITZ)	MALIGNANT MELANOMA
ATYPICAL MELANOCYTIC PROLIFERATION	MALIGNANT MELANOMA
BENIGN NEVUS	MALIGNANT MELANOMA
BENIGN NEVUS	MALIGNANT MELANOMA
MALIGNANT MELANOMA	BENIGN NEVUS (DYSPLASTIC)
MALIGNANT MELANOMA	BENIGN NEVUS (DYSPLASTIC)
MALIGNANT MELANOMA	BENIGN NEVUS (SPITZ)
BENIGN NEVUS (SPITZ)	MALIGNANT MELANOMA
BENIGN NEVUS (SPITZ)	MALIGNANT MELANOMA
BENIGN NEVUS	MALIGNANT MELANOMA
BIPHASIC NEOPLASM	MALIGNANT MELANOMA
MALIGNANT MELANOMA	BENIGN NEVUS (SPITZ)
BENIGN NEVUS (SPITZ)	MALIGNANT MELANOMA
BENIGN NEVUS (DESMOPLASTIC)	MALIGNANT MELANOMA
MALIGNANT MELANOMA	BENIGN NEVUS
BENIGN NEVUS (SPITZ)	MALIGNANT MELANOMA
BENIGN NEVUS	MALIGNANT MELANOMA
MALIGNANT MELANOMA	BENIGN NEVUS (DYSPLASTIC)
BENIGN NEVUS	MALIGNANT MELANOMA
ATYPICAL MELANOCYTIC PROLIFERATION	MALIGNANT MELANOMA
BENIGN NEVUS	MALIGNANT MELANOMA
BENIGN NEVUS	MALIGNANT MELANOMA
BENIGN NEVUS	MALIGNANT MELANOMA (DESMOPLASTIC)
BENIGN NEVUS	MALIGNANT MELANOMA

The composite diagnostic algorithm was applied to these twenty-four lesions with the following results.

DSSA-GENERATED DIAGNOSTIC CONCLUSION	CORRECT DIAGNOSIS OF LESION BENIGN	MALIGNANT	TOTAL
DYSPLASTIC CONFIRMED: 1-ATBDIFF<2	3	0	3
SPITZ CONFIRMED: FTBDIFF<0	1	0	1
SPITZ CONFIRMED: 3-WNT2TOP<2	1	0	1
DIAGNOSED BENIGN: WTBDIFF<0	0	3	3
DIAGNOSED MALIGNANT: WTBDIFF>=0	1	11	12
DIAGNOSED MALIGNANT: WNT2BOT>=2	0	2	2
DIAGNOSED BENIGN: OTBDIFF<0	0	2	2
TOTAL	6	18	24

Results of applying the summarized version of the composite algorithm to the same twenty-four initially misdiagnosed lesions are shown below.

DSSA-GENERATED DIAGNOSTIC CONCLUSION	CORRECT DIAGNOSIS OF LESION BENIGN	MALIGNANT	TOTAL
NEGATIVE TEST: INDICATES BENIGN	5	5	10
POSITIVE TEST: INDICATES MALIGNANT	1	13	14
TOTAL	6	18	24

Accuracy statistics were as follows.

1. DSSA produced a definite diagnostic conclusion for all lesions.
2. It successfully confirmed all three of the actually dysplastic nevi.
3. It successfully confirmed both of the actual Spitz nevi.
4. It achieved a sensitivity of 13/18 = 72.22 percent.
5. It achieved a specificity of 5/6 = 83.33 percent.
6. It made (13+5)/24 = 75.00 percent correct diagnoses.
7. It achieved an AUC of 0.7778.
8. The probability of achieving eighteen or more out of twenty-four correct reversals by chance alone (i.e., if determined by flipping a fair coin) would have been 0.0113.

Compared to the 600 lesions in the complete training sample these accuracy statistics are not as good. Nevertheless, the ability to correct three-quarters of the initial misdiagnoses via the composite DSSA diagnostic algorithm constructed solely from our five genes is more than just statistically significant. It is genuinely noteworthy.

5.10 Act IV: Using SPSA to Refine and Improve DSSA's Diagnostic Accuracy

Section 5.1 successfully validated the direction of impact of all five genes as originally indicated by the SAM analysis. To accomplish this validation the numeric measurement scale of each gene was optimally partitioned by means of cut points so as to facilitate its best univariate benign-versus-malignant discrimination through logistic regression. The raw measurement scale of each gene identified four levels of staining intensity as observed by the pathologist: absent (0); light (1); moderate (2); or intense (3).

For example, the optimal partitioning of the WNT2 scale was found to utilize all four scale values. No separate values were grouped together into the same subscale. This required three cut points: between 0 and 1; between 1 and 2; and between 2 and 3.

The optimal partitioning of the OPN (SPP1, also called osteopontin) scale was into three subscales (0 IF OPN=0 OR OPN=1 ELSE 1 IF OPN=2 ELSE 2 IF OPN=3). This required only two cut points: between 1 and 2; and between 2 and 3.

The optimal partitioning of the RGS1 scale was into two subscales (0 IF RGS1=0 OR RGS1=1 OR RGS1=2 ELSE 1 IF RGS1=3). This required only a single cut point between 2 and 3.

DSSA initially dichotomizes the numeric scale of each indicator it receives as input. It identifies the single best numeric cut point that maximizes diagnostic discrimination. SPSA can be used to refine the scale of each DSSA input indicator. SPSA mimics DSSA by initially identifying the same single best numeric cut point that maximizes diagnostic discrimination, but SPSA does not stop there. If the scale of any indicator can be usefully partitioned further, SPSA will accomplish that task. Thus, SPSA identifies any additional cut points that can improve diagnostic discrimination. A common reason to add cut points is when either extreme scale value of an indicator is especially useful in discriminating between a benign nevus and a malignant melanoma but the single best cut point lies in the interior of the scale.

All fifteen indicator inputs to DSSA were preprocessed by SPSA to identify additional useful cut points. The results were as follows.

1. WNT2TOP's best initial cut point was between 1 and 2, but a WNT2TOP value of 3 was especially discriminating. WNT2TOP was therefore replaced by WTOPCTP2 (cut point between 1 and 2) and WTOPCTP3 (cut point between 2 and 3).
2. WNT2BOT's best initial cut point was between 1 and 2, but WNT2BOT values of both 0 and 3 were especially discriminating. WNT2BOT was therefore replaced by WBOTCTP1 (cut point between 0 and 1), WBOTCTP2 (cut point between 1 and 2), and WBOTCTP3 (cut point between 2 and 3).
3. WTBDIFF could not be improved by SPSA. It was not replaced.
4. 3-ARPC2TOP could not be improved by SPSA. It was not replaced.
5. ARPC2BOT'S best initial cut point was between 2 and 3, but a ARPC2BOT value of 2 was especially discriminating. ARPC2BOT was therefore replaced by ABOTCTP2 (cut point between 1 and 2) and ABOTCTP3 (cut point between 2 and 3).
6. ATBDIFF could not be improved by SPSA. It was not replaced.
7. 3-OPNTOP's best initial cut point was between 1 and 2, but a 3-OPNTOP value of 0 was especially discriminating. 3-OPNTOP was therefore replaced by OTOPCTP1 (cut point between 0 and 1) and OTOPCTP2 (cut point between 1 and 2).
8. OPNBOT's best initial cut point was between 1 and 2, but a OPNBOT value of 3 was especially discriminating. OPNBOT was therefore replaced by OBOTCTP2 (cut point between 1 and 2) and OBOTCTP3 (cut point between 2 and 3).
9. OTBDIFF could not be improved by SPSA. It was not replaced.
10. 3-RGS1TOP could not be improved by SPSA. It was not replaced.
11. RGS1BOT could not be improved by SPSA. It was not replaced.
12. RTBDIFF could not be improved by SPSA. It was not replaced.
13. FN1TOP's best initial cut point was between 1 and 2, but a FN1TOP value of 0 was especially discriminating. FN1TOP was therefore replaced by FTOPCTP1 (cut point between 0 and 1) and FTOPCTP2 (cut point between 1 and 2).

14. FN1BOT could not be improved by SPSA. It was not replaced.
15. FTBDIFF could not be improved by SPSA. It was not replaced.

The combined result of SPSA improvements was to replace six original indicators (WNT2TOP, WNT2BOT, ARPC2BOT, 3-OPNTOP, OPNBOT, and FN1TOP) with thirteen refined indicators (WTOPCTP2, WTOPCTP3, WBOTCTP1, WBOTCTP2, WBOTCTP3, ABOTCTP2, ABOTCTP3, OTOPCTP1, OTOPCTP2, OBOTCTP2, OBOTCTP3, FTOPCTP1, and FTOPCTP2). A net increase of seven indicators (from fifteen to twenty-two) produced a net increase of fourteen discriminators (from thirty to forty-four).

There was no reason to improve DSSA's confirmatory diagnostic algorithms for dysplastic and Spitz nevi. Through judicious adjustments of the sensitivity weights DSSA achieved 100 percent accurate discrimination in both sets of training data.

DSSA was then applied to the homogenized 519-lesion training data with these twenty-two indicators. Once again, DSSA's weight on sensitivity was raised to 0.55 to nudge the diagnosis in the direction of slightly more sensitive than specific discriminations.

The two confirmatory algorithms previously produced were then merged with the homogenized algorithm generated by DSSA with the twenty-two indicators from the 519 training lesions to create the following improved final composite diagnostic training algorithm.

```
"DYSPLASTIC CONFIRMED: 1-ATBDIFF<2" IF TDX=DY AND 1-ATBDIFF<2 ELSE
"DYSPLASTIC CONFIRMED: 1-WTBDIFF<2.5" IF TDX=DY AND 1-WTBDIFF<2.5 ELSE
"DYSPLASTIC CONFIRMED: 1-OTBDIFF<2.5" IF TDX=DY AND 1-OTBDIFF<2.5 ELSE
"DYSPLASTIC CONFIRMED: 3-ARPC2TOP<2" IF TDX=DY AND 3-ARPC2TOP<2 ELSE
"DYSPLASTIC CONFIRMED: FN1TOP<3" IF TDX=DY AND FN1TOP<3 ELSE
"DYSPLASTIC CONFIRMED: FN1BOT<2" IF TDX=DY AND FN1BOT<2 ELSE
"DYSPLASTIC CONFIRMED: 3-ARPC2BOT<2" IF TDX=DY AND 3-ARPC2BOT<2 ELSE
"SPITZ CONFIRMED: FTBDIFF<0" IF TDX=SP AND FTBDIFF<0 ELSE
"SPITZ CONFIRMED: RTBDIFF<0" IF TDX=SP AND RTBDIFF<0 ELSE
"SPITZ CONFIRMED: WTBDIFF<-.5" IF TDX=SP AND WTBDIFF<-.5 ELSE
"SPITZ CONFIRMED: OTBDIFF<-1" IF TDX=SP AND OTBDIFF<-1 ELSE
"SPITZ CONFIRMED: 3-WNT2TOP<2" IF TDX=SP AND 3-WNT2TOP<2 ELSE
"SPITZ CONFIRMED: WNT2BOT<1" IF TDX=SP AND WNT2BOT<1 ELSE
"SPITZ CONFIRMED: RGS1BOT<2" IF TDX=SP AND RGS1BOT<2 ELSE
"SPITZ CONFIRMED: FN1BOT<1" IF TDX=SP AND FN1BOT<1 ELSE
"SPITZ CONFIRMED: OPNBOT<1.5" IF TDX=SP AND OPNBOT<1.5 ELSE
"DIAGNOSED BENIGN: WTBDIFF<0" IF WTBDIFF<0 ELSE
"DIAGNOSED MALIGNANT: WTBDIFF>=0" IF WTBDIFF>=0 ELSE
"DIAGNOSED MALIGNANT: WBOTCTP3>=3" IF WBOTCTP3>=3 ELSE
"DIAGNOSED MALIGNANT: WBOTCTP1>=1" IF WBOTCTP1>=1 ELSE
"DIAGNOSED MALIGNANT: WBOTCTP2>=2" IF WBOTCTP2>=2 ELSE
"DIAGNOSED BENIGN: OTBDIFF<0" IF OTBDIFF<0 ELSE
"DIAGNOSED BENIGN: RTBDIFF<0" IF RTBDIFF<0 ELSE
"DIAGNOSED MALIGNANT: FTOPCTP2>=2" IF FTOPCTP2>=2 ELSE
"DIAGNOSED MALIGNANT: 3-RGS1TOP>=2" IF 3-RGS1TOP>=2 ELSE
"DIAGNOSED BENIGN: FTBDIFF<0" IF FTBDIFF<0 ELSE
"DIAGNOSED BENIGN: ATBDIFF<0" IF ATBDIFF<0 ELSE
"DIAGNOSED MALIGNANT: WTOPCTP3>=3" IF WTOPCTP3>=3 ELSE
"DIAGNOSED BENIGN: OTOPCTP1<1" IF OTOPCTP1<1 ELSE
"DIAGNOSED MALIGNANT: 3-ARPC2TOP>=2" IF 3-ARPC2TOP>=2 ELSE
"DIAGNOSED MALIGNANT: RGS1BOT>=3" IF RGS1BOT>=3 ELSE
"DIAGNOSED BENIGN: OBOTCTP2<2" IF OBOTCTP2<2 ELSE
"DIAGNOSED MALIGNANT: FTOPCTP1>=1" IF FTOPCTP1>=1 ELSE
"DIAGNOSED BENIGN: WTOPCTP2<2" IF WTOPCTP2<2 ELSE
```

```
"DIAGNOSED MALIGNANT: OBOTCTP3>=3" IF OBOTCTP3>=3 ELSE
"DIAGNOSED MALIGNANT: RTBDIFF>=0" IF RTBDIFF>=0 ELSE
"DIAGNOSED MALIGNANT: OTOPCTP2>=2" IF OTOPCTP2>=2 ELSE
"DIAGNOSED BENIGN: OTOPCTP2<2" IF OTOPCTP2<2 ELSE
"DIAGNOSED MALIGNANT: FN1BOT>=1" IF FN1BOT>=1 ELSE
"DIAGNOSED MALIGNANT: OTBDIFF>=0" IF OTBDIFF>=0 ELSE
"DIAGNOSED MALIGNANT: OTOPCTP1>=1" IF OTOPCTP1>=1 ELSE
"DIAGNOSED BENIGN: RGS1BOT<3" IF RGS1BOT<3 ELSE
"DIAGNOSED MALIGNANT: OBOTCTP2>=2" IF OBOTCTP2>=2 ELSE
"DIAGNOSED MALIGNANT: WTOPCTP2>=2" IF WTOPCTP2>=2 ELSE
"DIAGNOSED MALIGNANT: ABOTCTP3>=3" IF ABOTCTP3>=3 ELSE
"DIAGNOSED BENIGN: 3-RGS1TOP<2" IF 3-RGS1TOP<2 ELSE
"DIAGNOSED BENIGN: WBOTCTP1<1" IF WBOTCTP1<1 ELSE
"DIAGNOSED BENIGN: WBOTCTP2<2" IF WBOTCTP2<2 ELSE
"DIAGNOSED BENIGN: WBOTCTP3<3" IF WBOTCTP3<3 ELSE
"DIAGNOSED BENIGN: WTOPCTP3<3" IF WTOPCTP3<3 ELSE
"DIAGNOSED BENIGN: ABOTCTP2<2" IF ABOTCTP2<2 ELSE
"DIAGNOSED BENIGN: OBOTCTP3<3" IF OBOTCTP3<3 ELSE
"DIAGNOSED BENIGN: 3-ARPC2TOP<2" IF 3-ARPC2TOP<2 ELSE
"DIAGNOSED MALIGNANT: FTBDIFF>=0" IF FTBDIFF>=0 ELSE
"DIAGNOSED MALIGNANT: ATBDIFF>=0" IF ATBDIFF>=0 ELSE
"DIAGNOSED BENIGN: ABOTCTP3<3" IF ABOTCTP3<3 ELSE
"DIAGNOSED BENIGN: FN1BOT<1" IF FN1BOT<1 ELSE
"DIAGNOSED MALIGNANT: ABOTCTP2>=2" IF ABOTCTP2>=2 ELSE
"DIAGNOSED BENIGN: FTOPCTP2<2" IF FTOPCTP2<2 ELSE
"DIAGNOSED BENIGN: FTOPCTP1<1" IF FTOPCTP1<1 ELSE
"NO DIAGNOSTIC CONCLUSION"
```

The improved final composite algorithm was applied to all 600 training lesions.
That produced the following results.

DSSA-GENERATED DIAGNOSTIC CONCLUSION	CORRECT DIAGNOSIS OF LESION		
	BENIGN	MALIGNANT	TOTAL
DYSPLASTIC CONFIRMED: 1-ATBDIFF<2	55	0	55
DYSPLASTIC CONFIRMED: 1-WTBDIFF<2.5	1	0	1
DYSPLASTIC CONFIRMED: 1-OTBDIFF<2.5	1	0	1
DYSPLASTIC CONFIRMED: 3-ARPC2TOP<2	2	0	2
DYSPLASTIC CONFIRMED: FN1TOP<3	1	0	1
SPITZ CONFIRMED: FTBDIFF<0	9	0	9
SPITZ CONFIRMED: RTBDIFF<0	3	0	3
SPITZ CONFIRMED: WTBDIFF<-.5	6	0	6
SPITZ CONFIRMED: OTBDIFF<-1	1	0	1
SPITZ CONFIRMED: 3-WNT2TOP<2	2	0	2
DIAGNOSED BENIGN: WTBDIFF<0	39	0	39
DIAGNOSED MALIGNANT: WTBDIFF>=0	0	105	105
DIAGNOSED MALIGNANT: WBOTCTP3>=3	0	57	57
DIAGNOSED MALIGNANT: WBOTCTP1>=1	0	167	167
DIAGNOSED BENIGN: OTBDIFF<0	17	0	17
DIAGNOSED BENIGN: RTBDIFF<0	4	0	4
DIAGNOSED MALIGNANT: FTOPCTP2>=2	0	9	9
DIAGNOSED MALIGNANT: 3-RGS1TOP>=2	0	13	13
DIAGNOSED BENIGN: FTBDIFF<0	2	0	2
DIAGNOSED BENIGN: ATBDIFF<0	5	0	5
DIAGNOSED MALIGNANT: WTOPCTP3>=3	0	6	6
DIAGNOSED BENIGN: OTOPCTP1<1	3	1	4
DIAGNOSED MALIGNANT: 3-ARPC2TOP>=2	1	11	12
DIAGNOSED MALIGNANT: RGS1BOT>=3	1	9	10
DIAGNOSED BENIGN: OBOTCTP2<2	11	4	15

DIAGNOSED MALIGNANT: FTOPCTP1>=1	1	7	8
DIAGNOSED BENIGN: WTOPCTP2<2	7	2	9
DIAGNOSED MALIGNANT: OBOTCTP3>=3	0	3	3
DIAGNOSED MALIGNANT: RTBDIFF>=0	0	2	2
DIAGNOSED MALIGNANT: OTOPCTP2>=2	0	2	2
DIAGNOSED BENIGN: OTOPCTP2<2	2	2	4
DIAGNOSED MALIGNANT: FN1BOT>=1	0	9	9
DIAGNOSED BENIGN: RGS1BOT<3	2	0	2
DIAGNOSED MALIGNANT: OBOTCTP2>=2	0	4	4
DIAGNOSED MALIGNANT: WTOPCTP2>=2	0	2	2
DIAGNOSED MALIGNANT: ABOTCTP3>=3	0	1	1
DIAGNOSED BENIGN: 3-ARPC2TOP<2	2	2	4
DIAGNOSED MALIGNANT: FTBDIFF>=0	0	1	1
DIAGNOSED BENIGN: ABOTCTP3<3	1	1	2
DIAGNOSED BENIGN: FTOPCTP2<2	0	1	1
TOTAL	179	421	600

A summarized version of the same improved final composite diagnostic algorithm was:

```
"NEGATIVE TEST: INDICATES BENIGN" IF TDX=DY AND 1-ATBDIFF<2 ELSE
"NEGATIVE TEST: INDICATES BENIGN" IF TDX=DY AND 1-WTBDIFF<2.5 ELSE
"NEGATIVE TEST: INDICATES BENIGN" IF TDX=DY AND 1-OTBDIFF<2.5 ELSE
"NEGATIVE TEST: INDICATES BENIGN" IF TDX=DY AND 3-ARPC2TOP<2 ELSE
"NEGATIVE TEST: INDICATES BENIGN" IF TDX=DY AND FN1TOP<3 ELSE
"NEGATIVE TEST: INDICATES BENIGN" IF TDX=DY AND FN1BOT<2 ELSE
"NEGATIVE TEST: INDICATES BENIGN" IF TDX=DY AND 3-ARPC2BOT<2 ELSE
"NEGATIVE TEST: INDICATES BENIGN" IF TDX=SP AND FTBDIFF<0 ELSE
"NEGATIVE TEST: INDICATES BENIGN" IF TDX=SP AND RTBDIFF<0 ELSE
"NEGATIVE TEST: INDICATES BENIGN" IF TDX=SP AND WTBDIFF<-.5 ELSE
"NEGATIVE TEST: INDICATES BENIGN" IF TDX=SP AND OTBDIFF<-1 ELSE
"NEGATIVE TEST: INDICATES BENIGN" IF TDX=SP AND 3-WNT2TOP<2 ELSE
"NEGATIVE TEST: INDICATES BENIGN" IF TDX=SP AND WNT2BOT<1 ELSE
"NEGATIVE TEST: INDICATES BENIGN" IF TDX=SP AND RGS1BOT<2 ELSE
"NEGATIVE TEST: INDICATES BENIGN" IF TDX=SP AND FN1BOT<1 ELSE
"NEGATIVE TEST: INDICATES BENIGN" IF TDX=SP AND OPNBOT<1.5 ELSE
"NEGATIVE TEST: INDICATES BENIGN" IF WTBDIFF<0 ELSE
"POSITIVE TEST: INDICATES MALIGNANT" IF WTBDIFF>=0 ELSE
"POSITIVE TEST: INDICATES MALIGNANT" IF WBOTCTP3>=3 ELSE
"POSITIVE TEST: INDICATES MALIGNANT" IF WBOTCTP1>=1 ELSE
"POSITIVE TEST: INDICATES MALIGNANT" IF WBOTCTP2>=2 ELSE
"NEGATIVE TEST: INDICATES BENIGN" IF OTBDIFF<0 ELSE
"NEGATIVE TEST: INDICATES BENIGN" IF RTBDIFF<0 ELSE
"POSITIVE TEST: INDICATES MALIGNANT" IF FTOPCTP2>=2 ELSE
"POSITIVE TEST: INDICATES MALIGNANT" IF 3-RGS1TOP>=2 ELSE
"NEGATIVE TEST: INDICATES BENIGN" IF FTBDIFF<0 ELSE
"NEGATIVE TEST: INDICATES BENIGN" IF ATBDIFF<0 ELSE
"POSITIVE TEST: INDICATES MALIGNANT" IF WTOPCTP3>=3 ELSE
"NEGATIVE TEST: INDICATES BENIGN" IF OTOPCTP1<1 ELSE
"POSITIVE TEST: INDICATES MALIGNANT" IF 3-ARPC2TOP>=2 ELSE
"POSITIVE TEST: INDICATES MALIGNANT" IF RGS1BOT>=3 ELSE
"NEGATIVE TEST: INDICATES BENIGN" IF OBOTCTP2<2 ELSE
"POSITIVE TEST: INDICATES MALIGNANT" IF FTOPCTP1>=1 ELSE
"NEGATIVE TEST: INDICATES BENIGN" IF WTOPCTP2<2 ELSE
"POSITIVE TEST: INDICATES MALIGNANT" IF OBOTCTP3>=3 ELSE
"POSITIVE TEST: INDICATES MALIGNANT" IF RTBDIFF>=0 ELSE
"POSITIVE TEST: INDICATES MALIGNANT" IF OTOPCTP2>=2 ELSE
"NEGATIVE TEST: INDICATES BENIGN" IF OTOPCTP2<2 ELSE
```

```
"POSITIVE TEST: INDICATES MALIGNANT" IF FN1BOT>=1 ELSE
"POSITIVE TEST: INDICATES MALIGNANT" IF OTBDIFF>=0 ELSE
"POSITIVE TEST: INDICATES MALIGNANT" IF OTOPCTP1>=1 ELSE
"NEGATIVE TEST: INDICATES BENIGN" IF RGS1BOT<3 ELSE
"POSITIVE TEST: INDICATES MALIGNANT" IF OBOTCTP2>=2 ELSE
"POSITIVE TEST: INDICATES MALIGNANT" IF WTOPCTP2>=2 ELSE
"POSITIVE TEST: INDICATES MALIGNANT" IF ABOTCTP3>=3 ELSE
"NEGATIVE TEST: INDICATES BENIGN" IF 3-RGS1TOP<2 ELSE
"NEGATIVE TEST: INDICATES BENIGN" IF WBOTCTP1<1 ELSE
"NEGATIVE TEST: INDICATES BENIGN" IF WBOTCTP2<2 ELSE
"NEGATIVE TEST: INDICATES BENIGN" IF WBOTCTP3<3 ELSE
"NEGATIVE TEST: INDICATES BENIGN" IF WTOPCTP3<3 ELSE
"NEGATIVE TEST: INDICATES BENIGN" IF ABOTCTP2<2 ELSE
"NEGATIVE TEST: INDICATES BENIGN" IF OBOTCTP3<3 ELSE
"NEGATIVE TEST: INDICATES BENIGN" IF 3-ARPC2TOP<2 ELSE
"POSITIVE TEST: INDICATES MALIGNANT" IF FTBDIFF>=0 ELSE
"POSITIVE TEST: INDICATES MALIGNANT" IF ATBDIFF>=0 ELSE
"NEGATIVE TEST: INDICATES BENIGN" IF ABOTCTP3<3 ELSE
"NEGATIVE TEST: INDICATES BENIGN" IF FN1BOT<1 ELSE
"POSITIVE TEST: INDICATES MALIGNANT" IF ABOTCTP2>=2 ELSE
"NEGATIVE TEST: INDICATES BENIGN" IF FTOPCTP2<2 ELSE
"NEGATIVE TEST: INDICATES BENIGN" IF FTOPCTP1<1 ELSE
"NO DIAGNOSTIC CONCLUSION"
```

Results of applying the summarized improved final composite algorithm to the same 600 lesions were:

DSSA-GENERATED DIAGNOSTIC CONCLUSION	CORRECT DIAGNOSIS OF LESION		
	BENIGN	MALIGNANT	TOTAL
NEGATIVE TEST: INDICATES BENIGN	176	13	189
POSITIVE TEST: INDICATES MALIGNANT	3	408	411
TOTAL	179	421	600

DSSA once again produced a definite diagnostic conclusion for all 600 training lesions, and it successfully confirmed all sixty dysplastic and all twenty-one Spitz nevi.

1. It achieved a sensitivity of 408/421 = 96.91 percent. This was an improvement compared to 93.82 percent without SPSA's refinements.
2. It achieved a specificity of 176/179 = 98.32 percent compared to 94.97 percent without SPSA's refinements.
3. It made (408+176)/600 = 97.33 percent correct diagnoses compared to 94.17 percent without SPSA's refinements.
4. It achieved an AUC of 0.9762 compared to 0.9440 without SPSA's refinements.

By every measure preprocessing DSSA's input indicators with SPSA produced noticeable improvements in diagnostic accuracy. If the increased accuracy persists when this improved final composite algorithm is subsequently applied to the two validation data sets we can have some confidence that it is not merely a reflection of statistical overfitting.

Results of applying the improved final composite algorithm to the seventy-five lesions in the thirty-seven matched pairs of melanomas arising from a nevus are shown on the next page.

DSSA-GENERATED DIAGNOSTIC CONCLUSION	CORRECT DIAGNOSIS OF LESION		
	BENIGN	MALIGNANT	TOTAL
DYSPLASTIC CONFIRMED: 1-ATBDIFF<2	3	0	3
DYSPLASTIC CONFIRMED: 1-OTBDIFF<2.5	1	0	1
DIAGNOSED BENIGN: WTBDIFF<0	26	0	26
DIAGNOSED MALIGNANT: WTBDIFF>=0	0	35	35
DIAGNOSED MALIGNANT: WBOTCTP1>=1	2	0	2
DIAGNOSED BENIGN: OTBDIFF<0	2	0	2
DIAGNOSED BENIGN: RTBDIFF<0	2	0	2
DIAGNOSED MALIGNANT: FTOPCTP2>=2	0	1	1
DIAGNOSED MALIGNANT: RTBDIFF>=0	0	1	1
DIAGNOSED BENIGN: WBOTCTP1<1	2	0	2
TOTAL	38	37	75

Results of applying the summarized version of the improved final composite algorithm to the same seventy-five lesions in the thirty-seven matched pairs are shown below.

DSSA-GENERATED DIAGNOSTIC CONCLUSION	CORRECT DIAGNOSIS OF LESION		
	BENIGN	MALIGNANT	TOTAL
NEGATIVE TEST: INDICATES BENIGN	36	0	36
POSITIVE TEST: INDICATES MALIGNANT	2	37	39
TOTAL	38	37	75

Accuracy statistics comparable to our previous analyses can be obtained by regarding diagnoses of the seventy-five lesions separately.

1. DSSA produced a definite diagnostic conclusion for all seventy-five evaluable validation lesions.
2. It successfully confirmed all four of the dysplastic nevi.
3. It achieved a sensitivity of 37/37 = 100.00 percent.
4. It achieved a specificity of 36/38 = 94.74 percent.
5. It made (37+36)/75 = 97.33 percent correct diagnoses.
6. It achieved an AUC of 0.9737.

Since only two of the seventy-five lesions were misdiagnosed, at least thirty-five of the thirty-seven matched pairs must have been diagnosed with complete accuracy. A sign test based on the random hypothesis that complete accuracy is 50 percent likely on each matched pair still assigned a p value less than 0.00005 to the observed or any more accurate diagnostic result. Once again, a hypothesized less-than-50-percent likelihood would have been far more reasonable. If used, it would have generated an even more convincing (i.e., more significant) p value.

All accuracy statistics either remained the same or improved as a result of preprocessing DSSA's input indicators with SPSA. The statistical significance achieved was also improved and quite compelling. One can hardly attribute this to statistical overfitting.

The improved final composite diagnostic algorithm was applied to the twenty-four initially misdiagnosed lesions with the results shown on the following page.

DSSA-GENERATED DIAGNOSTIC CONCLUSION	CORRECT DIAGNOSIS OF LESION		
	BENIGN	MALIGNANT	TOTAL
DYSPLASTIC CONFIRMED: 1-ATBDIFF<2	3	0	3
SPITZ CONFIRMED: FTBDIFF<0	1	0	1
SPITZ CONFIRMED: 3-WNT2TOP<2	1	0	1
DIAGNOSED BENIGN: WTBDIFF<0	0	3	3
DIAGNOSED MALIGNANT: WTBDIFF>=0	1	11	12
DIAGNOSED MALIGNANT: WBOTCTP3>=3	0	1	1
DIAGNOSED MALIGNANT: WBOTCTP1>=1	0	2	2
DIAGNOSED BENIGN: OTBDIFF<0	0	1	1
TOTAL	6	18	24

Results of applying the summarized version of the improved final composite algorithm to the same twenty-four lesions are shown below.

DSSA-GENERATED DIAGNOSTIC CONCLUSION	CORRECT DIAGNOSIS OF LESION		
	BENIGN	MALIGNANT	TOTAL
NEGATIVE TEST: INDICATES BENIGN	5	4	9
POSITIVE TEST: INDICATES MALIGNANT	1	14	15
TOTAL	6	18	24

Accuracy statistics were as follows.

1. DSSA produced a definite diagnostic conclusion for all lesions.
2. It successfully confirmed all three of the actually dysplastic nevi.
3. It successfully confirmed both of the actual Spitz nevi.
4. It achieved a sensitivity of 14/18 = 77.78 percent.
5. It achieved a specificity of 5/6 = 83.33 percent.
6. It made (14+5)/24 = 79.17 percent correct diagnoses.
7. It achieved an AUC of 0.8056.
8. The probability of achieving nineteen or more out of twenty-four correct reversals by chance alone (i.e., if determined by flipping a fair coin) would have been 0.0033.

DSSA succeeded in correcting more than three-quarters of the initial misdiagnoses with the final composite diagnostic algorithm constructed solely from our five genes and improved via SPSA preprocessing. This was, once again, statistically significant. Combined with similar results obtained from the previous seventy-five-lesion validation analysis it seems virtually impossible to attribute any of these improvements to statistical overfitting. That makes it even more noteworthy.

Everything described in this section constitutes a reanalysis of exactly the same data obtained from exactly the same 699 patients previously reported in "A Multi-Marker Assay to Distinguish Malignant Melanomas from Benign Nevi," **PNAS**, 2009, 106(15), doi:10.1073/pnas.0901185106 (entry 13, "ANNOTATED REFERENCES").

A reanalysis was required because the PCM methodology had not yet been developed when the original PNAS article was published. The purpose of the reanalysis was to incorporate PCM's accuracy-improving devices explicitly into the procedures implementing DSSA.

Almost nothing changed in Act I, since it did not involve DSSA. An additional six patients were reclassified as admissible in anticipation of the revised manner in which DSSA would be executed. Data obtained from these six patients had originally been excluded. Consequently, the training sample size increased from 513 to 519, and the total sample size increased from 693 to 699 patients.

Almost nothing changed in Act II. It was executed in the same manner as before, but on 519 instead of 513 patients.

However, Act III was substantially redesigned.

1. In the original analysis twenty-one of the sixty dysplastic nevi were used to train the DSSA algorithm. The remaining thirty-nine dysplastic nevi and all twenty-one Spitz nevi were used, along with the thirty-eight melanomas arising from a nevus and the twenty-four misdiagnosed lesions, to validate it.
2. All eighty-one dysplastic and Spitz nevi were used for training purposes in the reanalysis. Minimum sample size requirements made this necessary in order to perform separate training analyses of dysplastic, Spitz, and other benign nevi. By so doing the homogenizing impact of PCM's initial partitioning feature was explicitly introduced into the DSSA procedure. That substantially improved diagnostic accuracy, as documented in section 5.4.

Act IV applied SPSA uniformly to all training and validation data in the reanalysis. This served to refine and to improve further DSSA's diagnostic accuracy, as documented in section 5.10.

Intensity of gene expression readings drawn from the twenty-one dysplastic nevi originally used for training purposes and from the other 519 benign and malignant lesions included in the reanalyzed training sample were obtained via immunohistochemical analysis of tissue microarrays (TMAs). Similar readings drawn from the remaining thirty-nine dysplastic nevi, from all twenty-one Spitz nevi, from the thirty-eight melanomas arising from a nevus (seventy-five evaluable lesions), and from the twenty-four misdiagnosed lesions were obtained via immunohistochemical analysis of tissue sections.

Although this difference in the way gene intensity readings were obtained might matter in some other context, it did not seem to matter here. Approximately five percentage points of sensitivity, specificity, and diagnostic correctness, respectively, were added by the reanalysis to the originally published training accuracy statistics. All nine of the dysplastic and Spitz nevi in the two validation samples were correctly confirmed, and both sets of accompanying diagnostic accuracy statistics were also improved.

A final comment seems in order. No claim is made that the rather extensive calculations executed both in generating a DSSA algorithm and in applying it to patient data can easily be performed by hand or on the back of an envelope. Some kind of computer is essential. Many people today either possess or have easy access to at least a personal computer (e.g., over the Internet). Nothing fancier is required.

163

Appendix A

Attributes of the 1,039 Melanoma Patients Diagnosed Between 1987
and 2007 Who Underwent Sentinel Lymph Node Biopsies (SLNBs)

In all the following tables "*" signifies undefined (missing) observations.

SUMMARY STATISTICS	ATTRIBUTE AGE
n DEFINED	1038
MINIMUM	8
MEDIAN	53
MAXIMUM	96
MEAN	53.0260
STD. DEV.	15.5838

VALUE OF DESIGNATED EXPRESSION	1	2	3	4	5	6	7	8	*	TOTAL
10 =< AGE < 20 years old	13	0	0	0	0	0	0	0	0	13
20 =< AGE < 30 years old	0	49	0	0	0	0	0	0	0	49
30 =< AGE < 40 years old	0	0	152	0	0	0	0	0	0	152
40 =< AGE < 50 years old	0	0	0	225	0	0	0	0	0	225
50 =< AGE < 60 years old	0	0	0	0	234	0	0	0	0	234
60 =< AGE < 70 years old	0	0	0	0	0	183	0	0	0	183
70 =< AGE < 80 years old	0	0	0	0	0	0	143	0	0	143
AGE >= 80 years old	0	0	0	0	0	0	0	38	0	38
*	0	0	0	0	0	0	0	0	2	2
TOTAL	13	49	152	225	234	183	143	38	2	1039

VALUE OF ATTRIBUTE AJCCAGE

Note: One of the two patients with undefined AJCCAGE was eight years old. The other patient's date of diagnosis (hence, AGE at diagnosis) was missing.

VALUE OF ATTRIBUTE AJCCAGE	ABSOLUTE FREQUENCIES (COUNTS)	RELATIVE FREQUENCIES (PROPORTIONS)	CUMULATIVE RELATIVE FREQUENCIES
1	13	.0125	.0125
2	49	.0473	.0598
3	152	.1466	.2064
4	225	.2170	.4233
5	234	.2257	.6490
6	183	.1765	.8255
7	143	.1379	.9634
8	38	.0366	1.0000
TOTAL	1037	1.0000	

VALUE OF ATTRIBUTE SEX	ABSOLUTE FREQUENCIES (COUNTS)	RELATIVE FREQUENCIES (PROPORTIONS)	CUMULATIVE RELATIVE FREQUENCIES
FEMALE	432	.4158	.4158
MALE	607	.5842	1.0000
TOTAL	1039	1.0000	

VALUE OF ATTRIBUTE SEX	VALUE OF ATTRIBUTE AJCCSEX		
	0	1	TOTAL
FEMALE	432	0	432
MALE	0	607	607
TOTAL	432	607	1039

Note: There were no missing observations of a patient's SEX or of AJCCSEX.

VALUE OF ATTRIBUTE TUMPLACE	ABSOLUTE FREQUENCIES (COUNTS)	RELATIVE FREQUENCIES (PROPORTIONS)	CUMULATIVE RELATIVE FREQUENCIES
HEADNECK	176	.1694	.1694
HIGHEXT	178	.1713	.3407
LOWEXT	243	.2339	.5746
TRUNK	442	.4254	1.0000
TOTAL	1039	1.0000	

Note: TUMPLACE designates the anatomical location of a patient's primary tumor. There were no missing observations of TUMPLACE or AJCCSITE.

VALUE OF ATTRIBUTE TUMPLACE	VALUE OF ATTRIBUTE AJCCSITE		
	0	1	TOTAL
HEADNECK	0	176	176
HIGHEXT	178	0	178
LOWEXT	243	0	243
TRUNK	0	442	442
TOTAL	421	618	1039

SUMMARY STATISTICS	ATTRIBUTE TUMTHICK
n DEFINED	1039
MINIMUM	.1500
MEDIAN	1.2000
MAXIMUM	35.0000
MEAN	2.1797
STD. DEV.	2.6940

VALUE OF DESIGNATED EXPRESSION	VALUE OF ATTRIBUTE AJCCTHIC				
	1	2	3	4	TOTAL
T1: 0 < TUMTHICK =< 1 mm.	483	0	0	0	483
T2: 1 < TUMTHICK =< 2 mm.	0	231	0	0	231
T3: 2 < TUMTHICK =< 4 mm.	0	0	178	0	178
T4: TUMTHICK > 4 mm.	0	0	0	147	147
TOTAL	483	231	178	147	1039

Note: TUMTHICK designates the thickness (Breslow depth) of a patient's primary tumor. There were no missing observations of TUMTHICK or AJCCTHIC.

VALUE OF ATTRIBUTE TUMTHICK	ABSOLUTE FREQUENCIES (COUNTS)	RELATIVE FREQUENCIES (PROPORTIONS)	CUMULATIVE RELATIVE FREQUENCIES
.15	1	.0010	.0010
.20	4	.0038	.0048
.25	1	.0010	.0058
.30	3	.0029	.0087
.35	5	.0048	.0135
.40	14	.0135	.0269
.45	4	.0038	.0308
.46	1	.0010	.0318
.50	23	.0221	.0539
.54	1	.0010	.0549
.55	12	.0115	.0664
.60	33	.0318	.0982
.65	11	.0106	.1088
.68	2	.0019	.1107
.70	44	.0423	.1530
.72	1	.0010	.1540
.75	17	.0164	.1704
.78	1	.0010	.1713
.80	48	.0462	.2175
.82	1	.0010	.2185
.83	1	.0010	.2194
.84	1	.0010	.2204
.85	18	.0173	.2377
.88	2	.0019	.2397
.89	1	.0010	.2406
.90	66	.0635	.3041
.92	2	.0019	.3061
.93	1	.0010	.3070
.94	1	.0010	.3080
.95	33	.0318	.3397
.96	1	.0010	.3407
.97	1	.0010	.3417
.98	2	.0019	.3436
1.00	126	.1213	.4649
1.05	1	.0010	.4658
1.10	22	.0212	.4870
1.15	1	.0010	.4880
1.17	1	.0010	.4889
1.20	28	.0269	.5159
1.25	6	.0058	.5217
1.28	1	.0010	.5226
1.30	29	.0279	.5505
1.35	2	.0019	.5525
1.40	21	.0202	.5727
1.45	4	.0038	.5765
1.50	18	.0173	.5938
1.55	2	.0019	.5958
1.56	1	.0010	.5967
1.60	22	.0212	.6179
1.65	4	.0038	.6218
1.67	1	.0010	.6227
1.70	20	.0192	.6420
1.75	3	.0029	.6449
1.80	18	.0173	.6622
1.90	6	.0058	.6679

1.95	1	.0010	.6689
2.00	19	.0183	.6872
2.02	1	.0010	.6882
2.10	11	.0106	.6987
2.15	2	.0019	.7007
2.20	19	.0183	.7190
2.25	2	.0019	.7209
2.30	9	.0087	.7295
2.35	1	.0010	.7305
2.37	1	.0010	.7315
2.40	8	.0077	.7392
2.50	18	.0173	.7565
2.60	7	.0067	.7632
2.64	1	.0010	.7642
2.65	1	.0010	.7652
2.70	10	.0096	.7748
2.75	3	.0029	.7777
2.80	9	.0087	.7863
2.90	2	.0019	.7883
3.00	13	.0125	.8008
3.10	4	.0038	.8046
3.20	11	.0106	.8152
3.30	2	.0019	.8171
3.40	3	.0029	.8200
3.50	16	.0154	.8354
3.60	5	.0048	.8402
3.70	2	.0019	.8422
3.80	3	.0029	.8450
4.00	14	.0135	.8585
4.10	7	.0067	.8653
4.20	12	.0115	.8768
4.30	9	.0087	.8855
4.40	3	.0029	.8884
4.50	11	.0106	.8989
4.60	5	.0048	.9038
4.80	4	.0038	.9076
5.00	12	.0115	.9192
5.10	1	.0010	.9201
5.20	1	.0010	.9211
5.50	10	.0096	.9307
5.70	1	.0010	.9317
5.80	3	.0029	.9346
5.90	1	.0010	.9355
6.00	12	.0115	.9471
6.40	1	.0010	.9480
6.50	5	.0048	.9528
7.00	8	.0077	.9605
7.20	1	.0010	.9615
7.50	5	.0048	.9663
7.70	1	.0010	.9673
8.00	4	.0038	.9711
9.00	3	.0029	.9740
9.10	2	.0019	.9759
9.50	4	.0038	.9798
9.80	1	.0010	.9808
10.00	3	.0029	.9836
10.50	1	.0010	.9846
11.00	4	.0038	.9884
11.50	1	.0010	.9894

12.00	2	.0019	.9913
13.00	1	.0010	.9923
14.00	1	.0010	.9933
14.50	1	.0010	.9942
15.00	2	.0019	.9961
19.00	1	.0010	.9971
30.00	2	.0019	.9990
35.00	1	.0010	1.0000
TOTAL	1039	1.0000	

VALUE OF ATTRIBUTE CLARKLEV	ABSOLUTE FREQUENCIES (COUNTS)	RELATIVE FREQUENCIES (PROPORTIONS)	CUMULATIVE RELATIVE FREQUENCIES
I	1	.0010	.0010
II	37	.0356	.0366
III	390	.3754	.4119
IV	430	.4139	.8258
V	53	.0510	.8768
*	128	.1232	1.0000
TOTAL	1039	1.0000	

Note: There were 128 missing observations of each primary tumor's Clark level (CLARKLEV) and of AJCCLARK.

VALUE OF DESIGNATED EXPRESSION	VALUE OF ATTRIBUTE AJCCLARK						
	1	2	3	4	5	*	TOTAL
CLARK LEVEL I	1	0	0	0	0	0	1
CLARK LEVEL II	0	37	0	0	0	0	37
CLARK LEVEL III	0	0	390	0	0	0	390
CLARK LEVEL IV	0	0	0	430	0	0	430
CLARK LEVEL V	0	0	0	0	53	0	53
*	0	0	0	0	0	128	128
TOTAL	1	37	390	430	53	128	1039

SUMMARY STATISTICS	ATTRIBUTE MITRATE
n DEFINED	654
MINIMUM	0
MEDIAN	3
MAXIMUM	28
MEAN	3.9006
STD. DEV.	3.3915

VALUE OF ATTRIBUTE MITRATE	ABSOLUTE FREQUENCIES (COUNTS)	RELATIVE FREQUENCIES (PROPORTIONS)	CUMULATIVE RELATIVE FREQUENCIES
0	51	.0491	.0491
1	108	.1039	.1530
2	129	.1242	.2772
3	78	.0751	.3523
4	71	.0683	.4206
5	70	.0674	.4880
6	19	.0183	.5063
7	42	.0404	.5467
8	33	.0318	.5784
9	6	.0058	.5842
10	16	.0154	.5996
12	18	.0173	.6169
13	1	.0010	.6179
14	2	.0019	.6198
15	4	.0038	.6237
16	2	.0019	.6256
18	3	.0029	.6285
28	1	.0010	.6295
*	385	.3705	1.0000
TOTAL	1039	1.0000	

Note: MITRATE (mitotic rate of the primary tumor) counts the number of mitoses observed in a high-powered microscopic field (hpf, defined as one square millimeter). There were 385 missing observations of MITRATE and AJCCMITR.

VALUE OF DESIGNATED EXPRESSION	VALUE OF ATTRIBUTE AJCCMITR			
	0	1	*	TOTAL
0 per hpf	51	0	0	51
1 per hpf	0	108	0	108
2 per hpf	0	129	0	129
3 per hpf	0	78	0	78
4 per hpf	0	71	0	71
5 per hpf	0	70	0	70
6 per hpf	0	19	0	19
7 per hpf	0	42	0	42
8 per hpf	0	33	0	33
9 per hpf	0	6	0	6
10 per hpf	0	16	0	16
12 per hpf	0	18	0	18
13 per hpf	0	1	0	1
14 per hpf	0	2	0	2
15 per hpf	0	4	0	4
16 per hpf	0	2	0	2
18 per hpf	0	3	0	3
28 per hpf	0	1	0	1
*	0	0	385	385
TOTAL	51	603	385	1039

Note: In 2009 the AJCC recommended that partitioning the mitotic rate scale in the dichotomous manner shown above was appropriate for staging patients.

VALUE OF ATTRIBUTE ULCERATN	ABSOLUTE FREQUENCIES (COUNTS)	RELATIVE FREQUENCIES (PROPORTIONS)	CUMULATIVE RELATIVE FREQUENCIES
NO	674	.6487	.6487
YES	216	.2079	.8566
*	149	.1434	1.0000
TOTAL	1039	1.0000	

Note: ULCERATN signifies presence or absence of ulceration of the primary tumor. There were 149 missing observations of ULCERATN and AJCCULC.

VALUE OF ATTRIBUTE ULCERATN	VALUE OF ATTRIBUTE AJCCULC			
	0	1	*	TOTAL
NO	674	0	0	674
YES	0	216	0	216
*	0	0	149	149
TOTAL	674	216	149	1039

VALUE OF ATTRIBUTE FIRSTAGE	ABSOLUTE FREQUENCIES (COUNTS)	RELATIVE FREQUENCIES (PROPORTIONS)	CUMULATIVE RELATIVE FREQUENCIES
1a	117	.1126	.1126
1b	385	.3705	.4832
2a	93	.0895	.5727
2b	70	.0674	.6400
2c	36	.0346	.6747
3a	61	.0587	.7334
3b	100	.0962	.8296
3c	67	.0645	.8941
4	4	.0038	.8980
*	106	.1020	1.0000
TOTAL	1039	1.0000	

Note: FIRSTAGE is AJCC Stage at the time of initial patient diagnosis. There were 106 missing observations of FIRSTAGE.

VALUE OF ATTRIBUTE TUMTYPE	ABSOLUTE FREQUENCIES (COUNTS)	RELATIVE FREQUENCIES (PROPORTIONS)	CUMULATIVE RELATIVE FREQUENCIES
ACRAL	38	.0366	.0366
AMELANOTIC	2	.0019	.0385
DESMOPLASTIC	41	.0395	.0780
LENTIGO MALIGNANT MELANOMA	15	.0144	.0924
MALIGNANT MELANOMA IN NEVUS	1	.0010	.0934
MELANOMA IN PIGMENTED NEVUS	3	.0029	.0962
NODULAR	164	.1578	.2541
SPINDLE CELL	3	.0029	.2570
SUPERFICIAL SPREADING	357	.3436	.6006
OTHER OR NOT OTHERWISE CLASSIFIED	198	.1906	.7911
*	217	.2089	1.0000
TOTAL	1039	1.0000	

Note: TUMTYPE designates the histologic type of a patient's primary tumor. There were 217 missing observations of TUMTYPE.

VALUE OF ATTRIBUTE SLNSTATE	ABSOLUTE FREQUENCIES (COUNTS)	RELATIVE FREQUENCIES (PROPORTIONS)	CUMULATIVE RELATIVE FREQUENCIES
NEGATIVE	852	.8200	.8200
POSITIVE	187	.1800	1.0000
TOTAL	1039	1.0000	

Note: SLNSTATE designates the outcome of each patient's sentinel lymph node biopsy (SLNB). There were no missing observations of SLNSTATE.

Appendix B

A Split-Sample Reliability Analysis to Test for Statistical Overfitting

The 1,039 melanoma patients were randomly partitioned into a training subsample of 521 and a validation subsample of 518. The procedures described in sections 2.1 through 2.4 were then applied to the training subsample.

The goal of the split-sample analysis was to reproduce in the 521-patient training subsample PCM's superior predictive accuracy, as reported in section 2.5 for the complete sample, and then to use prediction algorithms generated from the training subsample to reproduce PCM's superior predictive accuracy in the validation subsample.

Three prediction algorithms were then generated from the 521-patient training subsample in the following manner.

1. The first algorithm (FCSLNPPR) produced individually tailored probabilities of SLNB positivity. These constituted the factor-centered base case. They emerged from a stepwise multivariate logistic regression analysis with backward elimination of the six traditional AJCC factor indexes, wherein missing observations of each index were replaced by the mean value of that index in the 521-patient training subsample.

    FCSLNPPR probabilities in the training subsample enabled 80.23 percent correct predictions. 81.81 percent correct predictions were enabled by the equivalent factor-centered base case algorithm derived from the complete 1,039-patient sample.

2. The second algorithm (PCSLNPPR) produced similar probabilities based on a PCM analysis of observations on the same six traditional AJCC factors, but not converted to AJCC factor indexes.

    PCSLNPPR probabilities in the training subsample enabled 83.69 percent correct predictions. 84.02 percent correct predictions were enabled by the equivalent PCSLNPPR algorithm derived from the complete sample.

3. The third algorithm (G2SLNPPR) produced similar probabilities based on a PCM analysis of observations on the same six traditional AJCC factors, augmented by sixteen additional nontraditional factors.

    G2SLNPPR probabilities in the training subsample enabled 87.14 percent correct predictions. 85.66 percent correct predictions were enabled by the equivalent G2SLNPPR algorithm derived from the complete sample.

4. Comparing PCSLNPPR probabilities to FCSLNPPR probabilities in the training subsample produced an index of error reduction = 0.4242. A Wilcoxon test performed on the corresponding 521 matched pairs of probabilistic prediction errors produced a normalized Z statistic = 7.05, with a two-tailed p value < 0.00005.

5. Comparing G2SLNPPR probabilities to PCSLNPPR probabilities in the training subsample produced an index of error reduction = 0.4012. A Wilcoxon test performed on the corresponding 521 matched pairs of probabilistic prediction errors produced a normalized Z statistic = 7.71, with a two-tailed p value < 0.00005.

Recall that the ultimate goal of split-sample reliability testing was to reproduce PCM's superior predictive accuracy in the validation subsample. This was accomplished in the following manner.

1. The factor-centered base case prediction algorithm (FCSLNPPR) produced from the 521-patient training subsample was applied to patients in the validation subsample. This yielded 518 SLNB positivity probabilities enabling 79.34 percent correct predictions.

2. The PCM-assessed base case prediction algorithm (PCSLNPPR) produced from the training subsample was also applied to patients in the validation subsample. This yielded a second set of 518 SLNB positivity probabilities enabling 82.02 percent correct predictions.

3. The PCM-assessed prediction algorithm (G2SLNPPR) produced from the training subsample was also applied to patients in the validation subsample. This yielded a third set of 518 SLNB positivity probabilities enabling 83.40 percent correct predictions.

4. Comparing PCSLNPPR probabilities to FCSLNPPR probabilities in the validation subsample produced an index of error reduction = 0.3514. A Wilcoxon test performed on the corresponding 518 matched pairs of probabilistic prediction errors produced a normalized Z statistic = 4.19, with a two-tailed p value < 0.00005.

5. Comparing G2SLNPPR probabilities to PCSLNPPR probabilities in the validation subsample produced an index of error reduction = 0.2741. A Wilcoxon test performed on the corresponding 518 matched pairs of probabilistic prediction errors produced a normalized Z statistic = 4.07, with a two-tailed p value < 0.00005.

The split-sample reliability analysis was successful. Its results are tabled in the following pages for easy reference.

Table C. Comparison of Accuracy Achieved in Predicting the
Outcome of a Sentinel Lymph Node Biopsy (SLNB) Through Differing
Predictive Methodologies and Differing Collections of Predictive
Factors (Complete Sample: N=1,039)

Pedictive Methodology	Correct Predictions	Index of Error Reduction	Wilcoxon Z Value	2-Tail P Value
Factor-Centered Base Case (six traditional AJCC factors)	81.81%	N/A	N/A	N/A
Patient-Centered Base Case (same six AJCC factors)	84.02%	0.3397	8.99	< 0.00005
Patient-Centered Methodology (same six AJCC + 16 more factors)	85.66%	0.2724	7.18	< 0.00005

Notes:

1. Results in the first row were produced by executing a multivariate logistic regression analysis of the six traditional factor indexes exactly as defined by and measured by the AJCC, except that missing observations of each index were uniformly replaced by the mean value of that index in the complete 1,039-patient sample. Factor indexes pointing in the "wrong" direction (i.e., possessing a negative regression coefficient) were first removed from the analysis. Then stepwise multiple logistic regression was performed with backward elimination.
2. Results in the second and third rows were produced by applying the Patient-Centered Methodology (PCM) to the same raw data observations (e.g., not transformed by the AJCC into factor indexes) of the same twenty-two predictive factors gathered from the same 1,039 patients. The second row reanalyzed just the same six traditional AJCC factors, but via PCM. The third row added seven histological factors and nine gene-based molecular factors and analyzed via PCM the total of twenty-two factors.
3. The PCM methodology first stratified the 1,039 patients into three separate risk subgroups according to their age when initially diagnosed with melanoma and the Breslow thickness of their primary tumors (in millimeters). None of the 1,039 patients presented with unidentified primary tumors.
4. Risk here is defined probabilistically as the anticipated likelihood of producing a positive test result from an SLNB.
5. The low-risk subgroup included all of the 483 T1 patients (tumor thickness no more than 1 millimeter), with a 6.83 percent actual prevalence of positive SLNBs.
6. The medium-risk subgroup included all T2 patients (tumor thickness more than 1, but no more than 2 millimeters) and all T3 patients (more than 2, but no more than 4 millimeters) who were at least fifty-two years old when initially diagnosed. These 327 patients experienced a 18.96 percent actual prevalence of positive SLNBs.
7. The high-risk subgroup included all T4 patients (tumor thickness more than 4 millimeters) and the remaining T3 patients initially diagnosed before reaching their fifty-second birthday. These 229 patients experienced a 40.17 percent actual prevalence of positive SLNBs.
8. Notice from the stratification into three risk subgroups that age at diagnosis exerted a reverse impact on SLNB positivity, opposite from that associated with popular survival outcomes (i.e., opposite with

respect to the conventional wisdom). Being diagnosed with melanoma at an earlier age produced a higher (not a lower) risk of a positive SLNB. Because some previously published research had reported this reverse impact (see entry 10 in "ANNOTATED REFERENCES"), PCM retained age as an admissible prognostic factor. Age was also the second most potent of all twenty-two predictors of SLNB outcome. Primary tumor thickness was the most potent.

9. After first stratifying patients into three separate risk subgroups, PCM then proceeded to analyze each subgroup independently. This generated separate predictive algorithms for each subgroup. The three algorithms were then merged across risk subgroups into a single, composite algorithm for making probabilistic predictions.

10. A different composite algorithm was produced in this manner for each separate collection of predictive factors. It was presumed that most patients would possess recorded values of the six traditional AJCC factors, but not many patients would possess values of the seven additional histological factors or of the nine additional gene-based molecular factors.

11. All three tabled predictive algorithms assigned an individually tailored probability of having a positive SLNB outcome to each of the 1,039 patients.

12. Correct Predictions in each table stands for the maximum percentage of correct predictions of SLNB outcomes enabled by the particular predictive methodology and factor collection tabled in each successive row.

13. Index of Error Reduction, Wilcoxon Z Value, and accompanying 2-Tail P Value refer to the results of Wilcoxon matched-pair, signed-rank tests performed on the accuracy of individually tailored probabilistic predictions made by the particular predictive methodology and factor collection tabled in each successive row, compared to comparable predictions made by the methodology and factor collection tabled in the row immediately above. Each Wilcoxon test was applied to 1,039 matched pairs of differences (usually reductions) in absolute-value probabilistic prediction errors. An individual patient's probabilistic prediction error is the difference between the predicted probability of a positive SLNB assigned to that patient and the actual biopsy outcome (zero for negative test result, one for positive test result).

14. The Index of Error Reduction is designed to mirror a correlation coefficient. It is calculated as the number of net error reductions (i.e., the number of reductions minus the number of increases) as a signed proportion of the total number of nonidentical matched-pair comparisons. The index ranges in value from -1.0, if all comparisons generate error increases, to +1.0, if all comparisons generate error reductions. As with a correlation coefficient, the index has a value of 0.0 if the number of error reductions is exactly counterbalanced by the number of error increases.

15. The distribution of differences between absolute probabilistic prediction errors can be quite skewed. It can also possess occasional outliers (extreme values). Because of this, matched pairs of error differences were tested by the Wilcoxon matched-pairs, signed-ranks test instead of by the more traditional matched-pairs t test. The t test assumes normally distributed data, while the Wilcoxon test makes no distributional assumptions. The Wilcoxon test is also less sensitive to outliers. Compared to the t test, the Wilcoxon test has a relative efficiency near 95 percent for small samples and slightly better than 95 percent for large samples. The Wilcoxon test produces exact one-tailed and two-tailed p values for sample sizes up to twenty-five. A normalized Z statistic

corresponding to the Wilcoxon T statistic is calculated for sample sizes greater than twenty-five. The Z value is then referred to the unit normal distribution to obtain appropriate p values.

16. As measured by the index of error reduction and tested by the Wilcoxon matched-pairs, signed-ranks tests, both of the tabled improvements were highly significant. Both showed two-tailed p values less than 0.00005.

17. Both of these Wilcoxon tests qualify as legitimate hypothesis tests in the classical (Neyman-Pearson) tradition. The Wilcoxon test is a randomization test whose null hypothesis simply states that no systematic differences exist between the two elements in a set of 1,039 matched pairs of absolute probabilistic prediction errors generated, respectively, by two different prediction methodologies. Pairs of errors are uniformly matched patient-by-patient.

18. Age at initial diagnosis and Breslow thickness of the primary tumor were the uniformly most potent predictive factors in both collections of predictive factors analyzed via PCM and in all three separate PCM analyses of the risk subgroups by each collection.

19. TIL level, histological tumor type, and anatomical location of the primary tumor were the second most potent factors (but only in the low-risk and the high-risk subgroups), followed by mitotic rate and vascular factors (but only in the medium-risk and the high-risk subgroups). Clark level of primary tumor invasion was important in only the low-risk subgroup. Selected gene-based molecular factors were important in the medium-risk and the high-risk subgroups. Intensity of NCOA3 expression was especially important in the high-risk subgroup. Insufficient data precluded assessing the impact of any molecular factors on SLNB outcome in the low-risk subgroup.

Table T. Comparison of Accuracy Achieved in Predicting the
Outcome of a Sentinel Lymph Node Biopsy (SLNB) Through Differing
Predictive Methodologies and Differing Collections of Predictive
Factors (Training Subsample: N=521)

Pedictive Methodology	Correct Predictions	Index of Error Reduction	Wilcoxon Z Value	2-Tail P Value
Factor-Centered Base Case (six traditional AJCC factors)	80.23%	N/A	N/A	N/A
Patient-Centered Base Case (same six AJCC factors)	83.69%	0.4242	7.05	< 0.00005
Patient-Centered Methodology (same six AJCC + 16 more factors)	87.14%	0.4012	7.71	< 0.00005

Notes:

1. Results in the first row were produced by executing a multivariate logistic regression analysis of the six traditional factor indexes exactly as defined by and measured by the AJCC, except that missing observations of each index were uniformly replaced by the mean value of that index in the 521-patient training subsample. Factor indexes pointing in the "wrong" direction (i.e., possessing a negative regression coefficient) were first removed from the analysis. Then stepwise multiple logistic regression was performed with backward elimination.

2. Results in the second and third rows were produced by applying the Patient-Centered Methodology (PCM) to the same raw data observations (e.g., not transformed by the AJCC into factor indexes) of the same twenty-two predictive factors gathered from the same 521 training patients. The second row reanalyzed just the same six traditional AJCC factors, but via PCM. The third row added seven histological factors and nine gene-based molecular factors and analyzed via PCM the total of twenty-two factors.

3. The PCM methodology first stratified the 521 training patients into three separate risk subgroups according to their age when initially diagnosed with melanoma and the Breslow thickness of their primary tumors (in millimeters).

4. Risk here is defined probabilistically as the anticipated likelihood of producing a positive test result from an SLNB.

5. After first stratifying patients into three separate risk subgroups, PCM proceeded to analyze each subgroup independently. This generated separate predictive algorithms for each subgroup. The three algorithms were then merged across risk subgroups into a single, composite algorithm for making probabilistic predictions.

6. A different composite algorithm was produced in this manner for each separate collection of predictive factors.

7. All three tabled predictive algorithms assigned an individually tailored probability of having a positive SLNB outcome to each of the 521 training patients.

8. Correct Predictions in each table stands for the maximum percentage of correct predictions of SLNB outcomes enabled by the particular predictive methodology and factor collection tabled in each successive row.

9. Index of Error Reduction, Wilcoxon Z Value, and accompanying 2-Tail P Value refer to the results of Wilcoxon matched-pair, signed-rank tests performed on the accuracy of individually tailored

probabilistic predictions made by the particular predictive methodology and factor collection tabled in each successive row, compared to comparable predictions made by the methodology and factor collection tabled in the row immediately above. Each Wilcoxon test was applied to 521 matched pairs of differences (usually reductions) in absolute-value probabilistic prediction errors. An individual patient's probabilistic prediction error is the difference between the predicted probability of a positive SLNB assigned to that patient and the actual biopsy outcome (zero for negative test result, one for positive test result).

Table V. Comparison of Accuracy Achieved in Predicting the Outcome of a Sentinel Lymph Node Biopsy (SLNB) Through Differing Predictive Methodologies and Differing Collections of Predictive Factors (Validation Subsample: N=518)

Pedictive Methodology	Correct Predictions	Index of Error Reduction	Wilcoxon Z Value	2-Tail P Value
Factor-Centered Base Case (six traditional AJCC factors)	79.34%	N/A	N/A	N/A
Patient-Centered Base Case (same six AJCC factors)	82.05%	0.3514	4.19	< 0.00005
Patient-Centered Methodology (same six AJCC + 16 more factors)	83.40%	0.2741	4.07	< 0.00005

Notes:

1. Results in each row of the table were produced by applying the particular predictive algorithm generated in that row from the 521-patient training subsample to the 518 patients in the validation subsample. Since training and validation subsamples shared no patients in common, no data from the 518 validation patients were used to generate any of the three training algorithms applied, respectively, to validation patients in the three rows of the table.
2. Each 521-patient-training-subsample-generated predictive algorithm assigned an individually tailored probability of having a positive SLNB outcome to each of the 518 validation patients.
3. Correct Predictions in each table stands for the maximum percentage of correct predictions of SLNB outcomes enabled by the particular predictive methodology and factor collection tabled in each successive row.
4. Index of Error Reduction, Wilcoxon Z Value, and accompanying 2-Tail P Value refer to the results of Wilcoxon matched-pair, signed-rank tests performed on the accuracy of individually tailored probabilistic predictions made by the particular predictive methodology and factor collection tabled in each successive row, compared to comparable predictions made by the methodology and factor collection tabled in the row immediately above. Each Wilcoxon test was applied to 518 matched pairs of differences (usually reductions) in absolute-value probabilistic prediction errors. An individual patient's probabilistic prediction error is the difference between the predicted probability of a positive SLNB assigned to that patient and the actual biopsy outcome (zero for negative test result, one for positive test result).

Appendix C

The Unusual Experience of a Patient Who Was Not Recommended
to Undergo an SLNB But Who Elected to Do So Anyway

PCM can show a seemingly low-risk patient (based on conventional risk factors)
to be at much higher risk of SLNB positivity than originally suspected. This
occurred with one of the 1,039 patients who did undergo an SLNB. His readings
on the twenty-two diagnostic factors analyzed via PCM are shown below. All
readings were made at the time of his initial diagnosis.

1. Age: 43
2. Sex: Male
3. Anatomical location of primary tumor: Leg
4. Thickness of primary tumor: 0.8 millimeters (in the T1 category)
5. Mitotic rate of primary tumor: 3 Mitoses per 1 square millimeter (hpf)
6. Ulceration: None
7. Primary tumor type: Malignant melanoma (not otherwise classified)
8. Clark level: Not recorded (missing data)
9. Tumor-Invading Lymphocyte (TIL) level: Absent
10. Vascularity of primary tumor (angiogenesis): Sparse
11. Vascular involvement of primary tumor: None
12. Microsatellites associated with primary tumor: Absent
13. Regression of primary tumor: None
14. Nine molecular (genetic) markers: None recorded (all data missing)

When initially diagnosed this patient did not meet the criteria to undergo an
SLNB. He was not recommended to do so, based on his thin melanoma (0.8
millimeters), coupled with the absence of any high-risk features as understood
according to the conventional wisdom prevailing at that time.

Being diagnosed at the relatively young age of 43 was then thought to indicate
low risk. For the more conventional end points such as distant metastasis and
disease-specific death that was and remains true. For SLNB positivity, however,
PCM has shown that T1 patients with thin primary tumors are at substantially
higher risk when diagnosed at age forty-three or younger.

Having the primary tumor located on the extremities was then thought to
indicate lower risk than having it located axially (i.e., on the head, neck, or
trunk). Again, for distant metastasis and disease-specific death that was and
remains true. However, PCM has shown that the riskiest anatomical location in
terms of SLNB positivity is on the legs.

PCM has also shown that possessing a TIL level of either absent or few
constitutes an important risk factor for SLNB positivity among patients with
thin primary tumors. That was not appreciated, either, when this patient was
initially diagnosed.

Because he possessed a thin primary tumor and because he presented with no
other features then understood to indicate high risk, this patient's positive
SLNB outcome probability was judged to be below 10 percent. That is why no SLNB
was recommended for him.

Interestingly, the probability assigned to him by the FCSLNPPR predictive
algorithm was 7.62 percent. FCSLNPPR reflects the then prevailing conventional
wisdom. No recommendation to undergo an SLNB was entirely consistent at that
point in time with the conventional perspective.

In contrast, all three PCM-based predictive algorithms assigned to him SLNB positivity probabilities above 20 percent. PCSLNPPR assigned a probability of 20.19 percent, and both G1SLNPPR and G2SLNPPR assigned 24.00 percent probabilities. Had PCM been available at the time of his initial diagnosis, his physician would very likely have recommended that he undergo an SLNB.

This patient elected to undergo an SLNB on his own initiative. He tested positive. A single lymph node "lit up." Following the lymph node dissection then recommended after his positive SLNB he has done quite well. To this day he has shown no further evidence of disease.

Appendix D

Attributes of the 301 Melanoma Patients Diagnosed Before or During
2007 Who Did Not Undergo a Sentinel Lymph Node Biopsy (SLNB)

In all the following tables "*" signifies undefined (missing) observations.

SUMMARY STATISTICS	ATTRIBUTE AGE
n DEFINED	301
MINIMUM	19
MEDIAN	48
MAXIMUM	87
MEAN	49.5349
STD. DEV.	15.3137

VALUE OF DESIGNATED EXPRESSION	1	2	3	4	5	6	7	8	TOTAL
10 =< AGE < 20 years old	2	0	0	0	0	0	0	0	2
20 =< AGE < 30 years old	0	25	0	0	0	0	0	0	25
30 =< AGE < 40 years old	0	0	60	0	0	0	0	0	60
40 =< AGE < 50 years old	0	0	0	76	0	0	0	0	76
50 =< AGE < 60 years old	0	0	0	0	52	0	0	0	52
60 =< AGE < 70 years old	0	0	0	0	0	51	0	0	51
70 =< AGE < 80 years old	0	0	0	0	0	0	29	0	29
AGE >= 80 years old	0	0	0	0	0	0	0	6	6

VALUE OF ATTRIBUTE AJCCAGE

Note: There were no missing observations of a patient's AGE or of AJCCAGE.

VALUE OF ATTRIBUTE AJCCAGE	ABSOLUTE FREQUENCIES (COUNTS)	RELATIVE FREQUENCIES (PROPORTIONS)	CUMULATIVE RELATIVE FREQUENCIES
1	2	.0066	.0066
2	25	.0831	.0897
3	60	.1993	.2890
4	76	.2525	.5415
5	52	.1728	.7143
6	51	.1694	.8837
7	29	.0963	.9801
8	6	.0199	1.0000
TOTAL	301	1.0000	

VALUE OF ATTRIBUTE SEX	ABSOLUTE FREQUENCIES (COUNTS)	RELATIVE FREQUENCIES (PROPORTIONS)	CUMULATIVE RELATIVE FREQUENCIES
FEMALE	151	.5017	.5017
MALE	150	.4983	1.0000
TOTAL	301	1.0000	

```
VALUE OF        VALUE OF ATTRIBUTE AJCCSEX
ATTRIBUTE
   SEX          0      1      TOTAL


   FEMALE      151      0      151
   MALE          0    150      150


   TOTAL       151    150      301
```

Note: There were no missing observations of a patient's SEX or of AJCCSEX.

VALUE OF ATTRIBUTE TUMPLACE	ABSOLUTE FREQUENCIES (COUNTS)	RELATIVE FREQUENCIES (PROPORTIONS)	CUMULATIVE RELATIVE FREQUENCIES
HEADNECK	64	.2126	.2126
HIGHEXT	40	.1329	.3455
LOWEXT	66	.2193	.5648
TRUNK	106	.3522	.9169
*	25	.0831	1.0000
TOTAL	301	1.0000	

Note: TUMPLACE designates the anatomical location of a patient's primary
tumor. Twenty-five observations of TUMPLACE and AJCCSITE were missing.

```
VALUE OF        VALUE OF ATTRIBUTE AJCCSITE
ATTRIBUTE
TUMPLACE        0      1      *      TOTAL


HEADNECK        0     64      0       64
HIGHEXT        40      0      0       40
LOWEXT         66      0      0       66
TRUNK           0    106      0      106
*               0      0     25       25


TOTAL         106    170     25      301
```

```
   SUMMARY          ATTRIBUTE
  STATISTICS        TUMTHICK


n DEFINED             245
MINIMUM              .0500
MEDIAN               .6000
MAXIMUM             4.0000
MEAN                 .7500
STD. DEV.            .5573
```

VALUE OF DESIGNATED EXPRESSION	VALUE OF ATTRIBUTE AJCCTHIC				
	1	2	3	*	TOTAL
T1: 0 < TUMTHICK =< 1 mm.	204	0	0	0	204
T2: 1 < TUMTHICK =< 2 mm.	0	32	0	0	32
T3: 2 < TUMTHICK =< 4 mm.	0	0	9	0	9
*	0	0	0	56	56
TOTAL	204	32	9	56	301

Note: TUMTHICK designates the thickness (Breslow depth) of a patient's primary
tumor. Fifty-six observations of TUMTHICK and AJCCTHIC were missing.

VALUE OF ATTRIBUTE TUMTHICK	ABSOLUTE FREQUENCIES (COUNTS)	RELATIVE FREQUENCIES (PROPORTIONS)	CUMULATIVE RELATIVE FREQUENCIES
.05	2	.0066	.0066
.15	4	.0133	.0199
.20	9	.0299	.0498
.25	7	.0233	.0731
.26	1	.0033	.0764
.27	1	.0033	.0797
.29	1	.0033	.0831
.30	16	.0532	.1362
.34	1	.0033	.1395
.35	10	.0332	.1728
.40	21	.0698	.2425
.42	1	.0033	.2458
.45	8	.0266	.2724
.50	18	.0598	.3322
.53	1	.0033	.3355
.55	7	.0233	.3588
.60	16	.0532	.4120
.62	1	.0033	.4153
.65	5	.0166	.4319
.68	1	.0033	.4352
.70	17	.0565	.4917
.72	2	.0066	.4983
.75	11	.0365	.5349
.76	2	.0066	.5415
.80	13	.0432	.5847
.85	8	.0266	.6113
.88	1	.0033	.6146
.90	7	.0233	.6379
.92	1	.0033	.6412
.95	3	.0100	.6512
1.00	8	.0266	.6777
1.03	1	.0033	.6811
1.10	6	.0199	.7010
1.20	3	.0100	.7110
1.30	5	.0166	.7276
1.35	2	.0066	.7342
1.40	2	.0066	.7409
1.45	1	.0033	.7442
1.50	4	.0133	.7575
1.70	1	.0033	.7608
1.80	1	.0033	.7641
1.85	1	.0033	.7674
1.90	1	.0033	.7708
2.00	4	.0133	.7841
2.40	1	.0033	.7874
2.50	6	.0199	.8073
3.50	1	.0033	.8106
4.00	1	.0033	.8140
*	56	.1860	1.0000
TOTAL	301	1.0000	

VALUE OF ATTRIBUTE CLARKLEV	ABSOLUTE FREQUENCIES (COUNTS)	RELATIVE FREQUENCIES (PROPORTIONS)	CUMULATIVE RELATIVE FREQUENCIES
I	4	.0133	.0133
II	91	.3023	.3156
III	98	.3256	.6412
*	108	.3588	1.0000
TOTAL	301	1.0000	

Note: There were 108 missing observations of each primary tumor's Clark level (CLARKLEV) and of AJCCLARK.

VALUE OF DESIGNATED EXPRESSION	VALUE OF ATTRIBUTE AJCCLARK				
	1	2	3	*	TOTAL
CLARK LEVEL I	4	0	0	0	4
CLARK LEVEL II	0	91	0	0	91
CLARK LEVEL III	0	0	98	0	98
*	0	0	0	108	108
TOTAL	4	91	98	108	301

SUMMARY STATISTICS	ATTRIBUTE MITRATE
n DEFINED	123
MINIMUM	0
MEDIAN	1
MAXIMUM	3
MEAN	1.0732
STD. DEV.	1.0135

VALUE OF ATTRIBUTE MITRATE	ABSOLUTE FREQUENCIES (COUNTS)	RELATIVE FREQUENCIES (PROPORTIONS)	CUMULATIVE RELATIVE FREQUENCIES
0	44	.1462	.1462
1	41	.1362	.2824
2	23	.0764	.3588
3	15	.0498	.4086
*	178	.5914	1.0000
TOTAL	301	1.0000	

Note: MITRATE (mitotic rate of the primary tumor) counts the number of mitoses observed in a high-powered microscopic field (hpf, defined as one square millimeter). There were 178 missing observations of MITRATE and AJCCMITR.

```
VALUE OF         VALUE OF ATTRIBUTE AJCCMITR
DESIGNATED
EXPRESSION        0     1      *      TOTAL

0 per hpf        44     0      0       44
1 per hpf         0    41      0       41
2 per hpf         0    23      0       23
3 per hpf         0    15      0       15
*                 0     0    178      178


TOTAL            44    79    178      301
```

Note: In 2009 the AJCC recommended that partitioning the mitotic rate scale in
the dichotomous manner shown above was appropriate for staging patients.

VALUE OF ATTRIBUTE ULCERATN	ABSOLUTE FREQUENCIES (COUNTS)	RELATIVE FREQUENCIES (PROPORTIONS)	CUMULATIVE RELATIVE FREQUENCIES
NO	174	.5781	.5781
*	127	.4219	1.0000
TOTAL	301	1.0000	

Note: ULCERATN signifies presence or absence of ulceration of the primary
tumor. There were 127 missing observations of ULCERATN and AJCCULC.

```
VALUE OF        VALUE OF ATTRIBUTE AJCCULC
ATTRIBUTE
ULCERATN         0      *     TOTAL

NO             174      0      174
*                0    127      127

TOTAL          174    127      301
```

VALUE OF ATTRIBUTE FIRSTAGE	ABSOLUTE FREQUENCIES (COUNTS)	RELATIVE FREQUENCIES (PROPORTIONS)	CUMULATIVE RELATIVE FREQUENCIES
1a	84	.2791	.2791
1b	76	.2525	.5316
2a	3	.0100	.5416
*	138	.4584	1.0000
TOTAL	301	1.0000	

Note: FIRSTAGE is AJCC Stage at the time of initial patient diagnosis. There
were 138 missing observations of FIRSTAGE.

VALUE OF ATTRIBUTE TUMTYPE	ABSOLUTE FREQUENCIES (COUNTS)	RELATIVE FREQUENCIES (PROPORTIONS)	CUMULATIVE RELATIVE FREQUENCIES
ACRAL	5	.0166	.0166
DESMOPLASTIC	1	.0033	.0199
LENTIGO MALIGNANT MELANOMA	9	.0299	.0498
NODULAR	5	.0166	.0664
SUPERFICIAL SPREADING	66	.2193	.2857
NOT OTHERWISE CLASSIFIED	5	.0166	.3023
*	210	.6977	1.0000
TOTAL	301	1.0000	

Note: TUMTYPE designates the histologic type of a patient's primary tumor. There were 210 missing observations of TUMTYPE.

VALUE OF ATTRIBUTE SLNSTATE	ABSOLUTE FREQUENCIES (COUNTS)	RELATIVE FREQUENCIES (PROPORTIONS)	CUMULATIVE RELATIVE FREQUENCIES
*	301	1.0000	1.0000
TOTAL	301	1.0000	

Note: SLNSTATE designates the outcome of each patient's sentinel lymph node biopsy (SLNB). All data were missing, since none of these 301 patients underwent an SLNB.

Appendix E

Attributes of the 173 Melanoma Patients Diagnosed
Between 2007 and 2014 Who Underwent FDG-PET/CT Scans

In all the following tables "*" signifies undefined (missing) observations.

SUMMARY STATISTICS	ATTRIBUTE AGEDIAG
n DEFINED	173
MINIMUM	19
MEDIAN	65
MAXIMUM	94
MEAN	62.0867
STD. DEV.	14.6961

Note: AGEDIAG designates patient age as of last birthday preceding initial diagnosis for cutaneous melanoma. There were no missing observations of AGEDIAG.

VALUE OF DESIGNATED EXPRESSION	VALUE OF ATTRIBUTE AJCCAGE								TOTAL
	1	2	3	4	5	6	7	8	
10 =< AGEDIAG < 20 years old	1	0	0	0	0	0	0	0	1
20 =< AGEDIAG < 30 years old	0	5	0	0	0	0	0	0	5
30 =< AGEDIAG < 40 years old	0	0	9	0	0	0	0	0	9
40 =< AGEDIAG < 50 years old	0	0	0	19	0	0	0	0	19
50 =< AGEDIAG < 60 years old	0	0	0	0	30	0	0	0	30
60 =< AGEDIAG < 70 years old	0	0	0	0	0	53	0	0	53
70 =< AGEDIAG < 80 years old	0	0	0	0	0	0	41	0	41
AGEDIAG >= 80 years old	0	0	0	0	0	0	0	15	15
TOTAL	1	5	9	19	30	53	41	15	173

Note: AJCCAGE designates patient age as of last birthday preceding initial diagnosis transformed into the conventional factor index recommended by the AJCC for prognostic purposes. Since there were no missing observations of AGEDIAG, there were no missing values of AJCCAGE.

VALUE OF ATTRIBUTE AJCCAGE	ABSOLUTE FREQUENCIES (COUNTS)	RELATIVE FREQUENCIES (PROPORTIONS)	CUMULATIVE RELATIVE FREQUENCIES
1	1	.0058	.0058
2	5	.0289	.0347
3	9	.0520	.0867
4	19	.1098	.1965
5	30	.1734	.3699
6	53	.3064	.6763
7	41	.2370	.9133
8	15	.0867	1.0000
TOTAL	173	1.0000	

VALUE OF ATTRIBUTE SEX	ABSOLUTE FREQUENCIES (COUNTS)	RELATIVE FREQUENCIES (PROPORTIONS)	CUMULATIVE RELATIVE FREQUENCIES
FEMALE	36	.2081	.2081
MALE	137	.7919	1.0000
TOTAL	173	1.0000	

Note: There were no missing observations of a patient's SEX (gender).

VALUE OF ATTRIBUTE SEX	VALUE OF ATTRIBUTE AJCCSEX		
	0	1	TOTAL
FEMALE	36	0	36
MALE	0	137	137
TOTAL	36	137	173

Note: AJCCSEX designates patient sex transformed into the conventional factor
index recommended by the AJCC for prognostic purposes. Since there were
no missing observations of SEX, there were no missing values of AJCCSEX.

VALUE OF ATTRIBUTE TUMPLACE	ABSOLUTE FREQUENCIES (COUNTS)	RELATIVE FREQUENCIES (PROPORTIONS)	CUMULATIVE RELATIVE FREQUENCIES
HEADNECK	59	.3410	.3410
HIGHEXT	25	.1445	.4855
LOWEXT	30	.1734	.6590
TRUNK	53	.3064	.9653
UNKNOWN PRIMARY	6	.0347	1.0000
TOTAL	173	1.0000	

Note: TUMPLACE designates the anatomical location of a patient's primary tumor
if a primary tumor was identified at the time of initial diagnosis. Six
patients presented with unknown primaries, so six values of the TUMPLACE
attribute were recorded as UNKNOWN PRIMARY.

VALUE OF ATTRIBUTE TUMPLACE	VALUE OF ATTRIBUTE AJCCSITE			
	0	1	*	TOTAL
HEADNECK	0	59	0	59
HIGHEXT	25	0	0	25
LOWEXT	30	0	0	30
TRUNK	0	53	0	53
UNKNOWN PRIMARY	0	0	6	6
TOTAL	55	112	6	173

Note: AJCCSITE designates the anatomical location of a patient's primary tumor
if a primary tumor was identified at the time of initial diagnosis,
transformed into the conventional factor index recommended by the AJCC
for prognostic purposes. Since six patients presented with unknown
primaries, there were six missing values of AJCCSITE.

SUMMARY STATISTICS	ATTRIBUTE TUMTHICK
n DEFINED	154
MINIMUM	.2000
MEDIAN	2.6000
MAXIMUM	12.0000
MEAN	3.5771
STD. DEV.	2.5619

Note: TUMTHICK designates the thickness (Breslow depth) of a patient's primary tumor in millimeters if a primary tumor was identified at the time of initial diagnosis. There were nineteen missing observations of TUMTHICK. These included missing observations for the six patients who presented with unknown primaries.

VALUE OF ATTRIBUTE TUMTHICK	ABSOLUTE FREQUENCIES (COUNTS)	RELATIVE FREQUENCIES (PROPORTIONS)	CUMULATIVE RELATIVE FREQUENCIES
.20	1	.0058	.0058
.35	1	.0058	.0116
.50	2	.0116	.0231
.60	1	.0058	.0289
.80	2	.0116	.0405
.90	3	.0173	.0578
.99	1	.0058	.0636
1.00	2	.0116	.0751
1.03	1	.0058	.0809
1.05	1	.0058	.0867
1.10	6	.0347	.1214
1.15	2	.0116	.1329
1.20	3	.0173	.1503
1.30	4	.0231	.1734
1.35	1	.0058	.1792
1.40	3	.0173	.1965
1.50	1	.0058	.2023
1.56	1	.0058	.2081
1.60	2	.0116	.2197
1.70	4	.0231	.2428
1.77	1	.0058	.2486
1.85	1	.0058	.2543
1.90	1	.0058	.2601
2.01	3	.0173	.2775
2.05	3	.0173	.2948
2.10	2	.0116	.3064
2.20	4	.0231	.3295
2.23	1	.0058	.3353
2.25	1	.0058	.3410
2.30	4	.0231	.3642
2.40	6	.0347	.3988
2.50	6	.0347	.4335
2.60	3	.0173	.4509
2.70	4	.0231	.4740
2.80	1	.0058	.4798
2.90	1	.0058	.4855
2.98	1	.0058	.4913
3.01	1	.0058	.4971
3.10	2	.0116	.5087

3.18	1	.0058	.5145
3.20	1	.0058	.5202
3.30	3	.0173	.5376
3.40	1	.0058	.5434
3.50	1	.0058	.5491
3.60	1	.0058	.5549
3.80	3	.0173	.5723
4.00	4	.0231	.5954
4.10	2	.0116	.6069
4.30	1	.0058	.6127
4.40	1	.0058	.6185
4.50	2	.0116	.6301
4.60	2	.0116	.6416
4.70	1	.0058	.6474
4.90	1	.0058	.6532
5.00	6	.0347	.6879
5.10	1	.0058	.6936
5.30	1	.0058	.6994
5.50	1	.0058	.7052
6.00	8	.0462	.7514
6.10	1	.0058	.7572
6.40	1	.0058	.7630
6.50	2	.0116	.7746
6.60	1	.0058	.7803
6.80	1	.0058	.7861
6.90	1	.0058	.7919
7.00	3	.0173	.8092
7.50	1	.0058	.8150
8.00	1	.0058	.8208
8.50	1	.0058	.8266
9.00	3	.0173	.8439
9.10	1	.0058	.8497
10.00	4	.0231	.8728
10.10	1	.0058	.8786
11.00	1	.0058	.8844
12.00	1	.0058	.8902
*	19	.1098	1.0000
TOTAL	173	1.0000	

VALUE OF DESIGNATED EXPRESSION	VALUE OF ATTRIBUTE AJCCTHIC					
	1	2	3	4	*	TOTAL
T1: 0 < TUMTHICK =< 1 mm.	13	0	0	0	0	13
T2: 1 < TUMTHICK =< 2 mm.	0	32	0	0	0	32
T3: 2 < TUMTHICK =< 4 mm.	0	0	58	0	0	58
T4: TUMTHICK > 4 mm.	0	0	0	51	0	51
*	0	0	0	0	19	19
TOTAL	13	32	58	51	19	173

Note: AJCCTHIC designates the thickness (Breslow depth) of a patient's primary
tumor if a primary tumor was identified at the time of initial diagnosis,
transformed into the conventional factor index recommended by the AJCC
for prognostic purposes. Since six patients presented with unknown
primaries, their values of AJCCTHIC were missing. In addition, thirteen
patients with known primaries had missing observations of TUMTHICK and,
therefore, missing values of AJCCTHIC.

VALUE OF ATTRIBUTE CLARKLEV	ABSOLUTE FREQUENCIES (COUNTS)	RELATIVE FREQUENCIES (PROPORTIONS)	CUMULATIVE RELATIVE FREQUENCIES
II	3	.0173	.0173
III	24	.1387	.1561
IV	88	.5087	.6647
V	18	.1040	.7688
*	40	.2312	1.0000
TOTAL	173	1.0000	

Note: CLARKLEV designates Clark's level of invasion of a patient's primary tumor if a primary tumor was identified at the time of initial diagnosis. There were forty missing observations of CLARKLEV. These included missing observations for the six patients who presented with unknown primaries.

VALUE OF DESIGNATED EXPRESSION	VALUE OF ATTRIBUTE AJCCLARK					
	2	3	4	5	*	TOTAL
CLARK LEVEL II	3	0	0	0	0	3
CLARK LEVEL III	0	24	0	0	0	24
CLARK LEVEL IV	0	0	88	0	0	88
CLARK LEVEL V	0	0	0	18	0	18
*	0	0	0	0	40	40
TOTAL	3	24	88	18	40	173

Note: AJCCLARK designates Clark's level of invasion of a patient's primary tumor if a primary tumor was identified at the time of initial diagnosis, transformed into the conventional factor index recommended by the AJCC for prognostic purposes. Since six patients presented with unknown primaries, their values of AJCCLARK were missing. In addition, thirty-four patients with known primaries had missing observations of CLARKLEV and, therefore, missing values of AJCCLARK.

SUMMARY STATISTICS	ATTRIBUTE MITRATE
n DEFINED	134
MINIMUM	0
MEDIAN	4
MAXIMUM	30
MEAN	5.5000
STD. DEV.	5.5594

VALUE OF ATTRIBUTE MITRATE	ABSOLUTE FREQUENCIES (COUNTS)	RELATIVE FREQUENCIES (PROPORTIONS)	CUMULATIVE RELATIVE FREQUENCIES
0	6	.0347	.0347
1	23	.1329	.1676
2	20	.1156	.2832
3	17	.0983	.3815
4	9	.0520	.4335
5	12	.0694	.5029
6	10	.0578	.5607
7	7	.0405	.6012

8	4	.0231	.6243
9	2	.0116	.6358
10	7	.0405	.6763
12	2	.0116	.6879
13	2	.0116	.6994
14	1	.0058	.7052
15	5	.0289	.7341
19	1	.0058	.7399
20	2	.0116	.7514
21	2	.0116	.7630
28	1	.0058	.7688
30	1	.0058	.7746
*	39	.2254	1.0000
TOTAL	173	1.0000	

Note: MITRATE (mitotic rate of the primary tumor) counts the number of mitoses observed in a high-powered microscopic field (hpf, defined as one square millimeter) if a primary tumor was identified at the time of initial diagnosis. There were thirty-nine missing observations of MITRATE. These included missing observations for the six patients who presented with unknown primaries.

VALUE OF DESIGNATED EXPRESSION	VALUE OF ATTRIBUTE AJCCMITR			
	0	1	*	TOTAL
0 per hpf	6	0	0	6
1 per hpf	0	23	0	23
2 per hpf	0	20	0	20
3 per hpf	0	17	0	17
4 per hpf	0	9	0	9
5 per hpf	0	12	0	12
6 per hpf	0	10	0	10
7 per hpf	0	7	0	7
8 per hpf	0	4	0	4
9 per hpf	0	2	0	2
10 per hpf	0	7	0	7
12 per hpf	0	2	0	2
13 per hpf	0	2	0	2
14 per hpf	0	1	0	1
15 per hpf	0	5	0	5
19 per hpf	0	1	0	1
20 per hpf	0	2	0	2
21 per hpf	0	2	0	2
28 per hpf	0	1	0	1
30 per hpf	0	1	0	1
*	0	0	39	39
TOTAL	6	128	39	173

Note: In 2009 the AJCC recommended that partitioning the mitotic rate scale in the dichotomous manner shown above was appropriate for staging patients (i.e., for distinguishing between stage 1a and stage 1b). AJCCMITR transforms MITRATE into this AJCC-recommended conventional factor index. Six patients presented with unknown primaries, so their values of AJCCMITR were missing. Also, thirty-three patients with known primaries had missing observations of MITRATE and, therefore, missing values of AJCCMITR.

VALUE OF ATTRIBUTE ULCERATN	ABSOLUTE FREQUENCIES (COUNTS)	RELATIVE FREQUENCIES (PROPORTIONS)	CUMULATIVE RELATIVE FREQUENCIES
NO	84	.4855	.4855
YES	61	.3526	.8382
*	28	.1618	1.0000
TOTAL	173	1.0000	

Note: ULCERATN designates presence or absence of any ulceration of a patient's primary tumor if a primary tumor was identified at the time of initial diagnosis. There were twenty-eight missing observations of ULCERATN. These included missing observations for the six patients who presented with unknown primaries.

VALUE OF ATTRIBUTE ULCERATN	VALUE OF ATTRIBUTE AJCCULC			
	0	1	*	TOTAL
NO	84	0	0	84
YES	0	61	0	61
*	0	0	28	28
TOTAL	84	61	28	173

Note: ACCULC designates presence or absence of any ulceration of a patient's primary tumor if a primary tumor was identified at the time of initial diagnosis, transformed into the conventional factor index recommended by the AJCC for prognostic purposes. Since six patients presented with unknown primaries, their values of AJCCULC were missing. In addition, twenty-two patients with known primaries had missing observations of ULCERATN and, therefore, missing values of AJCCULC.

VALUE OF ATTRIBUTE FIRSTAGE	ABSOLUTE FREQUENCIES (COUNTS)	RELATIVE FREQUENCIES (PROPORTIONS)	CUMULATIVE RELATIVE FREQUENCIES
1a	5	.0289	.0289
1b	25	.1445	.1734
2a	32	.1850	.3584
2b	33	.1908	.5491
2c	18	.1040	.6532
3	10	.0578	.7110
3a	7	.0405	.7514
3b	15	.0867	.8382
3c	9	.0520	.8902
4	3	.0173	.9075
*	16	.0925	1.0000
TOTAL	173	1.0000	

Note: FIRSTAGE designates AJCC Stage at the time of a patient's initial diagnosis. There were sixteen missing observations of FIRSTAGE. Of the six patients presenting with unknown primaries, three were initially staged 3b, two were initially staged 3c, and one possessed insufficient data to be properly staged.

VALUE OF ATTRIBUTE SLNSTATE	ABSOLUTE FREQUENCIES (COUNTS)	RELATIVE FREQUENCIES (PROPORTIONS)	CUMULATIVE RELATIVE FREQUENCIES
NEGATIVE	65	.3757	.3757
POSITIVE	65	.3757	.7514
*	43	.2486	1.0000
TOTAL	173	1.0000	

Note: SLNSTATE designates the outcome of each patient's sentinel lymph node biopsy (SLNB) if that biopsy was performed. There were no SLNB test results recorded (hence, missing observations) for forty-three patients. Of the six patients presenting with unknown primaries, only two underwent SLNBs. Both of their biopsies tested positive for melanoma. One of them was initially staged 3b, and the other was initially staged 3c.

VALUE OF ATTRIBUTE BLEEDING	ABSOLUTE FREQUENCIES (COUNTS)	RELATIVE FREQUENCIES (PROPORTIONS)	CUMULATIVE RELATIVE FREQUENCIES
NO	81	.4682	.4682
YES	59	.3410	.8092
*	33	.1908	1.0000
TOTAL	173	1.0000	

Note: BLEEDING designates whether or not each patient's primary tumor displayed some form of bleeding if a primary tumor was identified at the time of initial diagnosis. There were thirty-three missing observations of BLEEDING. These included missing observations for the six patients who presented with unknown primaries.

VALUE OF ATTRIBUTE BLISTER	ABSOLUTE FREQUENCIES (COUNTS)	RELATIVE FREQUENCIES (PROPORTIONS)	CUMULATIVE RELATIVE FREQUENCIES
NO	55	.3179	.3179
YES	97	.5607	.8786
*	21	.1214	1.0000
TOTAL	173	1.0000	

Note: BLISTER designates whether or not each patient experienced blistering of the skin due to sun exposure. There were twenty-one missing observations of BLISTER. Five of the six patients who presented with unknown primaries experienced blistering due to sun exposure.

VALUE OF ATTRIBUTE EYECOLOR	ABSOLUTE FREQUENCIES (COUNTS)	RELATIVE FREQUENCIES (PROPORTIONS)	CUMULATIVE RELATIVE FREQUENCIES
BLUE	66	.3815	.3815
BROWN	30	.1734	.5549
GREEN	7	.0405	.5954
HAZEL	17	.0983	.6936
*	53	.3064	1.0000
TOTAL	173	1.0000	

Note: EYECOLOR designates the color of the patient's eyes. There were fifty-three missing observations of EYECOLOR. Five of the six patients who presented with unknown primaries possessed recorded values of EYECOLOR. Of these five patients, three had blue eyes.

VALUE OF ATTRIBUTE LYMPHADY	ABSOLUTE FREQUENCIES (COUNTS)	RELATIVE FREQUENCIES (PROPORTIONS)	CUMULATIVE RELATIVE FREQUENCIES
NO	141	.8150	.8150
YES	30	.1734	.9884
*	2	.0116	1.0000
TOTAL	173	1.0000	

Note: LYMPHADY designates lymphadenopathy. There were two missing observations of LYMPHADY. All of the six patients who presented with unknown primaries had YES recorded for LYMPHADY.

Appendix F

Attributes of the Ninety-Six Plausible Candidates Diagnosed with Melanoma
Between 2007 and 2014 Who Did Not Undergo an FDG-PET/CT Scan

In all the following tables "*" signifies undefined (missing) observations.

SUMMARY STATISTICS	ATTRIBUTE AGEDIAG
n DEFINED	96
MINIMUM	6
MEDIAN	65
MAXIMUM	88
MEAN	62.1667
STD. DEV.	17.2359

Note: AGEDIAG designates patient age as of last birthday preceding initial
diagnosis for cutaneous melanoma. There were no missing observations of
AGEDIAG.

VALUE OF DESIGNATED EXPRESSION	VALUE OF ATTRIBUTE AJCCAGE								TOTAL
	2	3	4	5	6	7	8	*	
AGEDIAG < 10 years old	0	0	0	0	0	0	0	2	2
20 =< AGEDIAG < 30 years old	4	0	0	0	0	0	0	0	4
30 =< AGEDIAG < 40 years old	0	3	0	0	0	0	0	0	3
40 =< AGEDIAG < 50 years old	0	0	9	0	0	0	0	0	9
50 =< AGEDIAG < 60 years old	0	0	0	16	0	0	0	0	16
60 =< AGEDIAG < 70 years old	0	0	0	0	23	0	0	0	23
70 =< AGEDIAG < 80 years old	0	0	0	0	0	25	0	0	25
AGEDIAG >= 80 years old	0	0	0	0	0	0	14	0	14
TOTAL	4	3	9	16	23	25	14	2	96

Note: AJCCAGE designates patient age as of last birthday preceding initial
diagnosis transformed into the conventional factor index recommended by
the AJCC for prognostic purposes. Since the sample contained one patient
age six and one patient age nine but no patients between ten and twenty,
there were two missing values of AJCCAGE but no values of AJCCAGE = 1.

VALUE OF ATTRIBUTE AJCCAGE	ABSOLUTE FREQUENCIES (COUNTS)	RELATIVE FREQUENCIES (PROPORTIONS)	CUMULATIVE RELATIVE FREQUENCIES
2	4	.0417	.0417
3	3	.0313	.0729
4	9	.0938	.1667
5	16	.1667	.3333
6	23	.2396	.5729
7	25	.2604	.8333
8	14	.1458	.9792
*	2	.0208	1.0000
TOTAL	96	1.0000	

VALUE OF ATTRIBUTE SEX	ABSOLUTE FREQUENCIES (COUNTS)	RELATIVE FREQUENCIES (PROPORTIONS)	CUMULATIVE RELATIVE FREQUENCIES
FEMALE	33	.3438	.3438
MALE	63	.6562	1.0000
TOTAL	96	1.0000	

Note: There were no missing observations of a patient's SEX (gender).

VALUE OF ATTRIBUTE SEX	VALUE OF ATTRIBUTE AJCCSEX		
	0	1	TOTAL
FEMALE	33	0	33
MALE	0	63	63
TOTAL	33	63	96

Note: AJCCSEX designates patient sex transformed into the conventional factor index recommended by the AJCC for prognostic purposes. Since there were no missing observations of SEX, there were no missing values of AJCCSEX.

SUMMARY STATISTICS	ATTRIBUTE TUMTHICK
n DEFINED	96
MINIMUM	.7000
MEDIAN	2.0000
MAXIMUM	11.0000
MEAN	2.5040
STD. DEV.	1.7278

Note: TUMTHICK designates the thickness (Breslow depth) of a patient's primary tumor in millimeters if a primary tumor was identified at the time of initial diagnosis. There were no missing observations of TUMTHICK. All ninety-six patients presented with known primaries.

VALUE OF ATTRIBUTE TUMTHICK	ABSOLUTE FREQUENCIES (COUNTS)	RELATIVE FREQUENCIES (PROPORTIONS)	CUMULATIVE RELATIVE FREQUENCIES
.70	1	.0104	.0104
1.00	1	.0104	.0208
1.03	1	.0104	.0313
1.15	1	.0104	.0417
1.20	5	.0521	.0938
1.25	4	.0417	.1354
1.30	3	.0313	.1667
1.40	4	.0417	.2083
1.45	2	.0208	.2292
1.46	1	.0104	.2396
1.50	7	.0729	.3125
1.55	1	.0104	.3229
1.60	1	.0104	.3333
1.65	1	.0104	.3437
1.70	1	.0104	.3542
1.80	5	.0521	.4062

1.90	6	.0625	.4687
2.00	6	.0625	.5313
2.01	1	.0104	.5417
2.05	1	.0104	.5521
2.10	3	.0313	.5833
2.20	2	.0208	.6042
2.30	3	.0313	.6354
2.40	3	.0313	.6667
2.50	5	.0521	.7188
2.60	2	.0208	.7396
2.68	1	.0104	.7500
2.70	1	.0104	.7604
2.90	1	.0104	.7708
3.00	5	.0521	.8229
3.10	2	.0208	.8438
3.50	1	.0104	.8542
3.70	2	.0208	.8750
3.80	2	.0208	.8958
4.00	1	.0104	.9063
4.50	1	.0104	.9167
4.80	1	.0104	.9271
6.00	1	.0104	.9375
7.00	3	.0313	.9688
7.40	1	.0104	.9792
9.00	1	.0104	.9896
11.00	1	.0104	1.0000
TOTAL	96	1.0000	

VALUE OF DESIGNATED EXPRESSION	VALUE OF ATTRIBUTE AJCCTHIC				
	1	2	3	4	TOTAL
T1: 0 < TUMTHICK =< 1 mm.	2	0	0	0	2
T2: 1 < TUMTHICK =< 2 mm.	0	49	0	0	49
T3: 2 < TUMTHICK =< 4 mm.	0	0	36	0	36
T4: TUMTHICK > 4 mm.	0	0	0	9	9
TOTAL	2	49	36	9	96

Note: AJCCTHIC designates the thickness (Breslow depth) of a patient's primary tumor if a primary tumor was identified at the time of initial diagnosis, transformed into the conventional factor index recommended by the AJCC for prognostic purposes. Since there were no missing observations of TUMTHICK, there were no missing values of AJCCTHIC.

VALUE OF ATTRIBUTE FIRSTAGE	ABSOLUTE FREQUENCIES (COUNTS)	RELATIVE FREQUENCIES (PROPORTIONS)	CUMULATIVE RELATIVE FREQUENCIES
1b	38	.3958	.3958
2a	39	.4063	.8021
2b	12	.1250	.9271
2c	2	.0208	.9479
3	2	.0208	.9688
3a	1	.0104	.9792
3c	1	.0104	.9896
*	1	.0104	1.0000
TOTAL	96	1.0000	

Note: FIRSTAGE designates AJCC Stage at the time of a patient's initial diagnosis. There was one missing observation of FIRSTAGE. That patient possessed insufficient data to be properly staged.

VALUE OF ATTRIBUTE SLNSTATE	ABSOLUTE FREQUENCIES (COUNTS)	RELATIVE FREQUENCIES (PROPORTIONS)	CUMULATIVE RELATIVE FREQUENCIES
NEGATIVE	76	.7917	.7917
POSITIVE	7	.0729	.8646
*	13	.1354	1.0000
TOTAL	96	1.0000	

Note: SLNSTATE designates the outcome of each patient's sentinel lymph node biopsy (SLNB) if that biopsy was performed. There were no SLNB test results recorded (hence, missing observations) for thirteen patients.

VALUE OF ATTRIBUTE BLEEDING	ABSOLUTE FREQUENCIES (COUNTS)	RELATIVE FREQUENCIES (PROPORTIONS)	CUMULATIVE RELATIVE FREQUENCIES
NO	57	.5938	.5938
YES	31	.3229	.9167
*	8	.0833	1.0000
TOTAL	96	1.0000	

Note: BLEEDING designates whether or not each patient's primary tumor displayed some form of bleeding. There were eight missing observations of BLEEDING.

VALUE OF ATTRIBUTE BLISTER	ABSOLUTE FREQUENCIES (COUNTS)	RELATIVE FREQUENCIES (PROPORTIONS)	CUMULATIVE RELATIVE FREQUENCIES
NO	33	.3438	.3438
YES	58	.6042	.9479
*	5	.0521	1.0000
TOTAL	96	1.0000	

Note: BLISTER designates whether or not each patient experienced blistering of the skin due to sun exposure. There were five missing observations of BLISTER.

VALUE OF ATTRIBUTE EYECOLOR	ABSOLUTE FREQUENCIES (COUNTS)	RELATIVE FREQUENCIES (PROPORTIONS)	CUMULATIVE RELATIVE FREQUENCIES
BLUE	57	.5938	.5938
BROWN	19	.1979	.7917
GREEN	3	.0313	.8229
HAZEL	11	.1146	.9375
*	6	.0625	1.0000
TOTAL	96	1.0000	

Note: EYECOLOR designates the color of the patient's eyes. There were six missing observations of EYECOLOR.

VALUE OF ATTRIBUTE LYMPHADY	ABSOLUTE FREQUENCIES (COUNTS)	RELATIVE FREQUENCIES (PROPORTIONS)	CUMULATIVE RELATIVE FREQUENCIES
NO	91	.9479	.9479
YES	3	.0313	.9792
*	2	.0208	1.0000
TOTAL	96	1.0000	

Note: LYMPHADY designates lymphadenopathy. There were two missing observations of LYMPHADY.

ANNOTATED REFERENCES

1. Miller, James R. III, Mohammed Kashani-Sabet, and Richard W. Sagebiel. 2013. *Patient-Centered Prognosis: A Methodology to Improve Individually Tailored Prognostic Accuracy Illustrated in Two Cancers*. Bloomington, IN: iUniverse.

This was the first book in our series of books about using PCM to render various predictions of individual patient outcomes more accurate.

2. Kashani-Sabet, Mohammed, Richard W. Sagebiel, Heikki Joensuu, and James R. Miller III. 2013. "A Patient-Centered Methodology That Improves the Accuracy of Prognostic Predictions in Cancer." Published online February 2013 by *PLoS One*. plosone/article.0056435.

This journal article constitutes a condensed version of our first book. It introduces and describes PCM in some detail. Published shortly before the first book, it was directed toward the community of practicing physicians. Both the first book and this, our second book, were intended to serve as reference documentation for a methodologically oriented audience.

3. Miller, James R. III. 2001. "Assessing the Curative Impact of Medical Intervention." Stanford Business School Technical Report No. 85: Stanford, CA.

4. Miller, James R. III. 2002. "A Bayesian Assessment of the Curative Impact of Medical Intervention." Stanford Business School Technical Report No. 86: Stanford, CA.

These two monographs introduce a conceptual framework and a collection of facilitating procedures to assess, probabilistically, both the curative impact of a specified medical intervention and the likelihood that an individual patient has been cured following that intervention.

The logistic and Cox (proportional hazards) regression models are logically integrated by means of Bayes' theorem. Appropriately extended logistic regression supplies an individually tailored prior cure probability (prior to the intervention) for each patient. Appropriately extended Cox regression supplies an individually tailored conditional probability of survival time without further disease progression if the patient remains at risk. Then a Minimal Risk Partitioning Algorithm (MRPA) is constructed to assign an individually tailored posterior cure probability. It encapsulates the likelihood that each patient was actually cured following the intervention.

MRPA also estimates a specified medical intervention's cure rate for any given patient population.

Individually tailored posterior cure probabilities are a function of the time elapsed since the intervention with no evidence of further disease progression. In this sense they resemble survival probabilities, but with a critically important reversal in the direction of inference. A cure probability is defined as the conditional probability of having been cured (as opposed to remaining still at risk), given the duration of survival time free from further disease progression following some medical intervention. A survival probability is a reverse conditional probability. It indicates the likelihood of surviving for a specified period of time, given that the patient was not cured by the medical intervention and, therefore, remained still at risk following it and despite its curative potential.

It is through the application of Bayes' theorem that the direction of inference is successfully reversed. Reversing the direction of inference in this manner requires partitioning a set of patients who have undergone a potentially curative intervention into those who were and those who were not cured. This partitioning, in turn, reveals how failing to separate cured from noncured patients can sometimes lead to quite misleading conclusions. Performing a conventional Kaplan-Meier survival analysis on a sample containing a substantial proportion of cured patients was shown to distort the stable hazard rate over time characterizing the noncured patients. Any conventional survival analysis performed on a similarly mixed sample has the potential to produce the same false impression of a declining hazard rate. This was among the most compelling conclusions drawn from the MRPA analysis.

In terms of methodological lineage PCM is a direct descendant of MRPA. MRPA also begins by reconstructing conventional prognostic methodology to facilitate individual patient predictions. Both are designed to produce individually tailored focal event probabilities. In PCM, choice of the focal event is unrestricted. In MRPA, the focal event is always defined in terms of whether or not a particular patient has been transformed following a specified medical intervention from a prior state of being at risk to a posterior state of no longer remaining at substantial risk of further disease progression (i.e., to the state of now being cured).

Both PCM and MRPA were designed to exploit the facilities of and to execute within the same specialized software operating system (MDMS) employed and illustrated throughout both the first and this second book. Just like MRPA, PCM incorporates the logistic and the Cox regression models. Because PCM modifies both types of regression in the manner required by MRPA it also enhances the ability of MRPA to produce more accurate cure probabilities.

A third book is planned for the near future. It will describe MRPA and the Bayesian framework in which it is imbedded. It will use the MRPA algorithm to analyze several samples of cancer patients. MRPA's ability to assess both a specified medical intervention's cure rate and the likelihood that each individual patient who has undergone that intervention was actually cured will be demonstrated. It will also incorporate the analytical devices of PCM into the MRPA algorithm to enhance predictive accuracy.

5. Ware, James H. 2006. "The Limitations of Risk Factors as Prognostic Tools." *New England Journal of Medicine* 355:2615-17.

As described in the first book, this article by Dr. James H. Ware served as an inspirational trigger for the development of PCM.

6. Le, Chap T. 1997. *Applied Survival Analysis.* New York: John Wiley and Sons, Inc.

This book provides an excellent introduction to and summary of many of the analytical and statistical procedures executed in both our first and our second books.

7. *STATVIEW Reference Manual* (Third edition). 1999. Cary, NC: SAS Institute, Inc.

This reference manual and the accompanying user's manual were useful in validating for both logical and programming accuracy many of the procedures incorporated in the PCM methodology. Great care was taken to ensure that PCM procedures generated the same results as did STATVIEW when given the same input data to analyze.

8. Balch, Charles M. et al. 2001. "Prognostic Factors Analysis of 17,600 Melanoma Patients: Validation of the American Joint Committee on Cancer Melanoma Staging System." *Journal of Clinical Oncology* 19(16):3622-34.

9. Balch, Charles M. et al. 2009. "Final Version of 2009 AJCC Melanoma Staging and Classification." *Journal of Clinical Oncology* 27(36):6199-206.

These two journal articles identify the six traditional (i.e., routinely recorded) prognostic factors for melanoma as proposed by the American Joint Committee on Cancer (AJCC). The six AJCC factors and their recommended measurement indexes were used to construct factor-centered base case analyses against which to calibrate PCM's improved predictive accuracy for both the SLNB and the FDG-PET/CT scan outcomes. In 2009 the AJCC recommended substituting mitotic rate, when available, for Clark level of primary tumor invasion as one of the six traditional factors (to identify T1b patients).

10. Venna, Suraj S. et al. 2013. "Analysis of Sentinel Lymph Node Positivity in Patients With Thin Primary Melanoma." *Journal of the American Academy of Dermatology* 68(4):560-7.

This journal article reports that patient age at diagnosis points in the "wrong" direction as a predictor of SLNB positivity. It also reports that grouping anatomical locations of the primary tumor as axial (located on the head, neck, or trunk) versus peripheral (located on the upper or lower extremities) does not provide the most accurate predictions of SLNB positivity. Although the direction of age and the axial versus peripheral grouping of tumor locations (along with their respective measurement indexes) recommended by the AJCC are "right" when predicting popular survival measures, they are not so when predicting SLNB positivity.

These results were based on an analysis of 484 T1 patients with thin (no more than 1 millimeter thick) primary tumors who underwent SLNBs at the University of California at San Francisco (UCSF) before or during 2007. All but one of the 484 patients were included in the sample of 1,039 UCSF SLNB patients analyzed in this book.

The "right" predictive direction of age and the better anatomical grouping of upper body (head, neck, and upper extremities predicting lower SLNB positivity) versus lower body (trunk and lower extremities predicting higher SLNB positivity) were both confirmed for patients with intermediate and thick primary tumors in the complete sample of 1,039 SLNB patients.

All SLNB analyses of UCSF patients were originally performed in 2008.

11. Balch, Charles M. et al. 2014. "Age as a Predictor of Sentinel Node Metastasis Among Patients with Melanoma: An Inverse Correlation of Melanoma Mortality and Incidence of Sentinel Node Metastasis Among Young and Old Patients." *Annals of Surgical Oncology* 21(4):1075-81.

In this journal article the authors acknowledge that age at diagnosis and staging was inversely related to the incidence of sentinel node metastasis among the 7,756 patients in their expanded Melanoma Staging Database who had originally presented without clinical evidence of regional lymph node or distant metastasis and who then underwent an SLNB as a component of their staging workup. In contrast, increasing age continued to be directly related to poorer outcomes in terms of popular survival measures, just as previously reported.

The authors also acknowledge that grouping anatomical locations of the primary tumor as lower body versus upper body was more predictive of SLN metastasis than the traditional axial versus peripheral grouping, even though the traditional grouping still remained appropriate for predicting popular survival measures. These revised results applied to all 7,756 patients, not just to the subset of thin tumor (T1) patients.

The authors explained that the traditional direction and grouping were not based on any direct observation and analysis of SLNB outcomes. Rather, they were postulated on the basis of repeated, consistent observations related to predicting the more popular survival outcomes and other melanoma characteristics correlated therewith.

The authors do not report the "S-shaped" relationship linking mitotic rate to disease-specific death within five years of initial diagnosis (a popular survival measure) depicted in figure 4 of our first book. An "S-shaped" relationship also appears to link mitotic rate to SLNB positivity (as depicted in figure 3 of this book) and to FDG-PET/CT scan positivity (as depicted in figure 8 of this book). Perhaps no such "S-shaped" relationship exists in their expanded Melanoma Staging Database.

12. Haqq, Christopher et al. 2005. "The Gene Expression Signatures of Melanoma Progression." Published online April 2005 by *PNAS*. doi:10.1073/pnas.0501564102.

This journal article in the *Proceedings of the National Academy of Sciences (PNAS)* describes the pioneering effort to identify genes involved in the progression of melanoma and useful in distinguishing malignant melanomas from benign nevi. All but one of the five genes used in the differential diagnosis reported in this book were selected on the basis of the Significance Analysis of Microarrays (SAM) reported in the journal article.

13. Kashani-Sabet, Mohammed et al. 2006. "A Multi-Marker Assay to Distinguish Malignant Melanomas from Benign Nevi." Published online April 2009 by *PNAS*. doi:10.1073/pnas.0901185106.

This journal article in the *Proceedings of the National Academy of Sciences (PNAS)* reports the original analysis whose reanalysis of the same 699 melanoma patients is reported in this book.

The original analysis was noteworthy in three respects. It pioneered the use of five gene-based molecular markers to facilitate the diagnosis of melanoma. It showed that differences in the relative intensity of expression of all five genes between the top and bottom regions of a primary lesion were especially useful in making accurate differential diagnoses. It introduced DSSA and showed that its discriminating efficacy compared favorably with alternative diagnostic procedures.

A reanalysis was required because the PCM methodology had not yet been fully developed when the PNAS article was published. The purpose of the reanalysis was to incorporate PCM's accuracy-improving devices explicitly into the procedures implementing DSSA.

In the original analysis twenty-one of the sixty dysplastic nevi were used to train the DSSA algorithm. The remaining thirty-nine dysplastic nevi and all twenty-one Spitz nevi were used, along with the thirty-eight melanomas arising from a nevus and the twenty-four misdiagnosed lesions, to validate it.

All eighty-one dysplastic and Spitz nevi were used for training purposes in the reanalysis. Minimum sample size requirements made this necessary in order to perform separate training analyses of dysplastic, Spitz, and other benign nevi. By so doing the homogenizing impact of PCM's initial partitioning feature was explicitly introduced into the DSSA procedure. That substantially improved diagnostic accuracy.

SPSA was uniformly applied to all training and validation data in the reanalysis. This served to refine and to improve further DSSA's diagnostic accuracy.

Intensity of gene expression readings drawn from the twenty-one dysplastic nevi originally used for training purposes and from the other 519 benign and malignant lesions included in the reanalyzed training sample were obtained via immunohistochemical analysis of tissue microarrays (TMAs). Similar readings drawn from the remaining thirty-nine dysplastic nevi, from all twenty-one Spitz nevi, from the thirty-eight melanomas arising from a nevus (seventy-five evaluable lesions), and from the twenty-four misdiagnosed lesions were obtained via immunohistochemical analysis of tissue sections. Although this difference might matter in some other context, it did not seem to matter here. DSSA achieved in the original analysis a differential diagnosis with a sensitivity of 91 percent and a specificity of 95 percent. It made 92 percent correct discriminations. Modified by PCM, DSSA reanalyzed exactly the same data. This improved DSSA's diagnostic performance to a 97 percent sensitivity and to a 98 percent specificity, allowing it to make 97 percent correct discriminations.

AUTHOR BIOGRAPHIES

For more than thirty years James R. Miller III, PhD, was a professor at the Stanford Graduate School of Business. He has been doing full-time cancer research since his retirement in 1997 as Walter and Elise Haas Professor of Business Administration. He received a Bachelor's Degree from Princeton University, a Woodrow Wilson Fellowship (University of California at Berkeley), an MBA from the Harvard Business School, and a PhD from the Massachusetts Institute of Technology. He has previously published two books and more than 45 monographs and articles in professional journals. Professor Miller is the inventor of six United States software patents. He has served on more than a dozen boards of directors in the United States and Europe and as CEO of two start-up companies in the Silicon Valley. He has three daughters and six grandchildren.

Mohammed Kashani-Sabet, MD, is Medical Director of Cancer Programs at the California Pacific Medical Center (CPMC). He also serves as Director of the Center for Melanoma Research and Treatment and Senior Scientist at the CPMC Research Institute. Dr. Kashani-Sabet earned his medical degree from the State University of New York at Stony Brook, where he also completed an internship in internal medicine. He then completed a residency in dermatology at the University of California at San Francisco (UCSF), as well as a post-doctoral fellowship in cutaneous oncology, and received training in both dermatology and medical oncology. Dr. Kashani-Sabet maintains clinical interests in melanoma and cutaneous lymphoma and research interests in targeted therapy, ribozymes, siRNAs, tumor metastasis, prognostic factors, and tumor biomarkers for both diagnosis and prognosis.

Richard W. Sagebiel, MD, was born in Ohio in 1934. He received his Bachelor's Degree from Yale University in 1956 in Music and Literature. He did his medical studies at the Harvard Medical School, including a year of pathology and research between his second and third years at the Massachusetts General Hospital (MGH). After an intern year of general medicine he returned to MGH to study detmatopathology with Wallace H. Clark, MD. He completed his training in the Departments of Dermatology and Pathology at the University of Washington Medical School. In 1970 he joined the Clinical Faculty of the University of California at San Francisco (UCSF), working with M. Scott Blois, PhD, MD, and others to form a Clinical Cooperative Melanoma Group. This group included Drs. Clark, Fitzpatrick (Harvard), and Kopf (NYU). It stimulated the creation of similar melanoma groups throughout the country. From 1988 to 1998 Dr. Sagebiel was Director of the UCSF Melanoma Clinic. He then retired and became a Consulting Pathologist to that clinic and, later, to the CPMC Center for Melanoma Research and Treatment.

INDEX

Printed in the United States
By Bookmasters